New and Emerging Diseases: An Update

Editors

NICOLE R. WYRE
SUE CHEN

VETERINARY CLINICS OF NORTH AMERICA: EXOTIC ANIMAL PRACTICE

www.vetexotic.theclinics.com

Consulting Editor
JÖRG MAYER

May 2020 • Volume 23 • Number 2

ELSEVIER

1600 John F. Kennedy Boulevard • Suite 1800 • Philadelphia, Pennsylvania, 19103-2899
http://www.vetexotic.theclinics.com

VETERINARY CLINICS OF NORTH AMERICA: EXOTIC ANIMAL PRACTICE Volume 23, Number 2
May 2020 ISSN 1094-9194, ISBN-13: 978-0-323-75449-1

Editor: Colleen Dietzler
Developmental Editor: Nicole Congleton

Veterinary Clinics of North America: Exotic Animal Practice (ISSN 1094-9194) is published in January, May, and September by Elsevier, Inc., 360 Park Avenue South, New York, NY 10010-1710. Subscription prices are $287.00 per year for US individuals, $545.00 per year for US institutions, $100.00 per year for US students and residents, $338.00 per year for Canadian individuals, $657.00 per year for Canadian institutions, $352.00 per year for international individuals, $657.00 per year for international institutions, $100.00 per year Canadian students/residents, and $165.00 per year for international students/residents. To receive student/resident rate, orders must be accompanied by name of affiliated institution, date of term, and the *signature* of program/residency coordinator on institution letter-head. Orders will be billed at individual rate until proof of status is received. Foreign air speed delivery is included in all *Clinics* subscription prices. All prices are subject to change without notice. **POSTMASTER:** Send address changes to *Veterinary Clinics of North America: Exotic Animal Practice*, Elsevier Health Sciences Division, Subscription Customer Service, 3251 Riverport Lane, Maryland Heights, MO 63043. **Customer Service: Telephone: 1-800-654-2452** (U.S. and Canada); **1-314-447-8871** (outside U.S. and Canada). **Fax: 1-314-447-8029. E-mail: journalscustomerservice-usa@elsevier.com (for print support); journalsonlinesupport-usa@elsevier.com (for online support).**

Reprints. For copies of 100 or more of articles in this publication, please contact the Commercial Reprints Department, Elsevier Inc., 360 Park Avenue South, New York, New York 10010-1710. Tel.: 212-633-3874; Fax: 212-633-3820; E-mail: reprints@elsevier.com.

Veterinary Clinics of North America: Exotic Animal Practice is covered in *MEDLINE/PubMed (Index Medicus).*

Contributors

CONSULTING EDITOR

JÖRG MAYER, Dr med vet, MSc
Diplomate, American Board of Veterinary Practitioners (Exotic Companion Mammals); Diplomate, European College of Zoological Medicine (Small Mammals); Diplomate, American College of Zoological Medicine; Associate Professor of Zoological Medicine, Department of Small Animal Medicine and Surgery, University of Georgia College of Veterinary Medicine, Athens, Georgia, USA

EDITORS

NICOLE R. WYRE, DVM, CVA
Diplomate, American Board of Veterinary Practitioners (Avian Practice), Diplomate, American Board of Veterinary Practitioners (Exotic Companion Mammal); Head Veterinarian, Zodiac Pet & Exotic Hospital, Victoria Centre, Fortress Hill, Hong Kong

SUE CHEN, DVM
Diplomate, American Board of Veterinary Practitioners (Avian Practice); Department Lead, Avian & Exotics, Gulf Coast Veterinary Specialists, Houston, Texas, USA

AUTHORS

JEFFREY R. APPLEGATE, Jr, DVM
Diplomate, American College of Zoological Medicine; Adjunct Clinical Assistant Professor, Department of Clinical Sciences, North Carolina State University, College of Veterinary Medicine, Raleigh, North Carolina, USA

LAURA ADAMOVICZ, DVM, PhD
Wildlife Epidemiology Laboratory, University of Illinois College of Veterinary Medicine, Urbana, Illinois, USA

MATTHEW C. ALLENDER, DVM, MS, PhD
Diplomate, American College of Zoological Medicine; Wildlife Epidemiology Laboratory, University of Illinois College of Veterinary Medicine, Urbana, Illinois, USA

JOÃO BRANDÃO, LMV, MS
Diplomate, European College of Zoological Medicine (Avian); Department of Veterinary Clinical Sciences, College of Veterinary Medicine, Oklahoma State University, Stillwater, Oklahoma, USA

PETER M. DiGERONIMO, VMD, MSc
Adventure Aquarium, Camden, New Jersey, USA; Animal & Bird Health Care Center, Cherry Hill, New Jersey, USA

THOMAS DONNELLY, BVSc
Diplomate, American College of Laboratory Animal Medicine; Diplomate, American Board of Veterinary Practitioners (Small Mammals); Diplomate, European College of Zoological

Medicine; Exotic Pet Medicine Service, Alfort University Veterinary Teaching Hospital, Ecole Nationale Vétérinaire d'Alfort, Maisons-Alfort, France

PAUL M. GIBBONS, DVM, MS
Diplomate, American Board of Veterinary Practitioners (Reptiles and Amphibians); Avian and Exotic Veterinary Care, Portland, Oregon, USA

MOLLY GLEESON, DVM
Diplomate, American College of Zoological Medicine; Clinical Veterinarian, Department of Avian and Exotic Pets, ACCESS Specialty Animal Hospital, Culver City, California, USA

SHARMAN M. HOPPES, DVM
Diplomate, American Board of Veterinary Practitioners (Avian); Texas Avian and Exotic Hospital, Grapevine, Texas, USA; Professor Emerita, Texas A&M University, College of Veterinary Medicine, College Station, Texas, USA

EMMA KEEBLE, BVSc (Hons), MRCVS
Diplomate, ZooMed (Mammalian); RCVS Recognised Specialist in Zoo and Wildlife Medicine, Senior Lecturer in Rabbit, Exotic Animal and Wildlife Medicine and Surgery, Exotic Animal and Wildlife Clinician, Royal College of Veterinary Surgeons Specialist in Zoological Medicine, The University of Edinburgh, The Royal (Dick) School of Veterinary Studies, The Roslin Institute, Easter Bush Campus, Midlothian, United Kingdom

EMMA KEEBLE, BVSc (Hons), MRCVS
Diplomate, European College of Zoological Medicine (Mammalian); RCVS Recognised Specialist in Zoo and Wildlife Medicine, Senior Lecturer in Rabbit, Exotic Animal and Wildlife Medicine and Surgery, Exotic Animal and Wildlife Clinician, The University of Edinburgh, The Royal (Dick) School of Veterinary Studies, The Roslin Institute, Easter Bush Campus, Midlothian, United Kingdom

ERIC KLAPHAKE, DVM
Diplomate, American College of Zoological Medicine; Cheyenne Mountain Zoo, Colorado Springs, Colorado, USA

BRONWYN KOTERWAS, BA, BVM&S, MRCVS
Lecturer and Clinician in Rabbit, Exotic Animal and Wildlife Medicine and Surgery, Senior Clinical Scholar, European College of Zoological Medicine (Herpetology), The University of Edinburgh, The Royal (Dick) School of Veterinary Studies, The Roslin Institute, Easter Bush Campus, Midlothian, United Kingdom

LA'TOYA V. LATNEY, DVM
Diplomate, European College of Zoological Medicine; Diplomate, American Board of Veterinary Practitioners (Reptile/Amphibian); Avian and Exotic Medicine & Surgery, The Animal Medical Center, New York, New York, USA

CHRISTOPH MANS, Dr med vet
Diplomate, American College of Zoological Medicine; Diplomate, European College of Zoological Medicine; Department of Surgical Sciences, School of Veterinary Medicine, University of Wisconsin-Madison, Madison, Wisconsin, USA

ANNA MARTEL, DVM
Department of Surgical Sciences, School of Veterinary Medicine, University of Wisconsin-Madison, Madison, Wisconsin, USA

COLIN McDERMOTT, VMD, CertAqV
Zodiac Pet and Exotic Hospital, Victoria Centre, Fortress Hill, Hong Kong

GLENN H. OLSEN, DVM, MS, PhD
Veterinary Medical Officer, USGS Patuxent Wildlife Research Center, Laurel, Maryland, USA

REBECCA E. PACHECO, DVM
Gulf Coast Veterinary Specialists, Houston, Texas, USA

BRIAN PALMEIRO, VMD, CertAqV
Diplomate, American College of Veterinary Dermatology; Lehigh Valley Veterinary Dermatology & Fish Hospital, Pet Fish Doctor, Allentown, Pennsylvania, USA

OLIVIA A. PETRITZ, DVM
Diplomate, American College of Zoological Medicine; Assistant Professor of Avian and Exotic Animal Medicine, Department of Clinical Sciences, North Carolina State University, College of Veterinary Medicine, Raleigh, North Carolina, USA

ANTHONY A. PILNY, DVM
Diplomate, American Board of Veterinary Practitioners (Avian Practice); Arizona Exotic Animal Hospital, Phoenix, Arizona, USA

DRURY REAVILL, DVM
Diplomate, American Board of Veterinary Practitioners (Avian and Reptile/Amphibian Practice); Diplomate, American College of Veterinary Pathologists; ZNLabs, Salt Lake City, Utah, USA

H.L. SHIVAPRASAD, BVSc, MS, PhD, DACPVc
Diplomate, American College of Veterinary Pathologists; University of California Animal Health and Food Safety Laboratory System-Tulare, University of California, Davis, Tulare, California, USA

SUSAN J. TYSON-PELLO, VMD, MS
Exotics Department Head , Mount Laurel Animal Hospital, Mount Laurel, New Jersey, USA

JAMES F.X. WELLEHAN, DVM, MS, PhD
Diplomate, American College of Zoological Medicine, Diplomate, American College of Veterinary Microbiologists; Zoological Medicine Service, University of Florida College of Veterinary Medicine, Gainesville, Florida, USA

NICOLE R. WYRE, DVM, CVA
Diplomate, American Board of Veterinary Practitioners (Avian Practice), Diplomate, American Board of Veterinary Practitioners (Exotic Companion Mammal); Head Veterinarian, Zodiac Pet & Exotic Hospital, Victoria Centre, Fortress Hill, Hong Kong

Contents

> Recently, multiple infectious organisms have been identified as the cause of emerging diseases in lagomorphs. The most important of these emerging diseases is rabbit hemorrhagic disease virus (RHDV) type 2, a new variant with differences in pathogenicity to classical RHDV. Hepatitis E is considered an emerging zoonotic infectious disease, with widespread prevalence in many different rabbit populations. Mycobacteriosis has been recently reported in other captive domestic rabbit populations. This article provides a recent review of the published literature on emerging infectious diseases in rabbits, including farmed, laboratory, and pet rabbits, some of which have zoonotic potential.

> Chelonians are increasingly challenged by anthropogenic threats and disease. This article summarizes recent literature and clinical experiences regarding 4 emerging infectious diseases in turtles and tortoises: ranaviruses, cryptosporidiosis, intranuclear coccidiosis of Testudines, and Emydomyces testavorans.

> Most honeybee diseases are not newly emerging diseases; however, honeybee veterinary medicine and disease understanding are emerging concepts for veterinarians in the United States. Beekeepers in the hobby and commercial sectors need a prescription or veterinary feed directive from a veterinarian to obtain medically important antibiotics for administration to their honeybees. Medically important antibiotics such as oxytetracycline, lincomycin, and tylosin were removed from over-the-counter availability for use in honeybees. There are many other aspects of beekeeping that allow veterinarians to build a strong veterinarian-client patient relationship, and fulfill an integral role alongside apiarists.

> As veterinarians, we may be the first to diagnose emerging zoonotic diseases in ferrets and may be at increased risk of exposure. Pseudomonas luteola is a bacterial infection that causes respiratory disease, panniculitis, sialadenitis, and abscess formation. Hepatitis E virus can cause subclinical infection,

acute hepatitis, and persistent infection. Since the 2013 article discussing the 2009 influenza pandemic affecting ferrets, there has been an additional case of suspected anthroponotic infection in a pet ferret and experimental infection with influenza viruses from humans, cats, and dogs.

Urolithiasis in captive domestic ferrets has previously been predominantly struvite uroliths, although, more recent laboratory submissions show a shift to predominantly cystine uroliths. Genetic mutations for cystinuria have been identified in dogs, and it is suspected that underlying genetic mutations are partly responsible for this disease in ferrets. Currently, surgery remains the only definitive treatment of cystine urolithiasis in ferrets, since dietary dissolution protocols have not been thoroughly explored. Despite this, medical management with dietary and urinary manipulation should be considered for use in ferrets postoperatively based on principles of cystine urolithiasis management in dogs adapted for ferrets.

Chinchillas have been used mostly as fur animals and as animal models for human ontological diseases and only recently have been recognized as excellent, long-lived, and robust pet rodents. This review aims to provide updated information on emerging disease conditions in pet chinchillas, such as Streptococcus equi subsp zooepidemicus and Pseudomonas aeruginosa. Furthermore, this review article provides updated information on previously documented disorders, such as urolithiasis and middle ear disease, in chinchillas. This article is intended to serve as a complement to the current veterinary reference literature and to provide valuable and clinically relevant information for veterinarians treating chinchillas.

Avian bornavirus (ABV) is a neurotropic virus that can cause gastrointestinal and/or neurologic signs of disease in birds. The disease process is called proventricular dilatation disease (PDD). The characteristic lesions observed in birds include encephalitis and gross dilatation of the proventriculus. ABV is widely distributed in captive and wild bird populations. Most birds infected do not show clinical signs of disease. This article is an update of the Veterinary Clinics of North America article from 2013: Avian Bornavirus and Proventricular Dilatation Disease: Diagnostics, Pathology, Prevalence, and Control.

This article details emerging infectious diseases that have devastating impacts on captive and wild squamates. Treatment advances have been attempted for Cryptosporidium infections in squamates. Gram-positive bacteria, Devriesea agamarum and Austwickia chelonae, are contributing to severe disease in captive and now in wild reptiles, some critically endangered. Nannizziposis, Paranannizziopsis, and Ophidiomyces continue to cause fatal disease as primary pathogens in wild and captive populations of squamates and sphenodontids. Nidovirus, bornavirus, paramyxovirus, sunshine virus, and arenavirus have emerged to be significant causes of neurorespiratory disease in snakes. Controlled studies evaluating environmental stability, disinfection, transmission control, and treatment are lacking.

Updates on Thyroid Disease in Rabbits and Guinea Pigs

Peter M. DiGeronimo and João Brandão

Hyperthyroidism seems to be a rare, but likely underdiagnosed disease of guinea pigs (Cavia porcellus) and rabbits (Oryctolagus cuniculus). Diagnosis is confounded by nonspecific clinical signs, lack of validated assays, and species-specific reference intervals. With increasing English-language publications on the topic, naturally occurring thyroid disease is likely to be increasingly diagnosed in exotic small mammals. The most consistently observed clinical signs include weight loss with or without a change in appetite and a palpable cervical mass. Diagnosis is supported by elevated blood thyroxine concentrations. Treatment may include thyreostatic agents, radioactive iodine, or surgical thyroidectomy.

Emerging Diseases of Avian Wildlife

Susan J. Tyson-Pello and Glenn H. Olsen

Climate change and the interaction with humans and domestic species influences disease in avian wildlife. This article provides updated information on emerging disease conditions such as the spread of an Asian tick, Haemaphysalis longicornis, and its associated diseases among migratory birds in the eastern United States; lymphoproliferative disease virus in wild turkeys in the United States; and salmonellosis, particularly among passerines, which has zoonotic potential. In addition, it includes updated information on West Nile virus, Wellfleet Bay virus, and Avian Influenza and is intended to serve as a complement to the current veterinary literature for veterinarians treating avian wildlife species.

Selected Emerging Infectious Diseases of Amphibians

La'Toya V. Latney and Eric Klaphake

This article updates the understanding of three extirpation-driving infectious diseases, Batrachochytrium dendrobatidis and Batrachochytrium salamandrivorans, and Ranavirus. Experimental studies and dynamic, multifactorial population modeling have outlined the epidemiology and future population impacts of B dendrobatidis, B salamandrivorans, and Ranavirus. New genomic findings on divergent fungal and viral pathogens can help optimize control and disease management strategies. Although there have been major advances in knowledge of amphibian pathogens, controlled studies are needed to guide population recovery to elucidate and evaluate transmission routes for several pathogens, examine

VETERINARY CLINICS OF NORTH AMERICA: EXOTIC ANIMAL PRACTICE

SERIES OF RELATED INTEREST

Veterinary Clinics of North America: Small Animal Practice
Available at: https://www.vetsmall.theclinics.com/

THE CLINICS ARE NOW AVAILABLE ONLINE!
Access your subscription at:
www.theclinics.com

Preface

Exotic Animal Practice New and Emerging Diseases: An Update

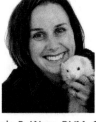
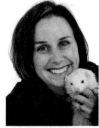

Nicole R. Wyre, DVM, CVA   Sue Chen, DVM
Editors

As discussed in our 2013 issue of emerging diseases of nontraditional exotic species, the "discovery" of new diseases not only encompasses newly reported pathogens and disease conditions but also includes known pathogens of 1 species that have spread to a novel host, pathogens that have new geographic ranges, and pathogens with changes in virulence, morbidity, and mortality. For example, Ranavirus has long plagued amphibian species, leading to global population decline, but has now been documented to infect chelonians with high morbidities and mortalities. Reports have now documented the potentially zoonotic pathogen *Pseudomonas luteola* in ferrets worldwide, thereby expanding its geographic range. *Streptococcus equi* subsp *zooepidemicus* is an emerging pathogen in chinchillas, while *Pseudomomas aeruginosa* continues to cause significant disease. Finally, new variants of some pathogens, such as Rabbit Hemorrhagic Disease virus 2, has led to increased morbidity and mortality in rabbits in Australia, and infection with 1 variant does not confer protection for the other.

Emerging diseases in our exotic species also have noninfectious causes. We have seen recent changes in the characterization of some diseases, such as the sudden switch of primarily struvite to cystine urolithasis in ferrets in the United States within the last decade. Bromethalin toxicosis, which has long been recognized in dogs and cats, has now been documented as the cause of neurologic signs in feral conures based on histologic lesions in the brain and positive fecal tests for desmethylbromethalin.

This issue also covers disease conditions of species that have not previously been well described in the veterinary literature, namely, honeybees and hedgehogs. Now that honeybees have been reclassified as food-producing animals, there is an increased need for knowledgeable veterinarians to develop a Veterinarian-Client Patient Relationship with apiarists to keep a hive healthy. As hedgehogs become

Vet Clin Exot Anim 23 (2020) xiii–xiv
https://doi.org/10.1016/j.cvex.2020.02.001
1094-9194/20/© 2020 Published by Elsevier Inc.   **vetexotic.theclinics.com**

popular pets worldwide, there is more information available on the common diseases, such as dermatologic, neoplastic, and gastrointestinal conditions, as well as information on zoonotic salmonellosis.

We also wanted to bring relevant updates on disease conditions described in the previous issue. Research on avian bornavirus and proventricular dilatation disease is ongoing, including efforts to produce a vaccine. Climate change affects many species and is particularly impacting disease spread in avian wildlife, squamates, and amphibians. Previously discussed thyroid disease in guinea pigs has now also been found in rabbits. In ornamental fish, the ability to detect and classify pathogens has improved, leading to the discovery that previously well-described pathogens have the potential to infect other species.

As with the previous issue, our goal was to compile the latest published information about these diseases in various exotics species, especially for those diseases not already well described. Our international group of contributing authors have distilled the veterinary literature to bring you the most recent information about these diseases as well as added their own personal observations and studies. We are grateful for their time and expertise in reviewing the latest literature to produce an updated issue on Emerging Diseases. We also want to thank Nicole Congleton for her guidance and assistance in putting this issue together.

Nicole R. Wyre, DVM, CVA
Zodiac Pet & Exotic Clinic
1/F, Victoria Centre
Fortress Hill, Hong Kong

Sue Chen, DVM
Avian & Exotics
Gulf Coast Veterinary Specialists
8042 Katy Freeway
Houston, TX 77024, USA

E-mail addresses:
wyredvm@gmail.com (N.R. Wyre)
sue.chen@gcvs.com (S. Chen)

Emerging Infectious Diseases of Rabbits

Molly Gleeson, DVM, DACZM[a], Olivia A. Petritz, DVM, DACZM[b],*

KEYWORDS

- Rabbit hemorrhagic disease virus • Zoonoses • Hepatitis E • Mycobacterium
- Parvovirus • Picornavirus

KEY POINTS

- A new subtype of rabbit hemorrhagic disease virus (RHDV-2) has emerged causing similar fatal viral hepatitis to classic RHDV strains. The new variant has evolved to be highly pathogenic and infects rabbits as young as 30 days old. RHDV-2 has now become the dominant subtype in endemic countries, and sporadic cases have been confirmed in North America.
- Mycobacteriosis in rabbits is rare; however, infections with both nontuberculosis and tuberculosis Mycobacterium have been reported in both wild and domestic rabbits.
- Hepatitis E is an emerging zoonotic disease in humans, and certain strains have a high prevalence in wild, farmed, and laboratory rabbits, which are often asymptomatic for the virus.
- A novel picornavirus has been detected in fecal samples of asymptomatic rabbits, demonstrating that they may act as hosts of kobuviruses.
- A novel bocaparvovirus was recently identified in rabbits with and without diarrhea, which expands the number of parvoviruses detected in this order than can contribute to clinical gastrointestinal disease.

INTRODUCTION

Recently, multiple infectious organisms have been identified as the cause of emerging diseases in lagomorphs. They have had widespread effects on wild, farmed, and domestic rabbit populations. The most important of these emerging diseases are rabbit hemorrhagic disease virus type 2 (RHDV-2), a new variant with differences in pathogenicity to classic RHDV. Hepatitis E is considered an emerging zoonotic infectious disease, with widespread prevalence in many different rabbit populations. Mycobacteriosis, classically described in captive pygmy rabbits in

[a] Department of Avian and Exotic Pets, ACCESS Specialty Animal Hospital, 9599 Jefferson Boulevard, Culver City, CA 90232, USA; [b] Department of Clinical Sciences, North Carolina State University, College of Veterinary Medicine, 1060 William Moore Drive, Raleigh, NC 27607, USA
* Corresponding author.
E-mail address: Olivia.dvm@gmail.com

Vet Clin Exot Anim 23 (2020) 249–261
https://doi.org/10.1016/j.cvex.2020.01.008
1094-9194/20/© 2020 Elsevier Inc. All rights reserved.

the Pacific northwest, has been recently reported in other captive domestic rabbit populations. With the increased use of metagenomics, novel viral diseases are being discovered in rabbits that also have the potential to play a role in disease. This article provides a recent review of the published literature on emerging infectious diseases in rabbits, including farmed, laboratory, and pet rabbits, some of which have zoonotic potential.

RABBIT HEMORRHAGIC DISEASE

Rabbit hemorrhagic disease (RHD) is a highly infectious, fatal viral hepatitis in rabbits. It has been an important cause of mortality in wild and domestic European rabbits (*Oryctolagus cuniculus*) worldwide and is considered a reportable disease by the World Organization for Animal Health (OIE).[1,2] A previous issue of Veterinary Clinics of North America[3] discussed in detail the pathogenesis and clinical disease associated with classic RHDVa. What follows is an update on RHD, with a specific focus on RHDV-2, a recently emerged variant, which has replaced RHDVa as the primary strain in populations across Europe and Australia.

Cause and Pathogenesis

RHD is caused by nonenveloped single-stranded RNA viruses belonging to the family *Caliciviridae*, genus *Lagovirus*. Rabbit lagoviruses include multiple related caliciviruses, including European brown hare syndrome virus, nonpathogenic rabbit caliciviruses, and RHDVa.[2,4–7] In 2010, a new antigenically distinct variant of RHDV was discovered and is now referred to as RHDV-2 or RHDVb.[8] This virus seems to have emerged separately in Europe rather than evolving from previously existing RHDVs, but the exact source is not known.[9] Both viruses causing RHD are extremely contagious. Transmission occurs via direct contact with infected animals, carcasses, bodily fluids (urine, feces, respiratory secretions), and hair. Fomites and vectors, both insect and animal, can contribute to viral spread.[1,2] Caliciviruses are highly resistant in the environment and can survive freezing for prolonged periods.[10] Virus can persist in frozen infected meat for months in addition to prolonged survival in decomposing carcasses. Importation of rabbit meat and products may be a major contributor to the spread to new geographic regions.[2]

There is generally high host specificity among lagoviruses.[11] Classic RHDVa has been restricted to the European rabbit *(O cuniculus)*,[1] a species widespread in Europe and from which the domestic rabbit is descended. This species is also 1 of 2 introduced lagomorphs in Australia.[11] Severe losses occur in wild and unvaccinated rabbits. Infection in other lagomorph species has not been seen. Studies have also shown that RHDVa cannot replicate in mice, even those with compromised immune systems.[12] The new variant RHDV-2 still has a narrow host range; however, in addition to the European rabbit, fatal RHD has been reported in various *Lepus* species, including Sardinian Cape hares,[13] Italian hares,[14] and most recently the European brown hare.[11]

RHD caused by classic RHDVa demonstrates high morbidity (up to 100%) and mortality (70%–90%) in adult rabbits. Young rabbits that are 6 to 8 weeks old are less likely to be infected, and kits younger than 30 days old remain unaffected.[2,3,5] The newly emerged RHDV-2 causes disease and death in animals as young as 15 to 20 days old, which has not previously been seen in RHD outbreaks. It seems to have more variably mortality (5%–70%) and has been confirmed as a cause of fatal disease in rabbits previously vaccinated for RHDV, demonstrating the distinct antigenic profiles between the 2 viruses. Mortality rates of early outbreaks of RHDV-2 averaged 20% to

30%, causing it to be classified as a mildly pathogenic calicivirus.[9] Since it was first detected in Italy, mortality rates have been increasing. Experimental infection of New Zealand white rabbits with various RHDV strains revealed a similar level of pathogenicity ($\geq$80% infection rate) between classic RHDVa and recently isolated RHDV-2.[9] Rapidly increasing fatality and infection rates suggest that RHDV-2 has evolved into a highly pathogenic calicivirus, similar to RHDVa.

Geographic Distribution

New variant RHDV-2 was first detected in France in 2010.[8] Within a short time span of 5 to 6 years, it had spread throughout Europe and reached Australia, Africa, and North America. Portugal,[15] Italy,[13] Spain,[16] the United Kingdom,[17,18] the Azorean islands,[19] and many other European countries have all reported disease caused by RHDV-2 since 2010. The most recent reports in 2017 to 2018 found the virus in Morocco, New Zealand, West Canada, the United States, and Israel. Rouco and colleagues[20] tracked the spread of this isolate since its emergence, noting that the rapid and large-scale geographic expansion is most consistent with the role of human movement and intervention in this recent epidemiology.

Both viruses are endemic in Europe and Australia, likely due to the abundance of susceptible hosts in the wild, on farms, and as domestic animals. Fatal disease has caused widespread losses affecting rabbitries and wild populations. Recently, RHDV-2 came to replace RHDVa as the primary viral strain in both Europe and Australia.[18,21,22] RHD is not currently endemic in the United States, as most European rabbits are kept as pets and no wild populations are found; however, periodic outbreaks of RHDVa in rabbitries have previously been identified. The first case of RHDV-2 reported in North America was seen in Québec, Canada during August 2016. Since then, additional fatalities in pet and feral European rabbits have been confirmed in British Columbia and around Vancouver Island, along the west coast of Canada.[23] In October 2018, the first case was confirmed in the United States in a domestic Ohio rabbit, involving a strain similar to that detected in Canada the same year.[24] The most recent cases in the United States were detected in a pet rabbit and 3 feral European rabbits on Orcas Island, Washington.[25] All confirmed cases in North America have involved European rabbits. It is unknown whether wild lagomorphs in North America are susceptible to RHDV-2, similar to *Lepus* species in Europe and Australia. Infection of wild rabbits could pose a significant risk for increased disease transmission in the United States, meaning rapid disease detection and protection from disease introduction is especially important.

Both European rabbits and European brown hares (*Lepus europaues*) were introduced in Australia as game species[11] but have since become overly abundant, resulting in impacts on the livestock industry and local ecosystems. Biological control agents were used in an attempt to control the abundant wild rabbit populations, including the introduction of RHDVa in 1995.[26,27] Substantial decreases in European rabbit population sizes were noted following release of this virus; however, partial recovery of some populations began about 8 years later.[21] Despite strict quarantine procedure, RHDV-2 was detected in Australia in 2015 and was not a planned introduction.[28] It was first detected in Canberra, located in Southeast Australia, and has since spread westward,[26] affecting both European rabbits and European brown hares.[11] RHDV-2 is now replacing RHDVa as the primary strain of RHD in Australia,[21,22] as it has in Europe, and is able to cause fatal disease even in rabbits with immunity to RHDVa from previous exposure.[29] Although in Europe and other areas of the world, outbreaks of RHD cause significant negative economic and wildlife impacts, the effects on the Australian populations are considered beneficial. Successful biological control of wild lagomorph populations have economic and conservation benefits, affecting the livestock industry and allowing for recovery of threatened small mammal species.[26] The arrival of RHDV-2 has led to almost 80% reduction in rabbit populations in some areas.[21]

Clinical Presentation

RHD manifests as a rapid course of fatal hepatitis. Whereas the incubation period of RHDVa is 1 to 2 days with death 12 to 48 hours after the onset of fever,[2,5] the clinical course of RHDV-2 is longer, with an incubation period of 3 to 5 days. More rabbits infected with RHDV-2 will show subacute to chronic signs and lesions.[10,30] Surviving rabbits may be contagious for up to 2 months, which is suspected to be similar in animals infected with either virus.

The clinical syndrome caused by RHDV-2 is similar to that described for RHDVa in previous publications.[3] Variable presentations have been seen. Rabbits with peracute disease generally experience sudden death without premonitory clinical signs. Individuals with acute disease will show brief lethargy and pyrexia (>40°C) before death but may also present with signs of circulatory shock. Subacute to chronic disease may manifest as protracted clinical disease, including lethargy, anorexia, weight loss, and jaundice. Gastrointestinal dilation, cardiac arrhythmia, heart murmur, and neurologic abnormalities have also been noted in rabbits affected by RHDV-2.[31] Death and progression of clinical signs is usually attributed to liver failure and may be preceded by icterus. Finally, subclinical carriers do occur and may continue to shed virus for months without obvious disease, acting as a source of infection for other individuals.[2,3,30] Surviving rabbits develop strong immunity to the specific viral variant causing infection, demonstrating that humoral immunity is important for protection from clinical RHD.[10,31]

Diagnosis

A presumptive diagnosis can be made based on clinical presentation, typical infection pattern within a population, and postmortem lesions, but viral detection is necessary for definitive diagnosis.[30] Most caliciviruses cannot be grown in cell culture, which means rabbit inoculation is the only way of isolating, propagating, and demonstrating infectivity of RHDVs.[2,32] Molecular and serologic methods are most often used for diagnosis. Premortem evaluation of blood samples may show leukopenia, thrombocytopenia, and elevated liver enzymes, despite normal erythrocyte counts.[5] A recent report of RHDV-2 in 2 pet rabbits demonstrated slightly different premortem clinical pathology findings, which may be due to the longer course of disease seen with this variant.[31] In addition to typical thrombocytopenia and elevated gamma-glutamyltransferase (GGT) and alkaline phosphatase , both rabbits also exhibited markedly decreased aspartate aminotransferase (AST) and alanine aminotransferase (ALT) activity, decreased fibrinogen, and prolonged prothrombin and activated partial thromboplastin times. Evidence of liver failure included hypoglycemia, elevated bile acids, elevated bilirubin, and hypocholesterolemia in one rabbit. Decreased AST/ALT was suspected to be related to massive hepatic necrosis, as is seen in humans. Urine was evaluated in both rabbits, which showed bilirubinuria, proteinuria, and high urinary GGT. Based on this report, rabbits infected with RHDV-2 may be more likely to present in the clinic than those with RHDVa, due to higher proportion of subacute disease, and it is important for clinicians to have viral hepatitis from RHD on their differential list in such cases, especially when multiple rabbits in the same household are affected or sudden death is seen.

Postmortem lesions

The primary pathologic lesion associated with RHD is extensive hepatic necrosis, but there may also be evidence of disseminated intravascular coagulation involving petechiation and hemorrhage of all organs and tissues[2] (**Fig. 1**). Jaundice is often apparent secondary to hepatic failure. Splenomegaly may be seen in some subacute to chronic cases, in addition to bronchopneumonia, pulmonary hemorrhage or edema, and cardiomyocyte necrosis.[30,31] In an outbreak of RHDV-2 in young rabbits on the Iberian peninsula, lesions noted on postmortem examination of kits aged 14 to 35 days included hemorrhages in the heart, trachea, thymus, lungs, liver, kidneys, and gut, with jaundice noted in most tissues.[16] The tissue of choice for molecular evaluation is fresh or frozen liver, as this usually contains the highest viral titers; however spleen and serum can also be used. Formalin fixed tissue can also be used for molecular evaluation, but fresh/frozen samples are preferred.[2]

Molecular testing

There are various methods available to detect RHD virus genome and virions from infected individuals. Reverse transcriptase polymerase chain reaction (RT-PCR) is a commonly used, rapid diagnostic with high sensitivity.[2] This is best performed on tissue samples as noted earlier but can also be evaluated on urine, feces, or serum.[30] Most body secretions will contain virus. When submitting swab samples, wooden handled or charcoal swabs should be avoided as they can inhibit the PCR reaction.[30]

The sequence regions of the major capsid protein (VP60) are used to type and classify strains following isolation,[16] but specific conventional and real time RT-PCRs have been developed for different RHDVstrains.[33] Specific monoclonal antibodies (Mab) have been produced to allow for subtyping of RHDV isolates, including both RHDVa and RHDV-2. This is important to distinguish the viral subtype causing an RHD outbreak.[6] An Mab-based enzyme-linked immunosorbent assay (ELISA) has been developed by the OIE Reference Laboratory for RHD diagnosis,[2] which can affect vaccination protocols. Other testing methods that are less commonly used include electron microscopy, immunostaining, Western blotting, and *in-situ* hybridization. See **Table 1** for a list of laboratories currently offering diagnostic testing for RHD.

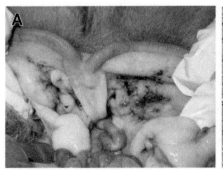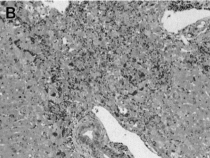

Fig. 1. (*A*) Gross image of hemorrhage within the abdominal fat surrounding the uterus in a rabbit affected by RHDV-2. (*B*) Histopathology of the liver of the same rabbit demonstrating centroacinar hepatocellular necrosis. H&E stain, 20x objective. (*From* Bonvehi C, Ardiaca M, Montesinos, A et al. Clinicopathologic findings of naturally occurring Rabbit Hemorrhagic Disease Virus 2 infection in pet rabbits. Vet ClinPathol. 2019; 48 (1):89-95; with permission.)

Table 1
Laboratories offering testing for rabbit hemorrhagic disease virus (RHDVa, RHDV-2)

Location	Laboratory	Tests Offered
United States	National Veterinary Services Laboratory (NVSL)	RHDVAb ELISA (serum)
		RHDV Ag ELISA (tissue)
	FADDL, Plum Island, NY	RHDV RT-PCR (tissue)
United Kingdom	BattLab	RT-PCR
	Laboklin	RT-PCR
	Pinmoore Animal Laboratory Services	RT-PCR

Serologic testing

The humoral response is an important factor in protection from RHD, as individuals surviving infection demonstrate immunity to reinfection with the same viral subtype. Serologic evaluation can be used to aid diagnosis in affected rabbits. Distinct antibody responses are detected to each antigenically distinct subtype. Use of specific Mab also allows differentiation between natural infection and vaccination.[2,32] Both indirect and competitive ELISAs have been developed and are more commonly used than hemagglutination inhibition (HI). Isotype-specific ELISAs are available to evaluate specific immunoglobulin responses, including IgM, IgA, and IgG.[2,10]

Treatment and Vaccination

There is no direct treatment of viral RHD, and treatment of affected rabbits should involve primarily supportive care. It is recommended to isolate any rabbits confirmed or suspected to be infected to due to high viral shedding.[30] Treatment is similar to RHDVa, which is discussed in depth in a previous issue.[3] Following the discovery of RHDVa, inactivated vaccines were developed that successfully reduce viral replication and clinical disease.[34] A combined RHDV and Myxoma vaccine available in Europe is most commonly used.[30] When RHDV-2 emerged, rabbits previously vaccinated or exposed to natural RHDVa infections still developed rapidly fatal disease, demonstrating a lack of cross-protection between these variants.[1,9,15] Vaccines specific for RHDV-2 have now been developed using isolates from livers of infected individuals, which appear highly protective in young rabbits.[35] Currently, 2 inactivated vaccines are available in Europe, including a monovalent RHDV2 vaccine (Eravac, Spain) and a bivalent RHDV, RHDV-2 vaccine (Filavac, VHD K C + V, France).[30] A recombinant vaccine that includes a modified myxoma virus with main RHDV protein has been developed and is now commercially available.[2] Studies have also been performed evaluating new DNA vaccinations with cytokine adjuvants (interleukin-2) to strengthen the immune response and have shown promising results.[36] Current recommendations in endemic countries are to vaccinate for both variants (RHDVa, RHDV-2), so it is important to be familiar with the specifics of each vaccine to develop an appropriate protocol. Maternal antibodies may impair vaccination success if performed early,[34] which should be taken into account when determining a vaccination schedule for RHDV-2. The Veterinary Medicines Directorate has made specific recommendations for vaccination protocols in Europe and the United Kingdom.[37] Vaccination is not currently a routine in the United States but would potentially be recommended in the case of an outbreak.[2]

Prevention and Control

Appropriate biosecurity and rapid diagnosis are the most important aspects of outbreak prevention. The OIE has published recommendations for control and prevention of RHD.[2]

- Unaffected countries: prevention of introduction is the most important strategy, which involves restriction on importation of animals or products from endemic areas.
- Endemic countries: as RHDV subtypes circulate in wild populations, eradication is not feasible in these locations. Control of disease is best achieved through appropriate sanitation/disinfection and the use of closed colonies and appropriate vaccination protocols.
- New outbreak: a combination of strict quarantine, depopulation, disinfection, surveillance, and vaccination should be used for eradication. Vaccination is recommended for all animals in an outbreak situation, as successful postexposure prophylaxis has been seen. Sentinel seronegative rabbits can be used to monitor for the persistence of virus on a premises following control of an outbreak.

Any suspect animal should be immediately isolated and barrier nursing techniques can be implemented in a breeding situation.[2,30] As noted previously, caliciviruses are very resistant in the environment. In the event of an outbreak, incineration of infected material and cremation of carcasses is recommended.[2] RHDV viruses can be inactivated using sodium hypochlorite (0.5%–1%, 10% household bleach), formalin (1%–2%), and chloramine. Higher concentrations of formalin (3%) are recommended for disinfecting pelts.[2,30]

MYCOBACTERIOSIS

The genus Mycobacterium contains more than 150 species of bacteria that include both obligate and opportunistic pathogens. They are gram-positive, aerobic, intracellular, acid-fast bacteria that are extremely resilient in even the harshest of environmental conditions. The mycobacteria species considered pathogenic in humans have been divided into 3 groups—Mycobacterium leprae, causative agent of leprosy or Hansen disease, Mycobacterium tuberculosis complex (such as Mycobacterium bovis and Mycobacterium caprae), and nontuberculosis mycobacteria. Bacteria in the tuberculosis mycobacteria complex are obligate pathogens and are spread directly from host to host, which include humans and a variety of animal species. Nontuberculosis mycobacteria are saprophytic bacteria, originating from the environment. Until recently, nontuberculosis mycobacteria, such as Mycobacterium avium, Mycobacterium kansasii, and Mycobacterium genovense, have been considered opportunistic pathogens, with infections being common in immunosuppressed people.[38] However, there are increasing reports of nontuberculosis mycobacterial infections in immunocompetent hosts.[39,40] At some point in history, rabbits have been used as an experimental model for all 3 groups of mycobacterium.[41] However, for the purposes of this review article, the authors focus on spontaneous or naturally occurring mycobacteriosis within lagomorphs.

As of this writing, there are no naturally occurring cases of leprosy (M leprae) in rabbits within the published literature. Spontaneous cases of tuberculosis mycobacteriosis are rare in rabbits, and some investigators have suggested this taxa may be resistant to infections with M bovis.[41] There are only a handful of reported cases of M bovis in rabbits, both wild rabbits[42,43] and farmed rabbits.[44] The investigators are not aware of any reported cases of tuberculosis mycobacteriosis in pet rabbits. A recently published report describes the first reported cases of M caprae, a mycobacterial species related to M bovis and within the tuberculosis group, in a group of farm-raised rabbits for meat in Spain.[45] The farm comprised more than 10,000 adult and offspring New Zealand white and California hybrid rabbits, individually housed exclusively indoors. Affected rabbits were does aged 1 to 1.5 years and showed progressive weight loss and generalized weakness. No antemortem diagnostics were reported. Gross necropsy findings of the first 10 clinically affected animals in this outbreak included multifocal white nodules in lungs, kidneys, sacculus rotundus, cecal appendix, and multiple lymph nodes. An additional 67 animals were also euthanized, and 70.6% had histopathologic evidence of mycobacteriosis. All of the initially affected animals as well as 44% of the subsequently euthanatized animals cultured positive for M caprae infection. Intradermal tuberculin testing with bovine purified protein derivative was also performed in affected rabbits, but this method requires further validation in this species.[45] Ultimately, the source of the outbreak was not determined, but it was suspected to arise from a nearby goat flock via fomite transfer. Although the rabbits in this outbreak were raised for meat production with minimal exposure to other animals, the breeds involved and the exposure risks hold true for many pet rabbits.

Although still considered rare, there are several reports of naturally occurring infections with nontuberculosis mycobacteriosis in rabbits. *Mycobacterium genavense* has been diagnosed in a dwarf rabbit with signs of dyspnea and suspected ascites.[46] The lungs were the primary organ affected, and a severe granulomatous pneumonia with acid-fast bacilli was found histologically. The investigators of that case report hypothesized an aerosol route of exposure for that rabbit. *M avium* was the most common cause of death in a captive population of adult pygmy rabbits in the Pacific northwest[47] (**Fig. 2**). Rabbits had a prolonged illness characterized by weight loss, anemia, and dyspnea secondary to granulomatous pneumonia. Lactation was also seen in nonpregnant does, which seems to be a unique clinical sign of mycobacteriosis in this species. There are also several studies that have found *M avium* subsp. *paratuberculosis* in wild rabbits, often in close proximity to infected cattle herds.[48–52] The exact epidemiology of this disease in wild rabbits as it pertains to cattle is still under investigation. Recently, there was a single case of *M avium* subsp. *hominissuis* infection in a 4-year-old pet rabbit that died acutely following intermittent diarrhea and weight loss over the previous couple of months.[53] Multifocal nodules were found throughout the small intestines and the mesenteric lymph nodes were enlarged. Acid-fast organisms were found in the small intestinal lesions, and PCR confirmed *M avium* subsp. *Hominissuis*, an opportunistic pathogen and potential zoonotic agent.

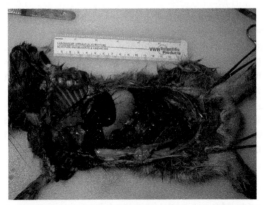

Fig. 2. This is a gross necropsy image of a pygmy rabbit (*Brachylagus idahoensis*) that died from mycobacteriosis. Multiple granulomas are visible throughout the thorax and abdomen. (*Courtesy of* Lisa Harrenstien, DVM, DACZM, Portland, OR. and Rodney D. Sayler, PhD, Pullman, WA.)

HEPATITIS E VIRUS

Hepatitis E virus (HEV) is an emerging zoonotic pathogen that has been isolated from several animals, including pigs and rabbits. HEV is in the family *Hepeviridae,* genera *Orthohepevirus,* and to date 8 genotypes have been identified.[54] Humans are typically infected via fecal-oral transmission in developing countries and via zoonotic transmission in developed countries.[55] The most prevalent genotype involved in zoonotic transmission is HEV3, and human infections are generally asymptomatic and self-limiting.[56] However, acute hepatitis can develop in patients with concurrent hepatic disease, and chronic hepatitis can occur in immunocompromised patients.[57] The mortality rate from hepatitis E in humans is approximately 2%, but mortality rates of greater than 20% have been reported in pregnant women infected with HEV.[58] Veterinarians, hunters, and slaughterhouse workers in numerous countries, particularly those who have contact with pigs and rabbits, have high reported seroprevalence to HEV.[59–63]

HEV has been identified in rabbits from countries all over the world, in many different environments including wild rabbits,[62,64,65] farmed rabbits,[62,66,67] laboratory rabbits (including specific pathogen-free animals),[68,69] and rabbits kept as pets.[64,70] Infected rabbits typically do not have any clinical signs; however, they often will have elevated serum ALT and histologic evidence of focal hepatocellular necrosis.[71] Chronic hepatitis and fibrosis has also been seen in specific pathogen-free rabbits experimentally infected with HEV.[72] High mortality rates and abortions have also been reported in pregnant does experimentally infected with rabbit HEV, confirming vertical transmission in this species.[73] Cynomolgus macaques have been successfully infected with rabbit HEV, and those monkeys developed hepatitis with viremia and shed virus in their feces.[74] In addition, there are several cases of humans infected with a strain of hepatitis E that is genetically similar to those found in rabbits.[55,75,76] Although the clinical signs of HEV infection in rabbits are minimal, veterinarians in contact with rabbits in any capacity should be familiar with this emerging disease and the possible zoonotic risk.

PICORNAVIRUS

Picornaviruses are small, nonenveloped, single-stranded RNA viruses that can infect a wide range of vertebrate species. Many significant veterinary viral diseases are included in this family, such as foot and mouth disease, encephalomyocarditis virus, and swine vesicular disease.[77] In 2016, following a viral metagenomic analysis, a novel picornavirus was identified in fecal samples of rabbits on multiple farms in Hungary.[78] These rabbits ranged in age from 6 weeks to 3 years and were shedding the virus in feces without any observable clinical signs. This is the first time that a picornavirus has been detected in a lagomorph species. Based on sequencing, the virus seems to group within the genus Kobuvirus and is most closely related to novel picornaviruses recently identified in bats. Kobuviruses have been reported in many mammalian species, including humans and rodents. They cause gastroenteritis in these hosts and are primarily detected in fecal samples.[77] It is unknown whether picornaviruses cause clinical disease in rabbits or if there is a potential for domestic rabbits to act as hosts of viruses with zoonotic potential, given their close association with humans.

PARVOVIRUS

Parvoviruses are nonenveloped, single-stranded DNA viruses that cause asymptomatic to severe gastrointestinal disease in a variety of mammalian species.[77] Viruses of the genus *Parvovirus* were first detected in rabbits exhibiting diarrhea in 1977.[79] Experimental infection in young rabbits demonstrated mild clinical signs and the presence of catarrhal enteritis, but virus was also detected in the liver, spleen, and mesenteric lymph nodes.[80] Recently, a novel parvovirus was identified in the feces of rabbits in Italy.[81] Based on genomic analysis, the virus groups within the genus *Bocaparvovirus* and is most closely related to porcine bocaparvoviruses. Using PCR, the new lapine bocaparvovirus was identified in both symptomatic and asymptomatic rabbits, with a prevalence of 20% to 40% in evaluated rabbit colonies. Further evaluation of this particular virus is needed, but it should be considered as a differential for diarrhea in rabbits, along with other rabbit parvoviruses.

DISCLOSURE

The authors have nothing to disclose.

REFERENCES

1. Terio KA, McAloose D, St Leger J. Pathology of wildlife and zoo animals. 1st edition. San Diego (CA): Elsevier; 2018.
2. Health. WOfA. Disease cards: Rabbit HemorrhagicDisease. Available at: https://www.oie.int/fileadmin/Home/eng/Animal_Health_in_the_World/docs/pdf/Disease_cards/RHD.pdf.
3. Kerr PJ, Donnelly TM. Viral infections of rabbits. Vet Clin North Am ExotAnimPract 2013;16:437–68.
4. Cox TE, Liu J, de Ven RV, et al. Different serological profiles to co-occurring pathogenic and nonpathogenic caliciviruses in wild European Rabbits (Oryctolagus-Cuniculus) across Australia. J Wildl Dis 2017;53:472–81.
5. Percy DHB, Stephen W. Pathology of laboratory rodents and rabbits. Oxford (UK): Blackwell Publishing; 2007.
6. Capucci L, Lavazza A. A brief update on rabbit hemorrhagic disease virus. Emerg Infect Dis 1998;4:343–4 [author reply: 345–6].
7. Ohlinger VF, Haas B, Meyers G, et al. Identification and characterization of the virus causing rabbit hemorrhagic disease. J Virol 1990;64:3331–6.
8. Le Gall-Recule G, Zwingelstein F, Boucher S, et al. Detection of a new variant of rabbit haemorrhagic disease virus in France. Vet Rec 2011;168:137–8.
9. Capucci L, Cavadini P, Schiavitto M, et al. Increased pathogenicity in rabbit haemorrhagic disease virus type 2 (RHDV2). Vet Rec 2017;180:426.
10. Spickler AR. Rabbit Hemorrhagic Disease. 2016. Available at: http://www.cfsph.iastate.edu/DiseaseInfo/factsheets.php.
11. Hall RN, Peacock DE, Kovaliski J, et al. Detection of RHDV2 in European brown hares (Lepuseuropaeus) in Australia. Vet Rec 2017;180:121.
12. Urakova N, Hall R, Strive T, et al. Restricted host specificity of rabbit hemorrhagic disease virus is supported by challenge experiments in immune-compromised mice (Musmusculus). J Wildl Dis 2019;55:218–22.
13. Puggioni G, Cavadini P, Maestrale C, et al. The new French 2010 rabbit hemorrhagic disease virus causes an RHD-like disease in the Sardinian Cape hare (Lepuscapensismediterraneus). Vet Res 2013;44:96.
14. Camarda A, Pugliese N, Cavadini P, et al. Detection of the new emerging rabbit haemorrhagic disease type 2 virus (RHDV2) in Sicily from rabbit (Oryctolaguscuniculus) and Italian hare (Lepuscorsicanus). Res Vet Sci 2014;97:642–5.
15. Abrantes J, Lopes AM, Dalton KP, et al. New variant of rabbit hemorrhagic disease virus, Portugal, 2012-2013. Emerg Infect Dis 2013;19:1900–2.
16. Dalton KP, Nicieza I, Balseiro A, et al. Variant rabbit hemorrhagic disease virus in young rabbits, Spain. Emerg Infect Dis 2012;18:2009–12.

17. Westcott DG, Choudhury B. Rabbit haemorrhagic disease virus 2-like variant in Great Britain. Vet Rec 2015;176:74.
18. Elliott S, Saunders R. Rabbit haemorrhagic disease in the UK. Vet Rec 2017; 181:516.
19. Duarte M, Henriques M, Barros SC, et al. Detection of RHDV variant 2 in the Azores. Vet Rec 2015;176:130.
20. Rouco C, Aguayo-Adan JA, Santoro S, et al. Worldwide rapid spread of the novel rabbit haemorrhagic disease virus (GI.2/RHDV2/b). TransboundEmerg Dis 2019; 66:1762–4.
21. Mutze G, De Preu N, Mooney T, et al. Substantial numerical decline in South Australian rabbit populations following the detection of rabbit haemorrhagic disease virus 2. Vet Rec 2018;182:574.
22. Mahar JE, Hall RN, Peacock D, et al. Rabbit hemorrhagic disease virus 2 (RHDV2; GI.2) is replacing endemic strains of RHDV in the Australian landscape within 18 months of its arrival. J Virol 2018;92(2).e01374–17.
23. AgricultureUSDo.Emerging Risk Notice - Animal Health 2018. Available at: https://www.aphis.usda.gov/animal_health/downloads/Rabbit-Hemorrhagic-Disease_062018.pdf.
24. United States Department of Agriculture AaPHISA. APHIS Detects Rabbit Hemorrhagic Disease Virus 2 (RHDV2) in a Domestic Ohio Rabbit, 2018. Available at: https://content.govdelivery.com/accounts/USDAAPHIS/bulletins/2109b9f.
25. AgricultureUSDo.Emerging Risk Notice - Rabbit Hemorrhagic Disease Virus, Serotype 2, 2019. Available at: https://www.aphis.usda.gov/animal_health/downloads/emerging-risk-notice-rabbit.pdf.
26. Cooke B. Long-term monitoring of disease impact: rabbit haemorrhagic disease as a biological control case study. Vet Rec 2018;182:571–2.
27. Cooke BD, Duncan RP, McDonald I, et al. Prior exposure to non-pathogenic calicivirusRCV-A1 reduces both infection rate and mortality from rabbit haemorrhagic disease in a population of wild rabbits in Australia. TransboundEmerg Dis 2018;65:e470–7.
28. Hall RN, Mahar JE, Haboury S, et al. Emerging rabbit hemorrhagic disease virus 2 (RHDVb), Australia. Emerg Infect Dis 2015;21:2276–8.
29. Peacock D, Kovaliski J, Sinclair R, et al. RHDV2 overcoming RHDV immunity in wild rabbits (Oryctolaguscuniculus) in Australia. Vet Rec 2017;180:280.
30. Rocchi M, Dagleish M. Diagnosis and prevention of RHVD2 infection. Vet Rec 2018;182:604–5.
31. Bonvehi C, Ardiaca M, Montesinos A, et al. Clinicopathologic findings of naturally occurring Rabbit Hemorrhagic Disease Virus 2 infection in pet rabbits. Vet Clin-Pathol 2019;48:89–95.
32. Barcena J, Guerra B, Angulo I, et al. Comparative analysis of rabbit hemorrhagic disease virus (RHDV) and new RHDV2 virus antigenicity, using specific virus-like particles. Vet Res 2015;46:106.
33. Dalton KP, Arnal JL, Benito AA, et al. Conventional and real time RT-PCR assays for the detection and differentiation of variant rabbit hemorrhagic disease virus (RHDVb) and its recombinants. J VirolMethods 2018;251:118–22.
34. Carvalho CL, Duarte EL, Monteiro M, et al. Challenges in the rabbit haemorrhagic disease 2 (RHDV2) molecular diagnosis of vaccinated rabbits. Vet Microbiol 2017;198:43–50.
35. Woodland DL. A vaccine against rabbit hemorrhagic disease virus. ViralImmunol 2016;29:535.

36. Deng Z, Geng Y, Wang K, et al. Adjuvant effects of interleukin-2 co-expression with VP60 in an oral vaccine delivered by attenuated Salmonella typhimurium against rabbit hemorrhagic disease. Vet Microbiol 2019;230:49–55.

37. Saunders R. Vaccinating rabbits against RVHD-2. Vet Rec 2016;178:100–1.

38. Henkle E, Winthrop KL. Nontuberculous mycobacteria infections in immunosuppressed hosts. ClinChest Med 2015;36:91–9.

39. Wu U-I, Holland SM. Host susceptibility to non-tuberculous mycobacterial infections. Lancet Infect Dis 2015;15:968–80.

40. Griffith DE, Aksamit T, Brown-Elliott BA, et al. An official ATS/IDSA statement: diagnosis, treatment, and prevention of nontuberculous mycobacterial diseases. Am J RespirCrit Care Med 2007;175:367–416.

41. Arrazuria R, Juste R, Elguezabal N. Mycobacterial infections in rabbits: from the wild to the laboratory. TransboundEmerg Dis 2017;64:1045–58.

42. Gill J, Jackson R. Tuberculosis in a rabbit: a case revisited. N Z Vet J 1993;41:147.

43. Delahay R, De Leeuw A, Barlow A, et al. The status of Mycobacterium bovis infection in UK wild mammals: a review. Vet J 2002;164:90–105.

44. Griffith A. Infections of wild animals with tubercle bacilli and other acid-fast bacilli: (Section of Comparative Medicine). Proc R Soc Med 1939;32(11):1405–12.

45. Sevilla IA, Arnal MC, Fuertes M, et al. Tuberculosis outbreak caused by Mycobacterium caprae in a rabbit farm in Spain. TransboundEmerg Dis 2020;67(1):431–41.

46. Ludwig E, Reischl U, Janik D, et al. Granulomatous pneumonia caused by Mycobacterium genavense in a dwarf rabbit (Oryctolaguscuniculus). Vet Pathol 2009; 46:1000–2.

47. Harrenstien LA, Finnegan MV, Woodford NL, et al. Mycobacterium avium in pygmy rabbits (Brachylagusidahoensis): 28 cases. J Zoo Wildl Med 2006;37:498–513.

48. Fox NJ, Caldow GL, Liebeschuetz H, et al. Counterintuitive increase in observed Mycobacterium avium subspecies paratuberculosis prevalence in sympatric rabbits following the introduction of paratuberculosis control measures in cattle. Vet Rec 2018;182:634–8.

49. Greig A, Stevenson K, Perez V, et al. Paratuberculosis in wild rabbits (Oryctolaguscuniculus). Vet Rec 1997;140:141–3.

50. Greig A, Stevenson K, Henderson D, et al. Epidemiological study of paratuberculosis in wild rabbits in Scotland. J ClinMicrobiol 1999;37:1746–51.

51. Beard P, Rhind S, Buxton D, et al. Natural paratuberculosis infection in rabbits in Scotland. J Comp Pathol 2001;124:290–9.

52. Daniels M, Henderson D, Greig A, et al. The potential role of wild rabbits Oryctolaguscuniculus in the epidemiology of paratuberculosis in domestic ruminants. Epidemiol Infect 2003;130:553–9.

53. Klotz D, Barth SA, Baumgärtner W, et al. Mycobacterium avium subsp. hominissuis Infection in a Domestic Rabbit, Germany. Emerg Infect Dis 2018;24:596.

54. Purdy MA, Harrison TJ, Jameel S, et al. ICTV virus taxonomy profile: hepeviridae. J Gen Virol 2017;98:2645.

55. Park W-J, Park B-J, Ahn H-S, et al. Hepatitis E virus as an emerging zoonotic pathogen. J Vet Sci 2016;17:1–11.

56. Abravanel F, Lhomme S, El Costa H, et al. Rabbit hepatitis E virus infections in humans, France. Emerg Infect Dis 2017;23:1191.

57. Kamar N, Dalton HR, Abravanel F, et al. Hepatitis E virus infection. ClinMicrobiol Rev 2014;27:116–38.

58. Kumar A, Beniwal M, Kar P, et al. Hepatitis E in pregnancy. Int J GynaecolObstet 2004;85:240–4.

59. Meng X, Wiseman B, Elvinger F, et al. Prevalence of antibodies to hepatitis E virus in veterinarians working with swine and in normal blood donors in the United States and other countries. J ClinMicrobiol 2002;40:117–22.
60. Chaussade H, Rigaud E, Allix A, et al. Hepatitis E virus seroprevalence and risk factors for individuals in working contact with animals. J ClinVirol 2013;58:504–8.
61. Kantala T, Kinnunen P, Oristo S, et al. Hepatitis E virus antibodies in Finnish veterinarians. ZoonosesPublic Health 2017;64:232–8.
62. Izopet J, Dubois M, Bertagnoli S, et al. Hepatitis E virus strains in rabbits and evidence of a closely related strain in humans, France. Emerg Infect Dis 2012;18:1274.
63. Geng Y, Zhao C, Geng K, et al. High seroprevalence of hepatitis E virus in rabbit slaughterhouse workers. TransboundEmerg Dis 2019;66:1085–9.
64. Burt SA, Veltman J, Hakze-van der Honing R, et al. Hepatitis E virus in farmed rabbits, wild rabbits and petting farm rabbits in the Netherlands. Food Environ Virol 2016;8:227–9.
65. Hammerschmidt F, Schwaiger K, Dähnert L, et al. Hepatitis E virus in wild rabbits and European brown hares in Germany. Zoonoses Public Health 2017;64:612–22.
66. Xia J, Zeng H, Liu L, et al. Swine and rabbits are the main reservoirs of hepatitis E virus in China: detection of HEV RNA in feces of farmed and wild animals. Arch Virol 2015;160:2791–8.
67. Ahn HS, Park BJ, Han SH, et al. Prevalence and genetic features of rabbit hepatitis E virus in Korea. J Med Virol 2017;89:1995–2002.
68. Han S-H, Park B-J, Ahn H-S, et al. Evidence of hepatitis E virus infection in specific pathogen-free rabbits in Korea. Virus Genes 2018;54:587–90.
69. Birke L, Cormier SA, You D, et al. Hepatitis E antibodies in laboratory rabbits from 2 US vendors. Emerg Infect Dis 2014;20:693.
70. Caruso C, Modesto P, Prato R, et al. Hepatitis E virus: first description in a pet house rabbit. A new transmission route for human? TransboundEmerg Dis 2015;62:229–32.
71. Ma H, Zheng L, Liu Y, et al. Experimental infection of rabbits with rabbit and genotypes 1 and 4 hepatitis E viruses. PLoS One 2010;5:e9160.
72. Han J, Lei Y, Liu L, et al. SPF rabbits infected with rabbit hepatitis E virus isolate experimentally showing the chronicity of hepatitis. PLoS One 2014;9:e99861.
73. Xia J, Liu L, Wang L, et al. Experimental infection of pregnant rabbits with hepatitis E virus demonstrating high mortality and vertical transmission. J Viral Hepat 2015;22:850–7.
74. Liu P, Bu Q-N, Wang L, et al. Transmission of hepatitis E virus from rabbits to cynomolgus macaques. Emerg Infect Dis 2013;19:559.
75. Sooryanarain H, Meng X-J. Hepatitis E virus: reasons for emergence in humans. CurrOpinVirol 2019;34:10–7.
76. Kaiser M, Delaune D, Chazouillères O, et al. A world health organization human hepatitis E virus reference strain related to similar strains isolated from rabbits. Genome Announc 2018;6 [pii:e00292-18].
77. MacLachlan NJ, Dubovi EJ. Fenner'sveterinary virology. 5th edition. Academic Press; 2016. p. 602.
78. Pankovics P, Boros A, Biro H, et al. Novel picornavirus in domestic rabbits (Oryctolaguscuniculus var. domestica). Infect Genet Evol 2016;37:117–22.
79. Matsunaga Y, Matsuno S, Mukoyama J. Isolation and characterization of a parvovirus of rabbits. Infect Immun 1977;18:495–500.
80. Matsunaga Y, Chino F. Experimental infection of young rabbits with rabbit parvovirus. Arch Virol 1981;68:257–64.
81. Lanave G, Martella V, Farkas SL, et al. Novel bocaparvoviruses in rabbits. Vet J 2015;206:131–5.

Emerging Infectious Diseases of Chelonians
An Update

Laura Adamovicz, DVM, PhD[a],*, Matthew C. Allender, DVM, MS, PhD, Dipl ACZM[a],
Paul M. Gibbons, DVM, MS, DABVP (Reptiles and Amphibians)[b]

KEYWORDS

- Testudines • Chelonian • Ranavirus • Intranuclear coccidiosis • Cryptosporidiosis
- *Emydomyces testavorans*

KEY POINTS

- Ranaviruses cause high morbidity and mortality and can be clinically indistinguishable from infection with herpesviruses or *Mycoplasma* spp. Recovered animals may become carriers, and treatment is not recommended.
- Cryptosporidiosis is associated with chronic diarrhea and weight loss in chelonians, although subclinical infections are also reported. There is no effective treatment.
- Intranuclear coccidiosis of Testudines causes a severe, systemic illness with high mortality. Treatment may not clear the organism, and recovered animals may become carriers.
- *Emydomyces testavorans* is associated with ulcerative skin and shell disease and may be underdiagnosed. Keratin inclusion cysts are a common feature of infection. Treatment protocols are currently being developed.

INTRODUCTION

Chelonians are one of the most imperiled vertebrate taxa, with more than 50% of the approximately 350 recognized species considered critically endangered, endangered, or vulnerable by the International Union for Conservation of Nature.[1] The primary causes of chelonian declines often include anthropogenic environmental changes, overharvesting, and direct mortality (e.g., roads, bycatch, lawn equipment); however, infectious diseases can affect survival and fecundity and may also threaten chelonian conservation efforts. Characterizing the epidemiology and clinical effects of emerging infectious diseases promotes the development of effective diagnostic, treatment, control, and preventive measures, ultimately supporting chelonian conservation goals and improving patient outcomes. This review provides an update on several clinically

[a] Wildlife Epidemiology Laboratory, University of Illinois College of Veterinary Medicine, 2001 South Lincoln Avenue, Urbana, IL 61802, USA; [b] Avian and Exotic Veterinary Care, 7826 Northeast Sandy Boulevard, Portland, OR 97213, USA
* Corresponding author.
E-mail address: adamovi2@illinois.edu

challenging emerging infectious diseases in chelonians, including ranaviruses, cryptosporidiosis, intranuclear coccidiosis, and *Emydomyces testavorans*.

RANAVIRUSES
Biology, Ecology, and Epidemiology

The family Iridoviridae comprises large, double-stranded DNA viruses with icosahedral virions, which can be enveloped or nonenveloped.[2] This family is divided into the subfamily Alphairidovirinae, which contains 3 genera infecting ectothermic vertebrates (*Ranavirus*, *Megalocytivirus*, and *Lymphocystivirus*) and the subfamily Betairidovirinae, which contains 3 genera infecting insects and crustaceans (*Iridovirus*, *Chloriridovirus*, and *Decapodiridovirus*).[2,3] Iridoviruses infecting reptiles belong to the genus *Ranavirus*, which includes 6 recognized species: frog virus 3 (FV3), *Ambystoma tigrinum* virus, epizootic hematopoietic necrosis virus, common midwife toad virus, Santee-Cooper ranavirus, and Singapore grouper iridovirus.[4] All chelonian ranavirus infections involve FV3 or FV3-like viruses, and Koch's postulates have been fulfilled in ornate box turtles (*Terrapene ornata ornata*) and red-eared sliders (*Trachemys scripta elegans*) using an FV3-like ranavirus.[2,5]

Ranavirus infections have been detected in more than 175 species of ectothermic vertebrates on 6 continents, and amphibian ranavirus infections are reportable to the World Organization for Animal Health.[6] The first chelonian ranavirus infection was identified in 1982, and since then reports of ranaviral disease in wild and managed-care chelonians have been steadily increasing in number.[7,8] Ranavirus-associated mortality (or susceptibility in challenge studies) has been documented in 21 chelonian species from 7 countries, including 15 states within the United States (**Table 1**), and it is likely that all turtles and tortoises are susceptible.

In nature, chelonian ranavirus infections occur as localized epizootics characterized by high morbidity and mortality (71%–100%).[32,34] Surveillance in several species has demonstrated low detection of ranaviral DNA (0%–3%), antibodies (0%–3.1%), and live virus (0%–3.4%) in blood, oral swabs, and cloacal swabs during nonoutbreak conditions, supporting the classification of ranavirus as an intermittent epidemic disease process in chelonians.[10,20,22,25,30,46–49] Ranaviral outbreaks have driven focal populations of eastern box turtles (*Terrapene carolina carolina*) to decline by 28% to 71%, especially when animals are artificially concentrated and/or outbreaks reoccur over several years.[21,23,32] Ranavirus outbreaks are concerning for the conservation of box turtles, and potentially for other threatened chelonian species.

The source of chelonian ranavirus infections is usually unknown, but many outbreaks are suspected to occur as spillover events from infected amphibians. This possibility is supported by experimental studies demonstrating ranavirus transmission between different classes of ectothermic vertebrate hosts, and by the anecdotal identification of sympatric chelonians and amphibians infected with the same virus.[9,24,34,37] Specific mechanisms of disease transmission are also unknown. Laboratory studies indicate that chelonians can become infected with ranavirus by bath immersion, sharing a water source with infected amphibians, oral inoculation, intramuscular administration, and intracoelomic injection, athough intramuscular and intracoelomic challenges produce the most consistent rates of infection and subsequent disease.[5,16,36,37,40,42,43] This may indicate that turtles can acquire infection via drinking, soaking, ingestion of infectious material such as carcasses, or via wounds; however, this has yet to be experimentally demonstrated and the success of each method likely depends on other factors such as dose, viral strain, age class, and temperature.[36,37,40,42–44] Because ranavirus has a systemic distribution during clinical

Table 1
Identity and location of chelonian species infected with ranaviruses

Species	Scientific Name	Location	References
Gopher tortoise	*Gopherus polyphemus*	USA: Florida, Georgia	7,9,10
Hermann's tortoise	*Testudo hermanni*	Switzerland, Germany	11–13
Egyptian tortoise	*Testudo kleinmanni*	Germany	13
Marginated tortoise	*Testudo marginata*	Germany	13
Russian tortoise	*Testudo horsfeldii*	USA	14
Leopard tortoise	*Stigmochelys pardalis*	Austria	15
Burmese star tortoise	*Geochelone platynota*	USA: Georgia	9
Chinese soft-shelled turtle	*Pelodiscus sinensis*	China	16
Eastern box turtle	*Terrapene carolina carolina*	USA: Alabama, Georgia, Indiana, Illinois, Kentucky, Maryland, North Carolina, New York, Pennsylvania, Tennessee, Texas, Virginia, West Virginia	10,14,17–35
Ornate box turtle	*Terrapene ornata ornata*	N/A	5
Florida box turtle	*Terrapene carolina bauri*	USA: Florida	9
Red-eared slider	*Trachemys scripta elegans*	N/A	5,36,37
Painted turtle	*Chrysemys picta picta*	USA: Indiana, Maryland, Virginia	35,38
Eastern mud turtle	*Kinosternon subrubrum*	USA: South Carolina	39
Krefft's river turtle	*Emydura macquarii krefftii*	N/A, Australia	40–42
Saw-shelled turtle	*Myuchelys latisternum*	N/A, Australia	40,41
Mississippi map turtle	*Graptemys pseudogeographica kohnii*	N/A	43,44
False map turtle	*Graptemys pseudogeographica*	N/A	44
Eastern river cooter	*Pseudemys concinna concinna*	N/A	43,44
Common snapping turtle	*Chelydra serpentina*	Canada: Ontario; USA: Pennsylvania	35,45
Florida softshell turtle	*Apalone ferox*	N/A	43

A location listed as N/A implies a challenge study.
Data from Refs.[5,7,9–45]

infection, invertebrate vectors such as mosquitoes, flies, midges, and leeches may also play a role in viral transmission. One study undertaken during a multiyear box turtle ranavirus outbreak in Indiana detected ranavirus DNA in mosquitoes using polymerase chain reaction (PCR) and sequencing.[50] However, the viability of this virus was not assessed and it is unknown whether mosquitoes may have served as competent vectors. Another study undertaken in Illinois under outbreak conditions failed to detect FV3 DNA in mosquitoes, suggesting that these vectors have a limited role in ranaviral epidemiology (Allender, personal communication, 2019).

Amphibians that survive ranavirus infection can become carriers, and are hypothesized to play a role in ranaviral persistence within wetlands over many years.[51] Although survival seems rare in ranavirus-infected chelonians, it has been documented in managed-care settings with survival rates ranging from 0% to 58% with treatment.[15,17,27,28,32] Eleven eastern box turtles survived ranavirus infection at the Maryland Zoo in Baltimore and tested negative for ranavirus on oral swabs for up to 5 months following brumation.[28] Seven of these animals were challenged with the same ranavirus whereby all became infected and one animal died.[27] Importantly, clinical signs either did not develop or were much milder in the reinfected animals and 86% of the reinoculated animals survived.[27] Viral shedding from the oral cavity persisted for at least 55 days after inoculation, raising concerns that reinfected survivors may represent a source of infection for naïve animals for prolonged periods of time. Furthermore, one sham-inoculated turtle had detectable FV3 DNA in splenic tissues more than a year after its initial infection, potentially indicating the presence of a carrier state in chelonian ranavirus survivors. The relatively mild clinical signs and prolonged shedding in reinfected turtles, and the potential for viral persistence in ranavirus survivors, has important implications for the treatment and rehabilitation of chelonians with ranavirus infections. In general, euthanasia of infected individuals is recommended to prevent disease transmission to other susceptible animals.

Clinical Signs

Various clinical signs have been reported in association with chelonian ranavirus infections, none of which are specific. The most consistently reported signs include lethargy, which is typically profound, anorexia, ophthalmic signs (conjunctivitis, blepharoedema, and ocular discharge), nasal discharge, oropharyngeal lesions (stomatitis, glossitis, pharyngitis, and esophagitis with ulceration and overlying oral plaques, occasional oral discharge or ptyalism), edema, and respiratory distress (**Fig. 1**).[5,7,9,11,15–20,23,24,26–29,32,34,36,39,42,44] Less commonly reported clinical signs include cutaneous ulceration or abscessation, diarrhea, cloacal plaques, cloacal discharge, exophthalmos, hyphema, fractures, and circling.[5,9,17,22,27,28,34,39,42,45] Mortality typically occurs within 30 days of development of clinical signs. Clinical signs of ranavirus infection are frequently indistinguishable from those of herpesvirus and *Mycoplasma* spp infections, emphasizing the importance of obtaining a definitive diagnosis when formulating a treatment plan. Coinfection with ranaviruses, herpesviruses, and *Mycoplasma* spp has also been documented, and detection of one pathogen does not rule out the presence of others.[15,27,28,34] As previously reviewed, clinical signs are mild in ranavirus survivors that become reinfected, and ranavirus testing should be considered for all cases of stomatitis and upper respiratory diseases in chelonians regardless of severity.[27]

Pathology

Chelonian ranavirus infection causes severe lesions with systemic distribution; death likely occurs because of multiorgan failure. Gross changes are variable, and may include conjunctivitis, ulceration of the oral, esophageal, and gastric mucosa (possibly obscured by yellow-tan caseous plaque material), pulmonary hyperemia, focal discolorations of the hepatic and splenic parenchyma, splenomegaly, and, less commonly, petechiae of the gastrointestinal (GI) tract and liver, GI hemorrhage, edema, and coelomic effusion.[5,7,11,12,16–18,36,42,45] Histologic lesions include multiorgan fibrinoid vasculitis, thrombosis, and necrosis (**Fig. 2**).[5,19,36,44] The spleen is typically one of

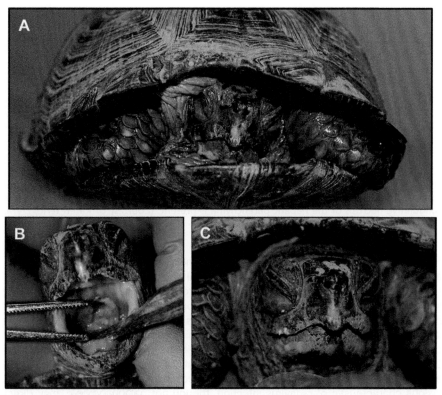

Fig. 1. Clinical signs of ranavirus infection in an eastern box turtle (*Terrapene carolina carolina*). (*A*) Left forelimb edema (note significant scale separation compared with right forelimb). (*B*) Oral plaque. (*C*) Blepharoedema, ocular discharge, and depressed mentation. (*Courtesy of* Laura Adamovicz, DVM, PhD, Urbana, IL.)

the most severely affected organs, and effacement of normal architecture and lymphoid depletion are commonly reported.[5,36,45] Necroulcerative stomatitis, glossitis, pharyngitis, and esophagitis are also common, and are thought to occur secondary to small-vessel thrombosis.[5,19] Hepatic lipidosis and sepsis are frequently identified in ranavirus-infected chelonians, and basophilic intracytoplasmic inclusion bodies are variably reported.[5,7,9,11,12,18,28,39,44]

Diagnosis

Chelonian ranaviruses can be diagnosed using several methods, including PCR (either quantitative or conventional followed by sequencing), virus isolation, and electron microscopy.[5,9,20,36,52] Recommended antemortem samples for ranavirus testing include blood and combined oral/cloacal swabs, which should be frozen for molecular testing or virus isolation (Allender, personal communication, 2019). Testing both blood and swabs increases diagnostic sensitivity, as several studies have demonstrated that ranavirus-infected chelonians are sometimes positive in one sample type but not the other.[22,27,32,36] Antemortem biopsies are also suitable, but many infected animals make extremely poor anesthetic candidates and these samples are infrequently presented for ranavirus testing.

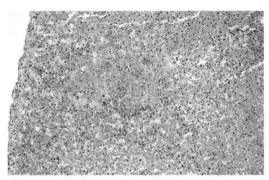

Fig. 2. Liver tissue from a red-eared slider (*Trachemys scripta elegans*) experimentally infected with frog virus 3. Magnification 200×; hematoxylin and eosin stain. Focally extensive coagulative necrosis of the hepatic parenchyma is present. (*Courtesy of* Karen Terio. DVM, PhD, Urbana, IL.)

Supportive testing for diagnosis of ranavirus includes clinical pathology, serology, and histopathology. Reported changes in clinical pathology during chelonian ranavirus infections include heterophilia, elevated heterophil/lymphocyte ratios, intermittent leukocytosis, and decreases in total protein, albumin, and α-globulins.[34,53,54] Toxic heterophils and intracytoplasmic inclusion bodies may also be identified within circulating heterophils and monocytes.[17,18] A serologic assay (ELISA) was developed for gopher tortoises (*Gopherus polyphemus*) and eastern box turtles; however, its clinical utility is debated owing to knowledge gaps about the occurrence and duration of an antibody response during chelonian ranavirus infections.[5,10] Identification of histologic lesions characteristic of ranavirus infection, though not pathognomonic, may direct additional confirmatory testing including PCR, immunohistochemistry, electron microscopy, or virus isolation.

Postmortem samples for ranavirus testing should include aseptically collected and frozen liver, spleen, kidney, and lung; however, ranavirus DNA, virions, and live virus have been successfully identified in many other organs including tongue, trachea, esophagus, stomach, intestine, pancreas, cloaca, gonad, and skeletal muscle, and these may also be suitable for testing if consistent histologic lesions are present.[9,12,17,19,36,40] Bone marrow can also be collected and tested for ranavirus via quantitative PCR in cases of advanced decomposition; as with tissue samples, marrow should be frozen after collection.[31]

Treatment

Treatment of chelonian ranavirus infections is frequently unrewarding and is generally not recommended because of the potential for survivors to become carriers. The decision to treat a ranavirus-infected animal should only be pursued after careful client counseling. Infected animals should be maintained in strict quarantine. Ranaviruses can be stable for 22 to 34 days in pond water, and for 30 to 48 days in soil at temperatures commonly encountered in vivaria; they also remain infectious following freezing.[55] Animals should therefore be maintained in cages that are easy to disinfect with paper substrates that are frequently changed. Waste from these cages should ideally be autoclaved, or alternatively exposed to an appropriate disinfectant and double-bagged before disposal. Effective disinfectants include chlorhexidine (at least 0.75%), sodium hypochlorite (bleach, at least 3%), and potassium peroxymonosulfate compounds (Virkon S, at least 1%) with a 1-minute contact time.[56]

Supportive care is the cornerstone of ranavirus treatment, including nutritional support, fluid therapy, and provision of an appropriate thermal gradient.[7,9,15,17,18,28] Ranaviruses do not produce infectious virions at temperatures higher than 32°C (90°F), and the authors have had anecdotal success with maintaining infected box turtles at the upper end of their preferred optimum temperature zone to promote survival.[57] Specific antiviral therapy has been attempted with acyclovir (80 mg/kg orally [PO] every 24 hours) and famciclovir (10, 20, or 30 mg/kg PO every 24 hours); however, the clinical efficacy of these drugs is unclear.[17,28] Other supportive therapies have included interferon (300 IU/kg PO every 24 hours), vitamin complex injections, parasiticides (pyrantel pamoate 5 mg/kg PO once), ocular treatments (flurbiprofen and ophthalmic ointments), and antibiotics.[9,17,18,28] Antibiotic therapy should be used judiciously because the underlying disease process is viral. However, many ranavirus-infected chelonians develop secondary sepsis, and antibiotics may be warranted on a case-by-base basis. Previous reports have used one or more of the following: enrofloxacin (5 mg/kg subcutaneously [SC] or intramuscularly [IM] every 24 hours, 10 mg/kg SC every 48 hours), clindamycin (10 mg/kg IM every 24 hours or 17.8 mg/kg IM every 72 hours), and ceftazidime (20 mg/kg IM every 72 hours).[7,17,18,28]

CRYPTOSPORIDIOSIS
Biology and Epidemiology

Cryptosporidium spp are apicomplexan coccidia in the family Cryptosporidiidae.[58] In reptiles *Cryptosporidium* spp infection is commonly associated with hypertrophic gastritis in snakes and hypertrophic or atrophic gastritis in lizards.[59] However, within the last 10 years, clinical and subclinical cryptosporidiosis has been diagnosed in chelonians.[60–64] Cases have been observed in 20 chelonian species from 6 countries (**Table 2**).

Three distinct species are described in tortoises with either intestinal tropism (*Cryptosporidium ducismarci*, also known as *Cryptosporidium* sp tortoise genotype II or *Cryptosporidium* sp CrIT20), gastric tropism (*Cryptosporidium tetudinis*, also known as *Cryptosporidium* sp tortoise 750 or *Cryptosporidium* sp tortoise genotype I), or unknown tissue tropism (*Cryptosporidium* sp tortoise genotype III).[60–62,64] A recent study demonstrated that *C ducismarci* is transmissible through fecal-oral contact.[64] The prepatent period for chelonian *Cryptosporidium* spp infections is 6 to 11 days and the patent period can last 200 days or longer.[64] The entire life cycle of *Cryptosporidium* spp is completed within a single host. Oocysts can persist in environmental substrates and water for months, especially in the presence of organic material.[75] Recent surveillance studies have been performed in client-owned and free-ranging chelonians and have produced prevalence estimates between 1% and 17%.[64,69,73,76]

Clinical Signs

Clinical signs are inconsistently reported in chelonians, but when present have consisted of chronic diarrhea with undigested food, pica, weight loss, weakness, and lethargy.[61,63,64,70,72] Many chelonians with *Cryptosporidium* spp infections exhibit no clinical signs and, as in other species, immunosuppression is proposed as an important antecedent cause of clinical cryptosporidiosis.[58,64] Concurrent infection with additional pathogens has been reported in chelonians, and concomitant infections may enhance disease progression.[61,72] A study of captive tortoises in Italy found that 7 of 21 tortoises (33.3%) tested positive for *Cryptosporidium* oocyst DNA in feces, 6 of which also had *Cryptosporidium*-like oocysts on light microscopy. Five of these individuals had concurrent intestinal nematodes, and 3 coinfected tortoises exhibited

Table 2
Identity and location of chelonian species infected with *Cryptosporidium* spp

Species	Scientific Name	Location	References
Radiated tortoise	*Astrochelys radiata*	USA	64,65
Indian star tortoise	*Geochelone elegans*	Portugal, Czech Republic, USA	60,64–68
Gopher tortoise	*Gopherus polyphemus*	USA	69
	Indotestudo sp	USA	67
Marginated tortoise	*Testudo marginata*	Italy, Czech Republic	61,64
Pancake tortoise	*Malacochersus tornieri*	Czech Republic, USA	64,70
African spurred tortoise	*Centrochelys sulcata*	Czech Republic	64
Red-footed tortoise	*Chelonoidis carbonaria*	Czech Republic	64
Chaco tortoise	*Chelonoidis chilensis*	Czech Republic	64
Angulate tortoise	*Chersina angulata*	Czech Republic	64
Bell's hinge-back tortoise	*Kinixys belliana*	Czech Republic	64
Serrated tortoise	*Psammobates oculifer*	Czech Republic	64
Leopard tortoise	*Stigmochelys pardalis*	Czech Republic	64
Hermann's tortoise	*Testudo hermanni*	Spain, UK, Czech Republic	64,71–73
Russian tortoise	*Testudo horsfeldii*	Czech Republic, USA	64,70
Egyptian tortoise	*Testudo kleinmanni*	Czech Republic, USA	64,68
Greek tortoise	*Testudo graeca*	Czech Republic	64
Green sea turtle	*Chelonia mydas*	USA	74
Bog turtle	*Clemmys muhlenbergi*	N/A	67
Box turtle	*Terrapene carolina*	Czech Republic	64

A location listed as N/A implies missing data.
Data from Refs.[60,61,64–74]

signs of gastrointestinal disease.[61] Robust estimates of morbidity and mortality rates associated with chelonian cryptosporidiosis are currently unavailable.

Pathology

Pathologic changes associated with *Cryptosporidium* spp infections in chelonians are infrequent. *C testudinis* infection has gastric mucosal tropism and can be associated with mild lymphocytic and heterophilic mucosal inflammation.[70] *C ducismarci* has intestinal mucosal tropism and may be associated with mixed inflammation (**Fig. 3**).[70] *Cryptosporidium* organisms are 1-5 μm amphophilic round structures with an eccentrically located dense basophilic internal structure in hematoxylin and eosin–stained tissue sections.[70]

Diagnosis

Diagnostic tests include morphologic characterization through microscopy (feces or biopsy), sugar flotation or formalin sedimentation, and acid-fast staining.[58] Wet-mount cytology with acid-fast staining, safranin-methylene blue, negative staining, or fluorescent staining techniques may also improve detection.[58] Oocytes are 4 to 5 μm (*C ducismarci*) or 6 to 7 μm (*C testudinis*) in a nearly spherical morphology with 4 sporozoites and no sporocyst.[64] Pathogen detection seems significantly more sensitive with the use of

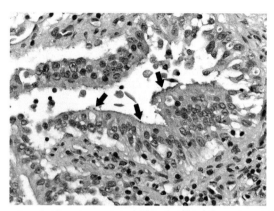

Fig. 3. Duodenum of an Indian star tortoise (*Geochelone elegans*) at 600× magnification, hematoxylin and eosin stain. *Cryptosporidium ducismarci* organisms (*arrows*) are present along the luminal surface of hyperplastic enterocytes, and mild to moderate lymphocytic and heterophilic inflammation is present in the lamina propria. (*Courtesy of* Robert Ossiboff, DVM, PhD, Gainesville, FL.)

molecular methods, such as fecal PCR, but the true sensitivity and specificity in detection of chelonian *Cryptosporidium* spp has not been determined.[64]

Treatment

There are no effective treatments published for cryptosporidiosis in chelonians, so effective management requires appropriate diagnosis, optimal husbandry, and management of concurrent disease.[63,77] Anticoccidial drugs, such as paromomycin (100 mg/kg PO every 24 hours × 7 days), toltrazuril, and ponazuril are proposed, but none eliminate disease.[63,72,77] A combination of paromomycin and supportive care has been shown to improve clinical signs and reduce shedding temporarily.[72]

Cryptosporidia are resistant to most disinfectants and survive well in the environment for many months.[75,77] Cresols, hydrogen peroxide (6%–10%), sodium hydroxide (2.5%) in windshield-washer fluid, formalin (10%), glutaraldehyde (2.65%), and 5% to 10% ammonia solution have demonstrated some efficacy after prolonged contact.[78–80] Hydrogen peroxide (6%–10%) is recommended for clean impermeable surfaces at room temperature because it greatly reduces infectivity of *Cryptosporidium* spp oocysts. Contact time should be 13 min with 6% hydrogen peroxide for good reduction of infectivity, with excellent decontamination expected for 10% hydrogen peroxide after 2 hours.[80,81] Several common disinfectants have proved to be inadequate, including chlorhexidine, ethanol, 3% hydrogen peroxide, iodophores, isopropanol, methanol, and sodium hypochlorite (bleach).[78,80,81]

INTRANUCLEAR COCCIDIOSIS OF TESTUDINES
Biology and Epidemiology

Intranuclear coccidiosis of Testudines (TINC) is associated with severe, multisystemic disease and has been detected in at least 18 species of chelonians in the United States, Europe, and China (**Table 3**).[85] The causative agent is a currently unnamed coccidian with a well-supported basal position relative to the Eimeriidae.[83,86,87] Like other coccidians, a challenge study has confirmed that TINC can be transmitted via the fecal-oral route.[87] Oocysts are shed in feces and sporulate after 3 to 4 days.

Table 3
Identity and location of chelonian species infected with intranuclear coccidiosis of Testudines

Species	Scientific Name	Location	Circumstances	References
Radiated tortoise	*Astrochelys radiata*	Germany, Spain, USA: Florida, Georgia	I, C, D	82–85
Sulawesi tortoise	*Indotestudo forstenii*	USA: New York	I, C	83,86
Leopard tortoise	*Stigmochelys pardalis*	Germany, Spain, Italy, Switzerland, Czech Republic, USA: Louisiana, New York	I, C, D	83,85,87
Bowsprit tortoise	*Chersina angulata*	United Kingdom, USA: Florida	I, C, D	83,85
Impressed tortoise	*Manouria impressa*	USA: Texas	I, C	83
Arakan Forest turtle	*Heosemys depressa*	N/A	D	88
Galapagos tortoise	*Chelonoidis niger becki*	N/A	D	88
Indian star tortoise	*Geochelone elegans*	Germany, Switzerland, Portugal	D	85,88
Eastern box Turtle	*Terrapene carolina carolina*	N/A	D	88
Flat-tailed tortoise	*Pyxis planicauda*	USA: California	I, C, D	88,89
Spider tortoise	*Pyxis arachnoides*	USA: California	I, C, D	88,89
Marginated tortoise	*Testudo marginata*	Germany, Spain	D	85
Hermann's tortoise	*Testudo hermanni*	Germany, Switzerland	I, D	85,87
Greek tortoise	*Testudo graeca*	N/A	I, C	87
Russian tortoise	*Testudo horsfeldii*	N/A	I	87
African spurred tortoise	*Centrochelys sulcata*	Austria, Spain	I, D	85,87
Yellow-footed tortoise	*Chelonoidis denticulatus*	Germany	D	85
Red-footed tortoise	*Chelonoidis carbonaria*	USA: Florida	I, C	90

A location listed as N/A either implies missing data or a challenge study.
Abbreviations: C, clinical signs; D, detection; I, infection.
Data from Refs.[82–90]

The prepatent period ranges from 30 to 47 days, and infected tortoises show extreme individual variability in the length of the patent period (43–133 days, or until death) and number of oocysts shed (<10–40,000 oocysts per gram of feces).[87] Previously infected tortoises can recover and become test negative; however, some of these individuals can later recrudesce, develop clinical signs, and become test positive, indicating the potential for a carrier state.[63]

The development of clinical disease may be species dependent, as Russian tortoises (*Testudo horsfeldii*), Hermann's tortoises (*Testudo hermanni*), and an African spurred tortoise (*Centrochelys sulcata*) failed to develop clinical signs following infection, while Greek tortoises (*Testudo graeca*) and leopard tortoises (*Stigmochelys pardalis*) developed fulminant disease resulting in death or euthanasia.[87] TINC cases appear to be overrepresented in radiated tortoises (*Astrochelys radiata*), although well-structured systematic prevalence studies have not been conducted and this may be an artifact of sampling bias.[82–85] All reported TINC cases have occurred in managed-care settings (including in recently imported animals), and this organism has yet to be identified in free-living chelonians.

Clinical Signs

Clinical signs associated with TINC are relatively nonspecific and include lethargy, anorexia, rapid weight loss or gain, weakness, oculonasal discharge, conjunctival or nasal erythema, oral discharge, respiratory distress, swollen erythematous vent, cloacal ulcers, edema, coelomic effusion, and diarrhea.[63,82–84,87,89,90] Illness tends to be severe and acute, with death occurring within a month of the development of clinical signs; however, some animals survive for a few months and others apparently recover.[63,82–84,87,89,90] Chronic rhinosinusitis and oronasal fistulae have also been reported in a series of Sulawesi tortoises (*Indotestudo forstenii*) infected with both TINC and *Mycoplasma* spp.[86]

Pathology

Gross necropsy findings may include thick oral mucus, pericloacal erythema, severely distended urinary bladder, hepatosplenomegaly, firm gray kidneys, pulmonary congestion or hemorrhage, pericardial effusion, epicardial petechiae, pseudomembrane formation within the GI tract, erythematous and edematous intestines with or without petechiation, and coelomic effusion.[63,82,84,89,90] Histopathologic changes include multisystemic necrosis, lymphocytic or lymphoplasmacytic inflammation, and variable epithelial hyperplasia, which can even occur in organs where TINC organisms are not visualized (**Fig. 4**).[82–84,86,90] TINC life stages are typically observed in the nuclei (rarely the cytoplasm or extracellular space) of multiple organs, and include trophozoites, meronts, merozoites, macrogametocytes, microgametocytes, and nonsporulated oocysts.[82–84] These organisms are easiest to identify using hematoxylin and eosin staining, and do not take up periodic acid–Schiff or Fite acid-fast stains.[83] Chelonians that die following treatment of TINC can present with fibrosis in areas previously infected by the organism, indicating that this pathogen may cause long-term tissue damage that compromises organ function.[63]

Diagnosis

TINC can be diagnosed using PCR (quantitative or conventional followed by sequencing), cytology, fecal flotation with Sheather solution, or histopathology.[88] Samples that have been successfully used for antemortem testing include blood (PCR), conjunctival swabs (PCR), nasal flushes (PCR or cytology), oral/cloacal swabs (PCR), feces (fecal float, PCR), and biopsies of the nasal and cloacal mucosa (PCR, cytology, or histopathology).[63,85,89,90] Cytologic impressions should be made and stained immediately (Wright-Giemsa, Fite acid-fast, or periodic acid–Schiff techniques have all been useful), samples collected for PCR should be frozen, and fecal samples should be refrigerated before flotation.[86] Fecal flotation for the diagnosis of TINC is challenging, partially because the oocysts are very small (6–7 μm), and high magnification (400–1000×) is necessary for visualization, and partially because the oocysts degrade within a few minutes of contact with the flotation solution.[87] It is therefore

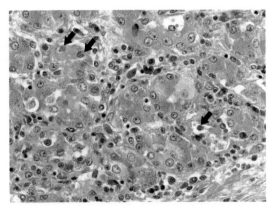

Fig. 4. Pancreas of a red-footed tortoise (*Chelonoidis carbonaria*) at 600× magnification, hematoxylin and eosin stain. Life stages of intranuclear coccidiosis of Testudines (TINC) are present (*arrows*) within the nucleus of exocrine pancreatic acinar cells and are associated with degeneration, necrosis, and active granulocytic and lymphoplasmacytic pancreatitis. (*Courtesy of* Robert Ossiboff, DVM, PhD, Gainesville, FL.)

recommended that fecal flotation be paired with PCR to improve diagnostic sensitivity.[87] Postmortem sampling should minimally include aseptically collected and frozen kidney, liver, pancreas, and intestine for molecular testing, although many other organs may also be PCR positive.[82,83,85,90] Samples for routine histopathology should include all major organs and the head (with calvaria partially opened to allow rapid penetration of formalin). TINC testing should be considered in all cases of severe systemic illness in chelonians.

Clinical pathologic changes in TINC-infected chelonians are nonspecific and reflect multiorgan dysfunction. Reported abnormalities include anemia, leukocytosis, hyperglycemia, hyponatremia, hyperkalemia, hypophosphatemia, hyperuricemia, and hypoalbuminemia.[82,90] Chelonians infected with TINC can be coinfected with *Mycoplasma* spp and herpesviruses. These pathogens should also be tested for if clinically indicated.[85,86]

Treatment

TINC treatment focuses on optimizing husbandry and minimizing stress. Infected individuals should be quarantined and fecal matter promptly removed to minimize the presence of infectious material. Nutritional support, fluid therapy, antibiotics, and broad-spectrum antiparasitics should be pursued on a case-by-case basis, if indicated. Specific antiprotozoal therapies include toltrazuril (15 mg/kg PO every 48 hours × 30–45 days) or ponazuril (20 mg/kg every 48 hours × 56 days).[63,90] Shorter courses of toltrazuril (<2 weeks) have been used and seem to reduce clinical signs; however, these treatment regimens have resulted in chronic infection and death after several months and are not recommended.[63,89] Neither toltrazuril nor ponazuril consistently clears TINC infection, although many animals clinically improve with treatment.[63,89,90] This may be attributable to delayed and variable oral absorption of ponazuril and the failure to achieve plasma levels considered coccidiocidal in mammalian infections at currently published doses.[91] Because chelonians that survive TINC infection may become carriers, the future exposure of treated animals to other chelonians must be considered and clients counseled appropriately.

EMYDOMYCES TESTAVORANS
Biology and Epidemiology

Emydomyces testavorans is a newly described keratinophilic fungal organism associated with ulcerative skin and shell disease in at least 10 species of chelonian (**Table 4**). *E testavorans* is a member of the order Onygenales, which includes primary reptile pathogens such as *Ophidiomyces* and *Nannizziopsis*.[94,95] The biology and epidemiology of *E testavorans* is almost completely uncharacterized, although it has been found in turtles in Illinois and Washington State and is considered a disease of conservation concern in Pacific pond turtles (*Actinemys marmarota*); it may be a contributing factor or cause of ulcerative shell disease in many chelonian species.[96] To date, the status of *E testavorans* as a primary pathogen has not been confirmed.

Clinical Signs

E testavorans has been found in association with common shell lesions including keratin discoloration, flaking and textural change, erosion, ulceration, and osteonecrosis (**Fig. 5**).[93,95,96] Keratin inclusion cysts associated with *Emydomyces* infection can expand into the coelomic cavity and compress viscera.[95] Bony lesions may be present even in the absence of apparent surface disease.[96] Juvenile alligator snapping turtles (*Macrochelys temminckii*) have a different clinical presentation including rhinitis, paronychia, nail loss, cutaneous ulceration, plastron ulceration, excessive shedding, and death (**Fig. 6**).[92] Infected alligator snapping turtles can resolve all clinical signs of *E testavorans* infection with proper husbandry, but still demonstrate excessive shedding and intermittent cutaneous ulceration associated with chronic infection.[92]

Pathology

Gross lesions associated with *E testavorans* include discoloration, flaking, pitting, and ulceration of the shell. Nodular lesions expanding into the coelom are occasionally noted (see **Fig. 5**).[95] Histologic findings include multilocular intradermal and intraosseous keratin inclusion cysts (present in more than 90% of *E testavorans* cases), ulceration, necrosis, inflammation, fibrosis, boney remodeling, squamous metaplasia, and hyperkeratosis (**Fig. 7**).[95] Fungi morphologically consistent with *E testavorans* are frequently visualized along the leading edge of lesions; however,

Table 4	
Chelonian species infected with *Emydomyces testavorans*	
Species	**Scientific Name**
Argentine snake-necked turtle	*Hydromedusa tectifera*
Western pond turtle	*Actinemys marmarota*
Savanna side-necked turtle	*Podocnemis vogli*
Spiny soft-shelled turtle	*Apalone spinifera*
Ringed map turtle	*Graptemys oculifera*
Alligator snapping turtle	*Macrochelys temminckii*
Red-eared slider	*Trachemys scripta elegans*
Red-bellied short-necked turtle	*Emydura subglobosa*
Mata mata	*Chelus fimbriatus*
Yellow-spotted river turtle	*Podocnemis unifilis*

Data from Refs.[92–95]

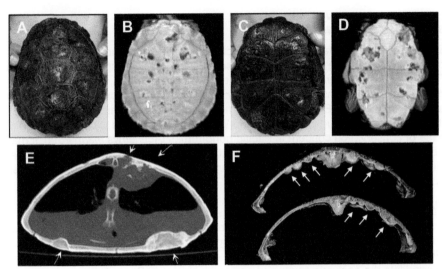

Fig. 5. Clinical signs, gross lesions, and computed tomographic appearance of shell disease in Pacific pond turtles (*Actinemys marmorata*, *A–E*) and a savanna side-necked turtle (*Podocnemis vogli*, *F*) testing PCR positive for *E testavorans*. (*A, C*) Discoloration, flaking, and pitting of the shell in a Pacific pond turtle with severe shell disease. (*B, D*) Computed tomographic 3-dimensional reconstruction of the carapace and plastron from the same individual, revealing multiple lytic boney lesions underlying areas of abnormal keratin. (*E*) Computed tomographic image of a Pacific pond turtle, mid-body axial view. Multiple lytic and proliferative lesions of the carapace and plastron (*arrows*) are present, and are expanding into the coelomic cavity. (*F*) Two cross-sectional views of the carapace of a savanna side-necked turtle. The bone is focally disrupted by multiple expansile nodules (*arrows*), which displace the coelomic membrane. Nodules are cystic and filled with brown caseous debris. (*Courtesy of [A–E]* Katherine Haman, DVM, Olympia, WA; and [*F*] Karen Terio. DVM, PhD, Urbana, IL.)

the histologic appearance of these fungi is not fully distinctive.[95] Secondary bacterial and fungal infections are frequently identified. In alligator snapping turtles, common histologic lesions include hyperkeratosis and ulcerative dermatitis/rhinitis with intralesional fungi.[92]

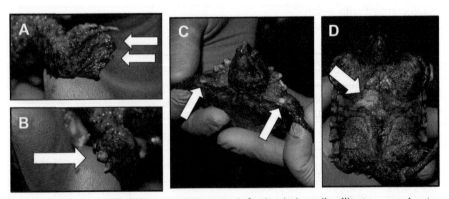

Fig. 6. Clinical signs of *Emydomyces testavorans* infection in juvenile alligator snapping turtles (*Macrochelys temminckii*). (*A*) Nail loss, (*B*) paronychia, (*C*) cutaneous ulceration, (*D*) scute ulceration. (*Courtesy of* Laura Adamovicz, DVM, PhD, Urbana, IL.)

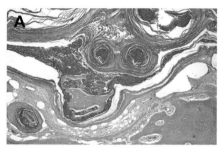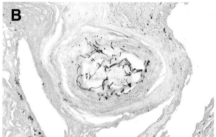

Fig. 7. Histologic appearance of shell disease in a savanna side-necked turtle (*Podocnemis vogli*) testing PCR positive for *Emydomyes testavorans*; same individual as in **Fig. 5**F. (*A*) Carapace at 100× magnification, hematoxylin and eosin stain. The dermal bone is replaced by multiple coalescing epithelial inclusion cysts containing whorls of keratin and necrotic cellular debris. (*B*) Carapace at 400× magnification, Grocott-Gomori methenamine silver stain. Numerous fungi morphologically consistent with *E testavorans* are associated with keratin layers within an epithelial inclusion cyst. (*Courtesy of* Karen Terio. DVM, PhD, Urbana, IL.)

Diagnosis

Diagnosis of *E testavorans* is accomplished through PCR (quantitative or conventional followed by sequencing) or culture. This fungus is keratinophilic, and requires specialized media enriched with reptile keratin for isolation.[94] Contamination with bacteria and fungi is common during culture attempts, and paired molecular testing is highly recommended. Recommended diagnostic samples include lesion swabs and biopsy material, which should be refrigerated for culture or frozen for molecular diagnostics.[93–95] Supportive diagnostics include histopathology and cytology showing compatible lesions and morphologically consistent fungi; however, these tests are inadequate for definitive diagnosis. Radiography (especially computed tomography) is useful to document the extent of disease, determine prognosis, and evaluate response to therapy (see **Fig. 5**).[93,96]

Treatment

E testavorans is susceptible to several antifungal drugs in vitro, but few reports of treatment are available.[94] A cohort of mildly affected Pacific pond turtles responded to management with lesion debridement, topical iodine, and terbinafine cream, and terbinafine nebulization is currently being explored (Adamovicz, personal communication, 2019).[93] Successful management will likely require husbandry improvements, supportive care, judicious use of topical or systemic antifungals, treatment of concurrent disease, and prolonged monitoring. Reported lesion resolution times in turtles with mild shell disease range from 3 to 16 months.[93] Environmental persistence and disinfectant protocols have not yet been explored for *E testavorans*, which is an important consideration for veterinary hospitals and clients with infected animals.

SUMMARY

The number of described pathogens in chelonians is increasing, and a solid understanding of available information is necessary to guide case management, especially for clinically challenging diseases such as ranavirosis, cryptosporidiosis, TINC, and emerging fungal pathogens (*Emydomyces*). Several important knowledge gaps remain for many chelonian pathogens, and ongoing research is necessary to fill them. Advances in diagnostics, therapeutics, and preventive protocols will continue to improve the quality of reptilian veterinary care and promote positive outcomes for chelonian patients.

DISCLOSURE

Two of the authors (L. Adamovicz and M.C. Allender) work in a laboratory that provides diagnostic testing for reptile clinicians. This role has not influenced the structure or content of this article.

REFERENCES

1. Rhodin AGJ, Stanford CB, van Dijk PP, et al. Global conservation status of turtles and tortoises (order Testudines). Chelonian Conservation and Biology 2018; 17(2):135–61.
2. Chinchar VG, Hick P, Ince IA, et al. ICTV virus taxonomy profile: Iridoviridae. J Gen Virol 2017;98:890–1.
3. Chinchar VG, Yang F, Huang J, et al. ICTV proposal 2018.004d: Short title: One new genus with one new species in the subfamily Betairidovirinae. 2018. Available at: https://talk.ictvonline.org/. Accessed November 1, 2019.
4. Chinchar VG, Hick P, Jancovich J, et al. ICTV proposal 2018.007D: Short title: 8 new species in the family Iridoviridae; removal of 3 existing species. 2019. Available at: https://talk.ictvonline.org/. Accessed November 1, 2019.
5. Johnson AJ, Pessier AP, Jacobson ER. Experimental transmission and induction of ranaviral disease in western ornate box turtles (*Terrapene ornata ornata*) and red-eared sliders (*Trachemys scripta elegans*). Vet Pathol 2007;44:285–97.
6. Duffus ALJ, Waltzek TB, Stöhr AC, et al. Distribution and host range of ranaviruses. In: Gray MJ, Chinchar VG, editors. Ranaviruses: lethal pathogens of ectothermic vertebrates. New York: Springer International Publishing; 2015. p. 9–57.
7. Westhouse RA, Jacobson ER, Harris RK, et al. Respiratory and pharyngoesophageal iridovirus infection in a gopher tortoise (*Gopherus polyphemus*). J Wildl Dis 1996;32:682–6.
8. Wirth W, Schwarzkopf L, Skerratt LF, et al. Ranaviruses and reptiles. PeerJ 2018; 6:e6083.
9. Johnson AJ, Pessier AP, Wellehan JF, et al. Ranavirus infection of free-ranging and captive box turtles and tortoises in the United States. J Wildl Dis 2008;44:851–63.
10. Johnson AJ, Wendland L, Norton TM, et al. Development and use of an indirect enzyme-linked immunosorbent assay for detection of iridovirus exposure in gopher tortoises (*Gopherus polyphemus*) and eastern box turtles (*Terrapene carolina carolina*). Vet Microbiol 2010;142:160–7.
11. Heldstab A, Bestetti G. Spontaneous viral hepatitis in a spur-tailed Mediterranean land tortoise (*Testudo hermanni*). J Zoo Anim Med 1982;13:113–20.
12. Marschang RE, Becher P, Posthaus H, et al. Isolation and characterization of an iridovirus from Hermann's tortoises (*Testudo hermanni*). Arch Virol 1999;144: 1909–22.
13. Blahak S, Uhlenbrok C. Ranavirus infections in European terrestrial tortoises in Germany. In: Öfner S, Weinzierl F, editors. Proceedings of the 1st international conference on reptile and amphibian medicine. Munich (Germany): Verlag Dr. Hut; 2010. p. 17–23.
14. Mao J, Hedrick RP, Chinchar VG. Molecular characterization, sequence analysis, and taxonomic position of newly isolated fish iridoviruses. Virology 1997;229: 212–20.

15. Benetka V, Grabensteiner E, Gumpenberger M, et al. First report of an iridovirus (genus Ranavirus) infection in a leopard tortoise (*Geochelone pardalis pardalis*). Wien Tierärztl Monatsschr 2007;9/10:243–8.

16. Chen ZX, Zheng JC, Jiang YL. A new iridovirus isolated from soft-shelled turtle. Virus Res 1999;63:147–51.

17. De Voe R, Geissler K, Elmore S, et al. Ranavirus associated morbidity and mortality in a group of captive eastern box turtles (*Terrapene carolina carolina*). J Zoo Wildl Med 2004;35:534–43.

18. Allender MC, Fry MM, Irizarry AR, et al. Intracytoplasmic inclusions in circulating leukocytes from an eastern box turtle (*Terrapene carolina carolina*) with iridoviral infection. J Wildl Dis 2006;42:677–84.

19. Ruder MG, Allison AB, Miller DL, et al. Pathology in practice: ranaviral disease in a box turtle. J Am Vet Med Assoc 2010;237:783–5.

20. Allender MC, Abd-Eldaim M, Schumacher J, et al. PCR prevalence of ranavirus in free-ranging eastern box turtles (*Terrapene carolina carolina*) at rehabilitation centers in three southeastern US States. J Wildl Dis 2011;47:759–64.

21. Belzer WR, Seibert S. A natural history of ranavirus in an eastern box turtle population. Turtle & Tortoise Newsletter 2011;15:18–25.

22. Allender MC, Mitchell MA, Mcruer D, et al. Prevalence, clinical signs, and natural history characteristics of frog virus 3-like infections in eastern box turtles (*Terrapene carolina carolina*). Herpetol Conserv Biol 2013;8:308–20.

23. Farnsworth SD, Seigel RA. Responses, movements, and survival of relocated box turtles during construction of the intercounty connector highway in Maryland. Transp Res Rec 2013;2362:1–8.

24. Currylow AF, Johnson AJ, Williams RN. Evidence of ranavirus infections among sympatric larval amphibians and box turtles. J Herpetol 2014;48:117–21.

25. Vannatta JM, Klukowski M, Wright S. Prevalence of ranavirus infection in the eastern box turtle, *Terrapene carolina carolina*, in an isolated, suburban wetland habitat of middle Tennessee. Herpetol Rev 2016;47:55–6.

26. Perpiñán D, Blas-Machado U, Sánchez S, et al. Concurrent phaeohyphomycosis and ranavirus infection in an eastern box turtle (*Terrapene carolina*) in Athens, Georgia, USA. J Wildl Dis 2016;52:742–5.

27. Hausmann JC, Wack AN, Allender MC, et al. Experimental challenge study of FV3-like ranavirus infection in previously FV3-like ranavirus infected eastern box turtles (*Terrapene carolina carolina*) to assess infection and survival. J Zoo Wildl Med 2015;46(4):732–46.

28. Sim RR, Allender MC, Crawford LK, et al. Ranavirus epizootic in captive eastern box turtles (*Terrapene carolina carolina*) with concurrent herpesvirus and mycoplasma infection: management and monitoring. J Zoo Wildl Med 2016;47:256–70.

29. Agha M, Price SJ, Nowakowski AJ, et al. Mass mortality of eastern box turtles with upper respiratory disease following atypical cold weather. Dis Aquat Organ 2017; 124:91–100.

30. Archer GA, Phillips CA, Adamovicz L, et al. Detection of copathogens in free-ranging eastern box turtles (*Terrapene carolina carolina*) in Illinois and Tennessee. J Zoo Wildl Med 2017;48:1127–34.

31. Butkus CE, Allender MC, Phillips CA, et al. Detection of ranavirus using bone marrow harvested from mortality events in eastern box turtles (*Terrapene carolina carolina*). J Zoo Wildl Med 2017;48:1210–4.

32. Kimble SJA, Johnson AJ, Williams RN, et al. A severe ranavirus outbreak in captive, wild-caught box turtles. Ecohealth 2017;14:810–5.

33. Goodman RM, Hargadon KM, Carter ED. Detection of ranavirus in eastern fence lizards and eastern box turtles in Central Virginia. Northeast Naturalist 2018;25: 391–8.
34. Adamovicz L, Allender MC, Archer G, et al. Investigation of multiple mortality events in eastern box turtles (*Terrapene carolina carolina*). PLoS One 2018; 13:1–20.
35. U.S. Geological Survey National Wildlife Health Center (NWHC). WHISPers (Wildlife Health Information Sharing Partnership—event reporting system). Available at: https://www.nwhc.usgs.gov/whispers/. Accessed October 20, 2019.
36. Allender MC, Mitchell MA, Torres T, et al. Pathogenicity of frog virus 3-like virus in red-eared slider turtles (*Trachemys scripta elegans*) at two environmental temperatures. J Comp Pathol 2013;149:356–67.
37. Brenes R, Gray MJ, Waltzek TB, et al. Transmission of ranavirus between ectothermic vertebrate hosts. PLoS One 2014;9:e92476.
38. Goodman RM, Miller DL, Ararso YT. Prevalence of ranavirus in Virginia turtles as detected by tail-clip sampling versus oral-cloacal swabbing. Northeast Naturalist 2013;20:325–32.
39. Winzeler ME, Hamilton MT, Tuberville TD, et al. First case of ranavirus and associated morbidity and mortality in an eastern mud turtle *Kinosternon subrubrum* in South Carolina. Dis Aquat Organ 2015;114:77–81.
40. Ariel E, Wirth W, Burgess G, et al. Pathogenicity in six Australian reptile species following experimental inoculation with bohle iridovirus. Dis Aquat Organ 2015; 115:203–12.
41. Ariel E, Elliott E, Meddings JI, et al. Serological survey of Australian native reptiles for exposure to ranavirus. Dis Aquat Organ 2017;126:173–83.
42. Wirth W, Schwarzkopf L, Skerratt LF, et al. Dose-dependent morbidity of freshwater turtle hatchlings, *Emydura macquarii krefftii*, inoculated with Ranavirus isolate (Bohle iridovirus, Iridoviridae). J Gen Virol 2019;100:1431–41.
43. Brenes R, Miller DL, Waltzek TB, et al. Susceptibility of fish and turtles to three ranaviruses isolated from different ectothermic vertebrate classes. J Aquat Anim Health 2014;26:118–26.
44. Allender MC, Barthel AC, Rayl JM, et al. Experimental transmission of frog virus 3-like ranavirus in juvenile chelonians at two temperatures. J Wildl Dis 2018;54(4): 716–25.
45. McKenzie CM, Piczak ML, Snyman HN, et al. First report of ranavirus mortality in a common snapping turtle *Chelydra serpentina*. Dis Aquat Organ 2019;132: 221–7.
46. Seimon TA, Horne BD, Tomaszewicz A, et al. Disease screening in southern river terrapins (*Batagur affinis edwardmolli*) in Cambodia. J Zoo Wildl Med 2017;48(4): 1242–6.
47. Winzeler ME, Haskins DL, Lance SL, et al. Survey of aquatic turtles on the savannah river site, South Carolina, USA, for prevalence of ranavirus. J Wildl Dis 2018;54:138–41.
48. Aplasca AC, Titus V, Ossiboff RJ, et al. Health assessment of free-ranging chelonians in an urban section of the Bronx river, New York, USA. J Wildl Dis 2019; 55(2):352–62.
49. Carstairs SJ. Evidence for low prevalence of ranaviruses in Ontario, Canada's freshwater turtle population. PeerJ 2019;7:e6987.
50. Kimble SA, Karna A, Johnson A, et al. Mosquitoes as a potential vector of ranavirus transmission in terrestrial turtles. Ecohealth 2014;12(2):334–8.

51. Robert J, Grayfer L, Edholm ES, et al. Inflammation-induced reactivation of the ranavirus frog VIRUS 3 in asymptomatic *Xenopus laevis*. PLoS One 2014;9: e112904.
52. Allender MC, Bunick D, Mitchell MA. Development and validation of TaqMan quantitative PCR for detection of frog virus 3-like virus in eastern box turtles (*Terrapene carolina carolina*). J Virol Methods 2013;188:121–5.
53. Allender MC, Mitchell MA. Hematologic response to experimental infections of frog virus 3-like virus in red-eared sliders (*Trachemys scripta elegans*). J Herpetol Med Surg 2013;23:25–31.
54. Moore AR, Allender MC, MacNeill AL. Effects of ranavirus infection of red-eared sliders (*Trachemys scripta elegans*) on plasma proteins. J Zoo Wildl Med 2014; 45(2):298–305.
55. Nazir J, Spengler M, Marschang RE. Environmental persistence of amphibian and reptilian ranaviruses. Dis Aquat Organ 2012;98:177–84.
56. Bryan LK, Baldwin CA, Gray MJ, et al. Efficacy of select disinfectants at inactivating ranavirus. Dis Aquat Organ 2009;84:89–94.
57. Tripier F, Braunwald J, Markovic L, et al. Frog virus 3 morphogenesis: effect of temperature and metabolic inhibitors. J Gen Virol 1977;37(1):39–52.
58. Vanathy K, Parija SC, Mandal J, et al. Cryptosporidiosis: a mini review. Trop Parasitol 2017;7(2):72–80.
59. Stacy BA, Pessier AP. Host response to infectious agents and identification of pathogens in tissue section. In: Jacobson ER, editor. Infectious diseases and pathology of reptiles. Boca Raton (FL): CRC Press; 2007. p. 257–97.
60. Xiao L, Ryan UM, Graczyk TK, et al. Genetic diversity of *Cryptosporidium* spp. in captive reptiles. Appl Environ Microbiol 2004;70(2):891–9.
61. Traversa D, Iorio R, Otranto D, et al. Cryptosporidium from tortoises: genetic characterisation, phylogeny and zoonotic implications. Mol Cell Probes 2008; 22(2):122.
62. Traversa D. Evidence for a new species of *Cryptosporidium* infecting tortoises: *Cryptosporidium ducismarci*. Parasit Vectors 2010;2010(3):21.
63. Gibbons PM, Steffes ZJ. Emerging infectious diseases of chelonians. Vet Clin North Am Exot Anim Pract 2013;16:303–17.
64. Ježková J, Horčičková M, Hlásková L, et al. *Cryptosporidium testudinis* sp. n., *Cryptosporidium ducismarci* Traversa, 2010 and *Cryptosporidium* tortoise genotype III (Apicomplexa: Cryptosporidiidae) in tortoises. Folia Parasitol (Praha) 2016;63:035.
65. Raphael B, Calle P, Gottdenker NL, et al. Clinical significance of Cryptosporidia in captive and free-ranging chelonians. In: Proceedings of the American Association of Zoo Veterinarians. Houston (TX): American Association of Zoo Veterinarians; 1997. p. 19–20.
66. Heuschele WP, Oosterhuis J, Janssen D, et al. Cryptosporidial infections in captive wild animals. J Wildl Dis 1986;22:493–6.
67. Graczyk TK, Cranfield MR. Experimental transmission of *Cryptosporidium* oocyst isolates from mammals, birds and reptiles to captive snakes. Vet Res 1998;29: 187–95.
68. Graczyk TK, Cranfield MR, Mann J, et al. Intestinal *Cryptosporidium* sp. infection in the Egyptian tortoise, *Testudo kleinmanni*. Int J Parasitol 1998;28(12):1885–8.
69. McGuire JL, Miller EA, Norton TM, et al. Intestinal parasites of the gopher tortoise (*Gopherus polyphemus*) from eight populations in Georgia. Parasitol Res 2013; 112:4205–10.

70. Griffin C, Reavill DR, Stacy BA, et al. Cryptosporidiosis caused by two distinct species in Russian tortoises and a pancake tortoise. Vet Parasitol 2010; 170(1–2):14–9.

71. Pedraza-Diaz S, Ortega-Mora LM, Carrion BA, et al. Molecular characterization of *Cryptosporidium* isolates from pet reptiles. Vet Parasitol 2009;160:204–10.

72. Richter B, Rasim R, Vrhovec MG, et al. Cryptosporidiosis outbreak in captive chelonians (*Testudo hermanni*) with identification of two *Cryptosporidium* genotypes. J Vet Diagn Invest 2012;24(3):591–5.

73. Hedley J, Eatwell K, Shaw DJ. Gastrointestinal parasitic burdens in UK tortoises: a survey of tortoise owners and potential risk factors. Vet Rec 2013. https://doi.org/10.1136/vr.101794.

74. Graczyk TK, Balazs GH, Work T, et al. *Cryptosporidium* sp. infections in green turtles, *Chelonia mydas*, as a potential source of marine waterborne oocysts in the Hawaiian Islands. Appl Environ Microbiol 1997;63:2925–7.

75. Alum A, Absar IM, Asaad H, et al. Impact of environmental conditions on the survival of *Cryptosporidium* and Giardia on environmental surfaces. Interdiscip Perspect Infect Dis 2014. https://doi.org/10.1155/2014/210385.

76. Huffman JN, Haizlett KS, Elhassani DK, et al. A survey of *Gopherus polyphemus* intestinal parasites in south Florida. J Parasitol Res 2018. https://doi.org/10.1155/2018/3048795.

77. Cranfield MR, Graczyk TK. Cryptosporidiosis. In: Mader DR, editor. Reptile medicine and surgery. 2nd edition. St Louis (MO): Saunders Elsevier; 2006. p. 756–62.

78. Campbell I, Tzipori S. Effects of disinfectants on survival of *Cryptosporidium* oocytes. Vet Rec 1982;111:414.

79. Jenkins MB, Bowman DD, Ghiorse WC. Inactivation of *Cryptosporidium parvum* oocysts by ammonia. Appl Environ Microbiol 1998;64(2):784–8.

80. Delling C, Holzhausen I, Daugschies A, et al. Inactivation of *Cryptosporidium parvum* under laboratory conditions. Parasitol Res 2016;115(2):863–6.

81. Weir SC, Pokorny NJ, Carreno RA, et al. Efficacy of common laboratory disinfectants on the infectivity of *Cryptosporidium parvum* oocysts in cell culture. Appl Environ Microbiol 2002;68(5):2576–9.

82. Jacobson ER, Schumacher J, Telford SR, et al. Intranuclear coccidiosis in radiated tortoises (*Geochelone radiata*). J Zoo Wildl Med 1994;25(1):95–102.

83. Garner MM, Gardiner CH, Wellehan JF, et al. Intranuclear coccidiosis in tortoises: nine cases. Vet Pathol 2006;43(3):311–20.

84. Schmidt V, Dyachenko V, Aupperle H, et al. Case report of systemic coccidiosis in a radiated tortoise (*Geochelone radiata*). Parasitol Res 2008;102(3):431–6.

85. Kolesnik E, Dietz J, Heckers KO, et al. Detection of intranuclear coccidiosis in tortoises in Europe and China. J Zoo Wildl Med 2017;48(2):328–34.

86. Innis CJ, Garner MM, Johnson AJ, et al. Antemortem diagnosis and characterization of nasal intranuclear coccidiosis in Sulawesi tortoises (*Indotestudo forsteni*). J Vet Diagn Invest 2007;19(6):660–7.

87. Hofmannová L, Kvičerová J, Bízková K, et al. Intranuclear coccidiosis in tortoises—discovery of its causative agent and transmission. Eur J Protistol 2019; 67:71–6.

88. Alvarez WA, Gibbons PM, Rivera S, et al. Development of a quantitative PCR for rapid and sensitive diagnosis of an intranuclear coccidian parasite in Testudines (TINC), and detection in the critically endangered Arakan Forest Turtle (*Heosemys depressa*). Vet Parasitol 2013;193(1–3):66–70.

89. Praschag P, Gibbons P, Boyer T, et al. An outbreak of intranuclear coccidiosis in Pyxis spp. tortoises. In: Presented at the 8th Annu Symp Conserv Biol Tortoises Freshwater Turtles. Orlando (FL): Turtle Survival Alliance; 2010. p. 42–3.
90. Stilwell JM, Stilwell NK, Stacy NI, et al. Extension of the known host range of intra-nuclear coccidia: infection in a group of red-footed tortoises (*Chelonoidis carbonaria*). J Zoo Wildl Med 2017;48(4):1165–71.
91. Benge SL, Heinrichs MT, Crevasse SE, et al. A preliminary analysis of prolonged absorption rate of ponazuril in red-footed tortoises, *Chelonoidis carbonaria*. J Zoo Wildl Med 2018;49(3):802–5.
92. Adamovicz L, Woodburn DB, Boers K, et al. Characterizing the clinical course of an emerging fungal pathogen (*Emydomyces testavorans*) in the state-endangered alligator snapping turtle (*Macrochelys temminckii*). In: Proceedings of the American Association of Zoo Veterinarians. St Louis (MO): American Association of Zoo Veterinarians; 2019. p. 34.
93. Browning GR, Wright L, Wack RF, et al. Fungal shell disease associated with *Emydomyces testavorans* in a zoo collection of western pond turtles (*Actinemys marmarota*). In: Proceedings of the American Association of Zoo Veterinarians. St Louis (MO): American Association of Zoo Veterinarians; 2019. p. 30.
94. Woodburn DB, Miller AN, Allender, et al. *Emydomyces testavorans*, a new genus and species of onygenalean fungus isolated from shell lesions of freshwater aquatic turtles. J Clin Microbiol 2019;57 [pii:00628-18].
95. Woodburn DB. *Emydomyces testavorans* infection in aquatic chelonians [PhD Dissertation]. Urbana (IL): University of Illinois; 2019.
96. Haman K, Hallock L, Schmidt T, et al. Shell disease in northwestern pond turtles (*Actinemys marmorata*) in Washington State, USA. Herpetol Rev 2019;50(3): 497–502.

Common and Emerging Infectious Diseases of Honeybees (*Apis mellifera*)

Jeffrey R. Applegate Jr, DVM, DACZM[a],*, Olivia A. Petritz, DVM, DACZM[b]

KEYWORDS

- Honeybees • American foulbrood • European foulbrood • *Nosema apis*
- *Nosema ceranae* • *Varroa destructor*

KEY POINTS

- Veterinary involvement in honeybee care has become a necessity following their reclassification as food-producing animals. Knowledge of honeybee disease and biosecurity helps develop a robust veterinary client patient relationship with apiarists.
- American foulbrood is a bacterial disease caused by *Paenibacillus larvae*, which is highly infectious and forms spores that can persist for years in the environment.
- European foulbrood is caused by a nonsporulating bacterium, *Melissococcus plutonius*, which is largely stress and nutrition related.
- Nosema is a microsporidial disease that affects the gastrointestinal tract of honeybees; prevention is important because there is no approved treatment to date.
- Varroosis, an infestation of *Varroa destructor*, is considered by many as the most important honeybee disease because of the severe impact it has on hive health and virus transmission.

INTRODUCTION

Most honeybee diseases are not newly emerging diseases; however, honeybee veterinary medicine and disease understanding are emerging concepts for veterinarians in the United States. As of January 1, 2017, beekeepers in the hobby and commercial sectors need a prescription or veterinary feed directive (VFD) from a veterinarian to obtain medically important antibiotics for administration to their honeybees, because they are now considered food-producing animals by the Food and Drug Administration (FDA) in the United States. Medically important antibiotics such as oxytetracycline, lincomycin, and tylosin were removed from over-the-counter availability for

[a] Department of Clinical Sciences, North Carolina State University, College of Veterinary Medicine, 602 Higgins Avenue, Suite 1-302, Brielle, NJ 08730, USA; [b] Department of Clinical Sciences, North Carolina State University, College of Veterinary Medicine, 1060 William Moore Drive, Raleigh, NC 27607, USA
* Corresponding author.
E-mail address: jrappleg@ncsu.edu

Vet Clin Exot Anim 23 (2020) 285–297
https://doi.org/10.1016/j.cvex.2020.01.001
1094-9194/20/© 2020 Elsevier Inc. All rights reserved.

use in honeybees. This change requires veterinarians and beekeepers to have an established veterinarian-client patient relationship (VCPR), and these requirements can vary state to state. Additional information about VCPRs can be found on the FDA's Web site (https://www.fda.gov/animal-veterinary/development-approval-process/does-state-or-federal-vcpr-definition-apply-lawful-vfd-my-state). Oxytetracycline (Terramycin) has been used for the control of American Foulbrood (AFB) and European foulbrood (EFB) in the United States and is available as a formulated powdered sugar with the incorporated antibiotic at a predetermined concentration. It can be obtained through approved commercial distributors with the use of a VFD or as a prescription. Tylosin and lincomycin, although rarely used, can be made available through prescription only. The VFD is completed by the veterinarian and the client fills the VFD at an authorized distributor. The VFD defines drug application timing and withdrawal times relative to nectar flow. Beyond the treatment of the bacterial diseases that require veterinary oversight, there are many other aspects of beekeeping, including a good understanding of husbandry and disease conditions, that allow veterinarians to build a strong VCPR, and fulfill an integral role alongside apiarists.

REVIEW OF THE SUPERORGANISM
Superorganism

Veterinarians have largely evolved to treat either individual animals and or those kept in herds. For honeybee veterinarians, a hive is considered a superorganism; a solitary colony that must be treated as a whole made up of thousands of adult individuals and a developing brood. Often it is the brood that is of the most concern and in need of being treated.

Queen

Within the superorganism, the caste members of the superorganism include the queen, the workers, and the drones. The queen is a unique individual in the hive. Under almost all circumstances, there is only 1 active queen per hive, and the hive depends on her for their survival. The queen's primary role is to lay eggs, and, in normal working order, she is the dam of all the workers and drones of that hive, provided there has not been a recent change of rule via swarm, supersedure, or queen death. In addition, she maintains control of the colony through pheromonal regulation. The queen can be identified by her long abdomen, short wings, and possibly an iatrogenic paint mark on her thorax indicating the year she was born.

Drone

The drones are the only haploid members of the superorganism. For eggs intended to be drones, the queen does not apply a sperm, which would have been gathered from distant drones on her single and only mating flight. The drones' only role is propagation of their queen's genetics to distant virgin queens. Once mated, the drone dies. All drones are eliminated from the superorganism in preparation for the winter. The drone can be identified by large eyes that meet dorsally and a thick, short, blunt, round abdomen.

Worker

The worker bees, all female and diploid, are the workhorses of the hive and responsible for all hive maintenance tasks. The role of the worker varies based on age and season. The queen has 6 to 10 nurse bees whose sole responsibility is to feed and care for the queen. Younger workers are responsible for hive care, such as sanitation, comb building, and temperature and humidity regulation. As they mature, the workers transition to foraging workers, who collect nectar and pollen. Additional worker tasks include mortuary duties, pollen packing, and guarding the hive. Winter workers are born with larger fat pads to survive the winter and have enhanced longevity. Their primary responsibilities include keeping the queen, brood, and cluster warm, and feeding the queen.

DISEASES
American Foulbrood

The term foulbrood is derived from the unpleasant odor produced by the infected brood, and most of these diseases are certainly not newly described. Aristotle first described a similar phenomenon of foul odors from presumably diseased bee hives in mid-300 BC.[1] The causal agent for AFB is *Paenibacillus larvae*, a gram-positive, spore-forming bacterium, whose whole genome has recently been sequenced.[2] This disease is found worldwide wherever honeybees in the genus *Apis* are maintained, despite having American in its name. This disease has one of the most significant economic impacts on the honeybee industry worldwide, and, therefore, AFB is a notifiable disease to the World Organization for Animal Health (OIE) and it is a reportable disease in certain states with the United States.[3] There has been significant work performed to identify the 4 genotypes of this bacterium to better evaluate the epidemiology of this disease.[4]

AFB only affects the larval stage of honeybees, and only the spores are infectious. These spores are extremely resistant in the environment and can remain potentially infectious for more than 10 years.[1] Larvae are most susceptible 12 to 36 hours after hatching from the egg, and 10 or fewer spores are considered a lethal dose.[4] The bacteria colonize the midgut of the bee larvae, and the infection eventually spreads throughout the host, leading to death. Bacterial proteases are responsible for the physical digestion of the larvae, which turns it into a semifluid state, the so-called ropey stage.[4] This stage dries out, and forms a hardened brown scale, also called the foulbrood scale. There are millions of *P larvae* spores within those scales, and they help facilitate transmission of the bacteria between colonies. Additional contributing factors for transmission of this bacterial infection include behaviors of the bees, such as robbing behavior, drifting behaviors between hives, and insufficient hygiene behaviors.[1]

The clinical signs of AFB disease are variable and overlap with other diseases. At a colony level, the distinct odor of AFB infection can be detected before even opening the hive in significant infections, and it has been described as something similar to decomposition and old gym socks.[3] Other bacterial infections of the brood also have an odor, but AFB is distinctive. AFB causes a spotty brood pattern, also called a shotgun or mottled brood pattern, which can be caused by any disease affecting the brood that causes larval death before capping.[3] The brood comb also has additional visible abnormalities, including perforated caps and sunken caps. Infected larvae can die with their developing proboscis extended, which sometimes is seen as a thin, linear, vertical attachment across the cell. This proboscis is referred to as a pupal tongue, and although uncommonly seen, is characteristic of AFB infection.[1]

Because of the characteristic ropey stage in this disease, the matchstick or rope test can be quickly performed in the field and is highly suggestive of AFB. A small, narrow object, such as a matchstick, is inserted into the affected cell and slowly removed, drawing out the cell's contents. A positive test occurs when the decayed larvae forms a viscous string that can be drawn out of the cell for 2 cm or more (**Fig. 1**). A negative test does not rule out AFB, because the larvae in that particular cell tested may be in a

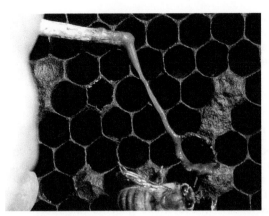

Fig. 1. A matchstick test of larval cell in an AFB-positive hive. The viscous, ropey nature of the material allows it to pull out 2 cm or more. (*Courtesy of* Don Hopkins, Raleigh NC.)

different stage of decay. There are several other field tests available for the detection of AFB, including the Holst milk test and a field enzyme-linked immunosorbent assay test.[3] Within the United States, samples (adult bees, comb/brood) can be submitted to the Bee Research Laboratory in Beltsville, Maryland, for AFB testing free of charge. Additional specifics on submission and testing specifications can be found on their Web site (https://www.ars.usda.gov/northeast-area/beltsville-md-barc/beltsville-agricultural-research-center/bee-research-laboratory/). Even if AFB is confirmed with a field test and reporting is not required in the state of residence, submission of known or highly suspect positive samples is still encouraged to help with national incidence data collection.

A large spectrum of treatment options are available for AFB depending on the location and strength of the hive, ranging from inducing a swarm to total depopulation and burning of the affected hive. Ultimately, the prognosis for a severely infected colony is guarded to poor. The shaking bee (shock swarm) method is a technique that has been recommended with mild cases of AFB in strong hives, especially in countries where treatment is illegal, such as the European Union.[1] Within the United States, similar to reporting requirements, treatment recommendations vary state to state, with some states requiring destruction of infected colonies.[3] Before initiating treatment or prescribing antibiotics, veterinarians should consult with their state apiarists to review the pertinent laws regarding treatment. If treatment is sanctioned by the state, it is recommended even with mild infections of AFB. Oxytetracycline, tylosin, and lincomycin are the only FDA-approved antibiotics for treatment of AFB in affected hives in approved states. Even then, there are specific limitations in place for what time of year these drugs can be administered, because they need to be consumed by the bees before the main honey flow to prevent contamination and antibiotic residues.[3] In addition, antibiotics are ineffective against the spores of *P larvae*. There are also several oxytetracycline-resistant strains of *P larvae* that have been identified within the United States,[5] and the Bee Research Laboratory can test for these strains. Because of the highly infectious nature and resistance of the bacterial spores, many states require that AFB-positive colonies are destroyed. Burning and gamma irradiation kill *P larvae* spores, whereas most other chemical disinfectants are completely ineffective.

It is imperative for veterinarians working with apiaries to understand the importance of biosecurity in the prevention of the spread of AFB. Exchange of frames and other materials between colonies, use of contaminated tools, inappropriate sanitation, and abandoned infected hives have all been implicated in the spread of this disease.[1,3] The bacterial spores are ubiquitous within the hive, and can be found in the honey, pollen, wax, wooden hive material, and on the adult honeybees.

Because of regulatory restrictions, increasing antibiotic resistance, and the potential for antibiotic residues in honey and other products, numerous alternative treatments for AFB are currently being investigated. These treatments include breeding for bees with increased immune response against AFB, biological control via antagonistic bacteria, and treatment with natural products that have antibacterial properties, such as essential oils.[4,6] Certain essential oils contain quorum-sensing inhibitor compounds, which, in simplified terms, act to limit bacterial cell-to-cell communication. Several of these have recently been evaluated in vitro against the proteases of *P larvae* with promising results.[7] Several studies have shown inhibitory effects of honeybee-specific lactic acid bacteria (hbs-LAB), which are naturally occurring bacteria within the honeybee gut microbiome, against *P larvae* bacterial infections.[8,9] However, in several recent studies, administration of hbs-LAB to infected colonies found that this bacterium did not have any significant effects on AFB symptoms or spore counts.[10,11] Those investigators stressed the importance of evaluating effects of treatments for honeybee diseases (for *P larvae* and others) on the whole colony, rather than the individual bees, because this could explain the difference between their findings and the previous studies. There is still a large amount of work that needs to be done to further evaluate the efficacy and safety of these proposed treatments before definitive recommendations can be made by veterinarians for treatment of infected hives.

European Foulbrood

Although the name foulbrood was originally coined in the late 1700s, it was not until 1912 that it was discovered to be 2 separate diseases, both affecting honeybee brood.[12] EFB is caused by the gram-positive bacterium *Melissococcus plutonius*, and, unlike *P larvae*, it is non--spore forming. EFB is also a notifiable disease in the OIE and is found worldwide, except in New Zealand.[1] There is often concurrent infection with other bacteria in EFB infections, including *Enterococcus faecalis* and *Paenibacillus alvei*, and their role in these infections remains unclear. A recent study evaluated these secondary invading bacteria as well as the genetic background of the host larvae after experimental infection in honeybee larvae with EFB.[13] Secondary invaders, such as *E faecalis* did not have any significant effect on larval survival or weight, and the investigators hypothesized that these concurrent infections may be colonization secondary to immunosuppression or death by EFB.[13]

M plutonius infects uncapped brood, and larvae usually succumb to the bacterial infection at 4 to 5 days of age. Clinical signs of EFB include a spotty brood pattern and larval discoloration (to a yellow or gray).[3] Affected larvae are also often deformed and in a twisted position rather than the standard C shape at the bottom of the cells (**Fig. 2**). As with all foulbrood diseases, there is also an odor produced from severely infected hives, which smells similar to sour milk. Similar to AFB, dead larvae may form dry scales inside the cells, but, unlike AFB, the scale is easy to remove. Most larvae die from EFB in the late spring to early summer, and colony collapse is uncommon but possible secondary to severe infections.[1] This disease has been associated with stressors to the colony, particularly when there is a deficiency in pollen, a vital protein source for bees. Additional stressors that predispose to EFB include prolonged confinement secondary to poor weather, an insufficient population of nurse bees,

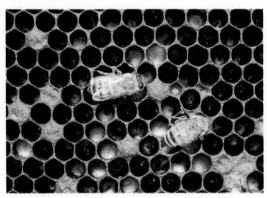

Fig. 2. Larvae from a hive that is positive with EFB. The larvae are dark in color, deformed, twisted, and dying. (*Courtesy of* Don Hopkins, Raleigh NC.)

and concurrent infections (eg, sacbrood bee virus and significant *Varroa destructor* infestation).[1]

There are commercial testing kits for EFB, and it can be confirmed in the United States by state and national laboratories. As with AFB, submission of samples is still highly recommended even if field testing is positive to help record national incidence data for this disease. The appearance of larvae infected with EFB is similar to AFB, but the matchstick test is negative. Instead of drawing out the larvae more than 2 cm, EFB-infected larvae do not form such a long string and break or snap back into place. In the United States, oxytetracycline is the only FDA-approved drug for treatment of EFB, and it now requires a VFD from a licensed veterinarian.[3] If antibiotics are used, they should be fed in the spring or fall and removed at least 6 weeks before the main honey flow to avoid drug residues. Unlike AFB, infections with EFB may resolve on their own, especially with stress reduction, feeding, and potentially replacing the queen in less severe infections. Infected frames can also be reused following storage or bleach sterilization, because *M plutonius* is non--spore forming.[3] Recently, a study explored the use of normal gut flora from the Japanese honeybee (*Apis cerana japonica*) against *M plutonius* and found that there was a reduction in infected larval mortality. Additional studies are needed to evaluate the effectiveness of that particular bacterial strain as a probiotic against EFB.[14]

Varroa Mites

Worldwide, varroosis is considered the leading risk to honeybee hive health. *Varroa* mites (*V destructor*) were initially host adapted to the Asian honeybee (*A cerana*) and species jumped to *Apis mellifera* in the mid--twentieth century. Varroa mites have been reported in the United States since 1987.

Varroa mites are hematophagous ectoparasites, belonging to the class Arachnida and order Mesostigmata, that feed on both adult and brood stock. Understanding the life cycle of the *Varroa* mite is essential in understanding its management and control. The reproductive phase of the life cycle is isolated to within the capped cell; however, the adult mites are found on adult honeybees during the phoretic (organism transport) phase. The mites that are counted during routine evaluations are typically the adult, exclusively female mites. It is during this phoretic period that the mites are spread to other hives through honeybee behaviors such as robbing, drifting, and swarming, and transported to the brood cells for progression of the reproductive phase. Once transported to a brood cell, with preference to drone brood, the female mother mite drops off the adult honeybee host and migrates past the larvae and into the larval jelly. She begins to feed on the hemolymph of the larvae and lays a single haploid male offspring. She then produces diploid female eggs every 30 hours resulting in 5 to 6 new mites per cell. The larvae hatch and progress through various molts until the immature adults feed on the maturing honeybee larvae (**Fig. 3**). At this point the mites are sexually mature and the male mates with the newly developing females.[1] The honeybee matures and emerges. Only the larger female *Varroa* mites survive, attached to the honeybee, and the cycle repeats.

Clinical signs of varroosis are nonspecific and include a weak hive, possible hive collapse, or a reduced number of workers going into the winter season. Colony weakness is more commonly seen later in the year. The most overt sign of *Varroa* mite infestation is to visualize the adult mites on the bees. The mites appear as red-brown, flat, oval discs, usually secured to the abdomen of the honeybee[15](**Fig. 4**). Another indication, specifically of *Varroa* mites, is identification of their droppings: guanine deposits on the side of the cell. When holding the frame in a horizontal orientation to evaluate the inside of the cell, these deposits produce a grainy appearance to the sides of the cell.[3]

Varroosis is likely more appropriately termed parasitic mite syndrome (PMS) because of disease transmission and conditions created by the *Varroa* mites that directly affect the health of the bees and, thus, hive health. Spotty brood pattern may be an indicator of *Varroa* mite infestation, including chewed pupae and melted larvae. Larval death may occur at virtual any stage because of PMS; death on emergence from cells may be the most obvious to the observer.

A variety of disorders have been associated with infestation of *Varroa* and PMS. Owing to the hematophagous nature of the *Varroa* mite, larval death, reduced hemolymph protein concentrations,[16,17] impaired immunity and decreased hemocyte concentration,[18,19] and reduction of lifespan[20] have been reported. Impaired flight, navigation, and successful return to the hive have also been documented in bees with PMS.[21,22] Secondary disorder caused by virus transmission may be identified, such as shortened abdomen and malformed wings, likely caused by transmission of deformed wing virus.[22] Other viruses for which *Varroa* is reported as a vector include acute bee paralysis virus, Kashmir bee virus, Israeli acute paralysis virus, and slow bee paralysis virus.[22]

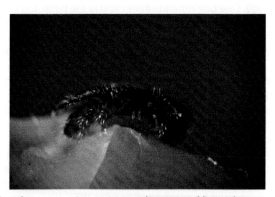

Fig. 3. An adult female *Varroa* mite on a recently emerged larva. (*Courtesy of* Don Hopkins, Raleigh NC.)

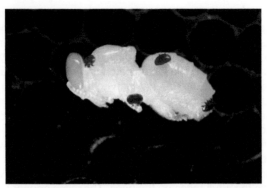

Fig. 4. Close up of *Varroa* mites feeding on a larva. Note the oval flat shape and red-brown coloration. (*Courtesy of* Don Hopkins, Raleigh NC.)

However, visual identification of mites alone should not be relied on for diagnosis. Sampling to establish a mite count and density of infestation should be completed at least once yearly, after the last honey harvest of the year. Multiple methods are described to establish mite counts. The sugar roll and alcohol shake (flotation method) are frequently used. The sugar roll is less likely to kill adult bees but is more likely to underestimate the mite count because of mites not falling from the bees. With either method, the typical procedure is to collect roughly 300 adult bees (100 mL or 0.42 cups). The collected bees should be young adults living on the brood frame, and it is important not to include the queen.

For the sugar roll, the collected bees are placed into a container with a screen top. The screen holes are large enough to allow the mites to fall through but retain the bees. Add a generous amount of powdered sugar into the container and roll to fully coat the bees. Allow the container to sit for 1 to 2 minutes. Then shake the contents of the container through the screen onto a light-colored plate. Return the bees to the hive. Add a small amount of water to the sugar on the plate to dissolve the sugar, but do not overflow the plate. Swirl gently and count mites. This method depends on the physical friction of the sugar to dislodge the mites and an exact ratio cannot be calculated because an accurate bee count is not possible.

During the alcohol wash method, both the bees and the mites die, which allows accurate counts to be completed. The sampling device consists of 2 cups that nestle tightly, a tight-fitting lid, a screen that allows mites to pass but not bees, and alcohol (ie, isopropyl, ethanol). One cup remains intact and is the base and collection chamber of the unit. About 2.5 cm (1 inch) of the bottom of the second cup should be cut and removed. A metal screen may be affixed to the bottom of the cut cup or a cloth screen can be draped over the intact cup and the cut cup inserted into the first intact cup, forcing the mesh into the intact cup and forming a net over the end of the inserted cut cup. The bees are placed into the upper cup, alcohol is added to cover the bees, and the top secured. Swirl the container for 1 minute. The bees remain in the upper section above the mesh, and the mites fall through to the collection chamber. Remove bees and count for accuracy. The mites may be counted through the bottom of a clear collection cup or poured out onto a light-colored plate.

Once shake/roll is completed, for the most precise answer, bees can be counted and the mite-to-bee percentage can be calculated. If the count is less than 5%, the hive is considered weakly parasitized and no immediate treatment is necessary; if 5% to 10%, treatment must be planned; if greater than 10%, then immediate treatment should be initiated.

Control of *V destructor* is paramount for long-term survival of the hive; without control, a hive is likely to collapse after a couple of years of infestation. The apiarist must design an active strategy to manage and treat for *Varroa* infestation to include surveillance, assessment, and treatment. Management begins with providing the tools to maintain a strong hive, sanitary hive conditions as directed by a sanitary queen, and good housekeeping practices.

Monitoring the colony parasite load can be completed via active spot checks or passively throughout the year. A mite collection board beneath the hive may help monitor natural mite fall throughout the year, and although a true mite count cannot be calculated, annual trends may be able to be monitored. Drone brood uncapping is a method designed to roughly evaluate the number of drone brood that are infected. Although *Varroa* are typically more attracted to drone brood, this method provides a bias sample of the potential brood affected. Evaluation of mite fall following miticide application can be completed. This technique is similar to the natural mite fall methodology with the added benefit of monitoring progression of mite treatment. Alcohol flotation and sugar roll provide the opportunity to perform objective mite counts.

Many options for treatment are available. Treatment is likely most effectively managed as an integrated pest management plan to include hive sanitation and some combination of various treatments, such as chemical miticides, organic acids, and essential oils. In the United States, *Varroa* treatment is largely under the purview of the apiarist, though a veterinarian's good working knowledge of the topic helps to develop a solid VCPR with an active apiarist. Antiparasitics are managed by veterinary prescription in the European Union and some other countries. With a good understanding of the treatment options, veterinary input may help prevent product residue in wax and honey, similar to that of antibiotics. All parasiticides should be used according to manufacturer recommendations to avoid residues and harm to the honeybees.

A productive treatment of *Varroa* must be effective against the phoretic mites and not toxic to the honeybees. Most miticides, apart from formic acid, are not effective against mites within capped cells. Miticides effective against *Varroa* include Amitraz (formamidine), tau-fluvalinate (pyrethroid), coumaphos (organophosphate), and flumethrin (pyrethroid). These synthetic acaricides need to be used as sustained release for good results because they are not effective against mites in capped cells. As seen in other veterinary venues, resistance and lack of efficacy have been described.[22,23] More organic options include thymol and organic acids (ie, formic, oxalic, lactic). Local regulations should be followed during administration of these compounds. In combination with chemical and organic methods, integrated pest management may be used adjunctively. These methods may include a 24-day duration of queen trapping to interrupt the brood and mite life cycle or encouraging the queen to lay drone brood using a specially designed drone brood frame. Because of the mites' preference to reproduce in drone cells, removing and euthanizing the entire frame of drone brood may help reduce the hive's mite load. The goal is to reduce the mite load immediately following the final honey harvest, thereby promoting overwinter health and reducing the possibility of residues in honey.

Nosema

Nosemosis is an infectious disease of the honeybee gastrointestinal system caused by *Nosema apis* and *Nosema ceranae*. *Nosema* spp are obligate intracellular, spore-forming, unicellular parasites, recently reclassified as fungi, that affect the midgut of all 3 castes of *A mellifera*.[1,24] *N ceranae* originated in the Asian honeybee (*A cerana*), but is not worldwide and can be considered an emerging disease in *A mellifera*. *N apis* has been recognized in the United States for many years, but it has been found that most are coinfections with *N ceranae*.[25–27]

Two clinical diseases are identified based on the infective organism: type A (*N apis*) or type C (*N ceranae*). Although mixed infections are common, type C infection seems to be asymptomatic in colonies and without a seasonality pattern.[28–34] Type A infections are opportunistic, affecting weak colonies and further weakening the hive. Hive confinement, such as during times of prolonged inclement weather, overwintering, and commercial-related practices, is considered a predisposing factor. Signs of nosemosis can be nonspecific or include weakness and mortality of worker bees, dysentery and excreta on combs or lighting boards, and workers crawling out of the hive (**Fig. 5**). Reproduction of the organism occurs within the ventricular walls, resulting in destruction of the epithelial cells. Resulting gastrointestinal inflammation leads to diarrhea or constipation depending on spore load, impaired nutrient uptake, and negative effects on the fat bodies and protein metabolism. Spores are shed in feces and transmission is subsequently associated with ingestion of spores, which is exacerbated by confinement and cleaning of diarrhea.

The standard for diagnosis is to estimate the number of spores in a sample of 50 to 100 bees.[35,36] Bees collected for sampling should be older mature workers, collected from the entrance or peripheral frames. According to the OIE, "for reliable diagnosis, a number of bees in a sample should be examined. For example, at least 60 bees examined in a composite sample will detect a 5% infection level with 95% probability."[36] Testing for spores requires microscopy and a laboratory that is comfortable testing for *Nosema* (**Fig. 6**). Species identification can be difficult based on visual identification alone; however, polymerase chain reaction is available and is the most sensitive method for distinguishing between species.[29]

There are no approved treatments for nosemosis. Over-the-counter Fumagilin Soluble Powder HS (Fumagilin-B, Medivet), is used by many beekeepers, but it is not approved for bees in the United States and not authorized in the European Union. Good housekeeping practices and keeping a strong hive are the best preventive measures.[1]

BIOSECURITY

As veterinarians become more integral in the care of honeybees in the United States, good management practices and hive health safety must be at the forefront of thought

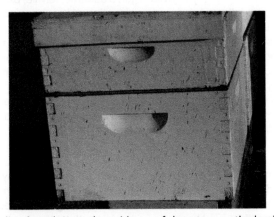

Fig. 5. A hive landing board. Note the evidence of dysentery on the landing board, an indicator of nosemosis. (*Courtesy of* Don Hopkins, Raleigh NC.)

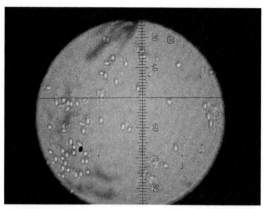

Fig. 6. Microscopic image of *Nosema* (light microspcopy at high dry (400×). (*Courtesy of Don Hopkins, Raleigh NC.*)

when working within an apiary. Biosecurity is paramount when working with food animals and should be accomplished as best as possible when working with honeybees. However, true biosecurity and quarantine are something of a utopia with regard to honeybees, because they forage and feed at their own volition for up to 5 km (3 miles) away from their hive. In addition, robbing, mating, swarming, and other such activities reduce the ability to maintain strict biosecurity.

Hive-side biosecurity should be designed to reduce the risk of introduction of biological pathogens or pests into a hive, decrease the risk of dissemination of a particular condition within the hive, and reduce subsequent spread of pathogens and pests outside of the existing hive. In so doing, contamination with toxic or harmful chemicals and physical hazards, such as harm to the queen, must also be considered.

Bioexclusion, the attempt to prevent pathogen introduction into a hive, and bio-compartmentalization, early diagnosis and treatment, quarantine, or euthanasia of an affected hive, are possibly the most important biosecurity tools that can be used to maintain biosafety of an apiary.[1] When approaching a hive in an apiary, tool management, proper personal protective equipment, and frame handling are paramount. Simple decisions, such as using the beekeeper's hive tool and smoker, reduce the possibility of transmitting disease to other apiaries via fomites. Allowing the beekeeper to open the hive and remove the frames decreases the veterinarian's contact with the structural hive, allowing more time for frame examination and reducing liability of harm to the queen by the veterinarian during frame removal. Wearing nitrile gloves and changing gloves between hives and apiaries virtually eliminates contamination of hives via fomites, such as leather reusable gloves.

DISCLOSURE

The authors have nothing to disclose.

REFERENCES

1. Vidal-Naquet N. Honeybee veterinary medicine: Apis mellifera L. Sheffield (United Kingdom): 5m Publishing; 2015.

2. Chan QW, Cornman RS, Birol I, et al. Updated genome assembly and annotation of Paenibacillus larvae, the agent of American foulbrood disease of honey bees. BMC Genomics 2011;12:450.

3. Honey bees: a guide for veterinarians. American Veterinary Medical Association; 2017 . Available at: https://www.avma.org/KB/Resources/Documents/honeybees-veterinary-medicine-guide-for-veterinarians.pdf. Accessed November 1, 2019.

4. Genersch E. American Foulbrood in honeybees and its causative agent, Paenibacillus larvae. J Invertebr Pathol 2010;103:S10–9.

5. Miyagi T, Peng CY, Chuang RY, et al. Verification of oxytetracycline-resistant American foulbrood pathogen Paenibacillus larvae in the United States. J Invertebr Pathol 2000;75:95–6.

6. González M, Marioli J. Antibacterial activity of water extracts and essential oils of various aromatic plants against Paenibacillus larvae, the causative agent of American Foulbrood. J Invertebr Pathol 2010;104:209–13.

7. Pellegrini MC, Zalazar L, Fuselli SR, et al. Inhibitory action of essential oils against proteases activity of Paenibacillus larvae, the etiological agent of American Foulbrood disease. Spanish Journal of Agricultural Research 2017;15(4):e0504.

8. Forsgren E, Olofsson TC, Váasquez A, et al. Novel lactic acid bacteria inhibiting Paenibacillus larvae in honey bee larvae. Apidologie 2010;41:99–108.

9. Killer J, Dubná S, Sedláček I, et al. Lactobacillus apis sp. nov., from the stomach of honeybees (Apis mellifera), having an in vitro inhibitory effect on the causative agents of American and European foulbrood. Int J Syst Evol Microbiol 2014;64: 152–7.

10. Lamei S, Stephan JG, Nilson B, et al. Feeding honeybee colonies with honeybee-specific lactic acid bacteria (Hbs-LAB) does not affect colony-level Hbs-LAB composition or paenibacillus larvae spore levels, although American Foulbrood affected colonies harbor a more diverse Hbs-LAB community. Microb Ecol 2019;1–13.

11. Stephan JG, Lamei S, Pettis JS, et al. Honeybee-specific lactic acid bacterium supplements have no effect on American Foulbrood-infected honeybee colonies. Appl Environ Microbiol 2019;85 [pii:e00606-19].

12. Forsgren E. European foulbrood in honey bees. J Invertebr Pathol 2010; 103:S5–9.

13. Lewkowski O, Erler S. Virulence of Melissococcus plutonius and secondary invaders associated with European foulbrood disease of the honey bee. Microbiologyopen 2019;8:e00649.

14. Wu M, Sugimura Y, Iwata K, et al. Inhibitory effect of gut bacteria from the Japanese honey bee, Apis cerana japonica, against Melissococcus plutonius, the causal agent of European foulbrood disease. J Insect Sci 2014;14:129.

15. De Jong D. Mites: Varroa and other PArasites of brood. In: Morse RA, Flottum K, editors. Honey bee pests, predators, and diseases. 3rd edition. Medina (Saudi Arabia): A.I. Root Company; 1997. p. 281–327.

16. Bowen-Walker PL, Gun A. The effect of the ectoparasitic mite, Varroa destructor on adult worker honeybee (Apis mellifera) emergence, weights, water, protein, carbohydrate, and lipid levels. Entomol Exp Appl 2001;101:207–17.

17. Boecking O, Genersch E. Varroosis - the ongoing crisis in bee keeping. J Verbrauch Lebensm 2008;3:221–8.

18. Amdam GV, Hartfelder K, Norberg K, et al. Altered physiology in worker honey bees (Hymenoptera: Apidae) infested with the mite Varroa destructor (Acari: Varroidae): a factor in colony loss during overwintering? J Econ Entomol 2004;97: 741–7.

19. Belaïd M, Doumandji. Effet du *Varroa destructor* sur la morphométrie alaire et sur les composants du système immunitaire de l'abeille ourière *Apis mellifera* intermissa. LSJ 2010;11:83–90.

20. Schneider P, Drescher W. EInfluss der Parasitierung durch die Milbe *Varroa jacobsoni* aus das Schlupfgewicht, die Gewichtsentwicklung, die Entwicklung der Hypopharynxdrusen und die Lebensdauer von Apis mellifera. Apidologie 1987;18:101–6.

21. Kralj J, Brockmann A, Fuchs S, et al. The parasitic mite *Varroa destructor* affects non-associative learning in honey bee foragers, *Apis mellifera* L. J Comp Physiol A Neuroethol Sens Neural Behav Physiol 2007;193:363–70.

22. Rosenkrantz P, Aumeier P, Ziegelmann B. Biology and control of *Varroa destructor*. J Invertebr Pathol 2010;103:96–119.

23. Mallick A. Action sanitaire en production apicole: gestion de la varroose face a l'apparition de resistance aux traitements chez *Varroa destructor*. Thèse pour obtenir le grade de Docteur Vétérinaire. Lyon (France): Vetagro Sup; 2013.

24. Fries I. Protozoa. In: Morse RA, Flottum K, editors. Honey bee pests, predators, and diseases. 3rd edition. Medina (Saudi Arabia): A.I. Root Company; 1997. p. 59–76.

25. Paxton RJ, Klee J, Korpela S, et al. *Nosema ceranae* has infected *Apis mellifera* in Europe since at least 1998 and may be more virulent than *Nosema apis*. Apidologie 2007;38:558–65.

26. Chen Y, Evans JD, Zhou L, et al. Assymetrical coexistence of Nosema ceranae and Nosema apis in honey bees. J Invertebr Pathol 2009;101:204–9.

27. Forsgren E, Fries I. Comparative virulence of Nosema ceranae and Nosema apis in individual European honey bees. Vet Parasitol 2010;170:212–7.

28. Fernandez JM, Puerta F, Cousinou M, et al. Asymptomatic presence of *Nosema* spp. in Spanish commercial apiaries. J Invertebr Pathol 2012;111:106–10.

29. Traver BE, Williams MR, Fell RD. Comparison of within hive sampling seasonal activity of Nosema ceranae in honey bee colonies. J Invertebr Pathol 2012;109: 187–93.

30. Fries I. Microsporidia. In: Ritter W, editor. Bee heath and veterinarians. Paris: OIE; 2014. p. 125–9.

31. Martin-Hernández R, Meana A, Prieto L, et al. Outcome of colonization of *Apis mellifera* by *Nosema ceranae*. Appl Environ Microbiol 2007;73(20):6331–8.

32. Martin- Hernández R, Botias C, Bailón EG, et al. Microsporidia infecting *Apis mellifera*: coexistence or competition. Is *Nosema ceranae* replacing *Nosema apis*? Environ Microbiol 2012;14:2127–38.

33. Traver BE, Fell RD. Prevalence and infection intensity of *Nosema* in honey bee (*Apis mellifera* L.) colonies in Virginia. J Invertebr Pathol 2011;107:43–9.

34. Higes M, Meana A, Bartolomé C, et al. *Nosema ceranae* (Microsporidia), a controversial 21st century honey bee pathogen. Environ Microbiol Rep 2013; 5(1):17–29.

35. Goblirsch M, Huang ZY, Spivak M. Physiological and behavioral changes in honey bees (Apis mellifera) Induced by Nosema ceranae infection. PLoS One 2013; 8(3):e58165.

36. OIE Terrestrial Manual. Nosemosis of honey bees Chapter 3.2.4. 2018. Available at: https://www.oie.int/fileadmin/Home/eng/Health_standards/tahm/3.02.04_NOSE MOSIS_FINAL.pdf. Accessed November 15, 2019.

Emerging Zoonotic Diseases in Ferrets

Nicole R. Wyre, DVM, DABVP (Avian), DABVP (Exotic Companion Mammal), CVA

KEYWORDS

- Ferrets • *P luteola* • Hepatitis E virus • Influenza • Zoonotic

KEY POINTS

- *P luteola* is a bacterial infection causing respiratory disease and abscess formation that has been reported in ferrets in Spain, Finland, Austria, Australia, France, and the United States.
- Hepatitis E virus can cause 3 patterns of infection and has been reported in ferrets in the Netherlands, United States, Canada, Japan, and China.
- Influenza causes natural and experimentally induced infection in ferrets.
- Influenza is a proven zoonotic and anthroponotic disease. Both *P luteola* and hepatitis E virus have zoonotic potential and are emerging in ferrets worldwide.

PSEUDOMONAS LUTEOLA
Etiology and Disease in Other Species

Pseudomonas luteola (previously *Chryseomonas luteola*) is a gram-negative, rod-shaped bacterium with a nonstaining capsule that is ubiquitous in damp environments, soil, and water.[1] It is a rare cause of disease in humans and animals. In humans, it is generally found to cause disease in immunosuppressed patients or associated with medical implants, indwelling catheters, and peritoneal dialysis.[2] In fish, it causes septicemia in rainbow trout,[3] whereas it is part of the normal flora of zebra fish.[4] This disease is rarely reported in mammals, but has been found in cats, dogs, and sheep.[5] This infection was first reported in 3 ferrets in Spain[6] in 2012 and since then infection in ferrets has been reported in Finland, Austria, Australia, France, and the United States.

Pathogenesis in Ferrets

The disease in ferrets seems to take several forms and causes significant morbidity and mortality. It causes respiratory disease, panniculitis, sialadenitis, and abscess formation. At present, it has been diagnosed in 12 ferrets[5–8] and suspected in several others.[5] The disease is thought to have a subcutaneous,[8] respiratory,[6] or oral[7] route of infection.

Different from the disease in humans, none of the ferrets had obvious immunosuppressive diseases or medical implants/catheters as a source of the infection. In humans, the incubation period of this infection is variable.[1] If this same variable

Zodiac Pet & Exotic Hospital, Victoria Centre, Shop 101A, 1/F, Fortress Hill, Hong Kong
E-mail address: wyredvm@gmail.com

Vet Clin Exot Anim 23 (2020) 299–308
https://doi.org/10.1016/j.cvex.2020.01.012
1094-9194/20/© 2020 Elsevier Inc. All rights reserved.

incubation time is true in ferrets, an initial trauma or injury may have healed by the time the disease was recognized in them. Because this disease has also been reported in humans with respiratory disease, the infection may have a predilection for human and ferret respiratory tracts.[6] In ferrets with respiratory infection, transmission electronic microscope examination showed white blood cell recruitment in the area of infection, but no phagocytosis. This led the authors to postulate that the bacteria were able to elude the ferret's natural anti-inflammatory response.[6] If this is true, it may explain why this infection is seen in ferrets with no obvious immunosuppression, trauma, or medical implants.

Clinical Presentation

Clinical signs are dependent on the location of the infection and can include respiratory signs or subcutaneous swelling (inguinal or cranial cervical) (**Table 1**). As expected with a bacterial infection, fever, dehydration, lethargy, and anorexia have been reported. One ferret with a cranial cervical mass had ptyalism and a head tilt.[7]

Diagnostic Testing

Diagnostic imaging (radiographs, ultrasound, computed tomography) results depend on the location of the infection and can include mediastinal masses and pleural effusion with respiratory infections,[5,6] abdominal effusion, and lymphadenopathy, with subcutaneous masses in the inguinal/femoral region[5,8] and heterogeneous mixed soft tissue and fluid attenuating masses with cranial cervical/salivary gland infections[7] (see **Table 1**).

Complete blood counts and serum biochemical examinations were only available for 3 ferrets[6,7] and included anemia, leukocytosis with neutrophilia and toxic changes, hyperglycemia, hypoproteinemia, hypoalbuminemia, hyperglobulinemia, hyperbilirubinemia, and low alanine aminotransferase (ALT). All 3 ferrets had anemia and hypoalbuminemia.

Definitive diagnosis of *P luteola* requires collection of infected tissue for culture and sensitivity or molecular analysis. This can be acquired surgically or with fine needle aspiration. Fine needle aspiration of any mass (subcutaneous, mediastinal, lymph node) can be helpful for an initial diagnosis while awaiting culture and sensitivity results. With Romanowsky stain, *P luteola* has the distinct appearance of a rod-shaped microorganism (2–3 μm) with a clear to basophilic halo.[6,8] Pyogranulomatous inflammation is usually seen surrounding these microorganisms.

Treatment and Prognosis

Initial treatment involves stabilizing any dyspneic patient with oxygen therapy and performing thoracocentesis or abscess drainage for patients with pleural effusion/abscesses compressing the trachea. Intravenous catheter placement with fluid therapy and analgesia is also recommended. If *P luteola* is suspected, intravenous antibiotic therapy should be initiated.

P luteola is reported to be sensitive to third-generation cephalosporins, aminoglycosides, and fluoroquinolones; therefore, systemic antimicrobials in these classes should be chosen while awaiting final culture and sensitivity results.[9] Aminoglycosides are not recommended in ferrets with dehydration as they could potentiate the nephrotoxicity of these drugs.[10] *P luteola* is reported to be resistant to first- and second-generation cephalosporins, tetracyclines, and ampicillin.[9] Therefore, antibiotics in these classes are not a prudent first choice.

In general, *P luteola* infections in ferrets carries a grave prognosis, with only 2 of 12 ferrets surviving a confirmed infection (see **Table 1**).

Table 1
Reported cases of *Pseudomonas luteola* in domestic ferrets

Age	Sex	Country	Clinical Signs/PE	Diagnostic Results	Surgery	Antibiotic	Outcome	Reference
3 y	MC	Spain	Dyspnea, fever	Mediastinal mass, pleural effusion, anemia, hypoalbuminemia, neutrophilic leukocytosis, hyperglycemia		Enrofloxacin, metronidazole, clindamycin	Died 2–5 d after presentation	Martínez et al,[6] 2012
3 y	MI	Spain	Dyspnea, fever	Mediastinal mass, pleural effusion, anemia, hypoalbuminemia, hyperglobulinemia, neutrophilic leukocytosis, hyperglycemia		Enrofloxacin, metronidazole, clindamycin	Died 2–5 d after presentation	Martínez et al,[6] 2012
2 y	MI	Spain	Dyspnea	Mediastinal mass, pleural effusion			Euthanized immediately	Martínez et al,[6] 2012
1 y	MI	Finland	Inguinal abscess		Surgical removal of abscess		Died postoperatively	Baum et al,[8] 2015
4.5 y	FS	Austria	Femoral swelling, fever	Purulent bronchopneumonia and multisystemic pyogranulomas (postmortem)	Surgical removal of abscess and lymph nodes		Euthanized postoperatively	Baum et al,[8] 2015
3 y	MC	Austria	Preputial swelling, fever		Surgical removal of abscess and lymph nodes		Euthanized 3 d postoperatively	Baum et al,[8] 2015

(continued on next page)

Table 1
(continued)

Age	Sex	Country	Clinical Signs/PE	Diagnostic Results	Surgery	Antibiotic	Outcome	Reference
4.5 y	MC	USA	Cranial cervical swelling	Anemia, hypoalbuminemia, hyperbilirubinemia, and low alanine aminotransferase	Abscess and salivary gland removed	Clindamycin, enrofloxacin × 6 wk	Alive 11 mo postoperatively	Schmidt et al,[7] 2019
5 y	FS	USA	Mandibular swelling, head tilt, ptylism, tachypnea, fever			Amoxicillin-clavulanic acid, enrofloxacin	Euthanized 25 d after initial presentation	Schmidt et al,[7] 2019
8 mo	MI	France	Respiratory distress, fever	Pleural effusion, cranial mediastinal mass		Enrofloxacin, marbofloxacin, ceftazadime, clindamycin	Died 14 d after emergency presentation; 7 mo after initial respiratory signs	Coignet,[5] 2012
2 y	MI	France	Diarrhea, inguinal abscess, fever	Peritonitis	Surgical debridement twice	Amoxicillin-clavulanic acid	Alive, stopped antibiotics 40 d after second surgery	Coignet,[5] 2012
U	U	Australia	Respiratory distress				Died	Coignet,[5] 2012
U	U	Australia	Respiratory distress				Died	Coignet,[5] 2012

Abbreviations: FI, female intact; FS, female spayed; MC, male castrated; MI, male intact; PE, physical examination; U, not reported.
Data from Refs.[5-8]

Surgical removal of infected abscesses in the cranial cervical region may be helpful. In the 2 ferrets with cranial cervical abscesses, the one that had surgical removal of the infected salivary gland survived but the other that was medically managed died within 25 days of presentation.[7]

Surgical removal of caudal abscesses may not be as successful. Three ferrets with subcutaneous abscesses (preputial, inguinal, femoral) died or were euthanized post-operatively,[8] with only one surviving (inguinal) after 2 debridement procedures.[5]

All ferrets with respiratory disease died despite antibiotic therapy,[6,8] making this a worse prognosis that those with subcutaneous swellings.

HEPATITIS E VIRUS
Etiology and Epidemiology

Hepatitis E virus (HEV) is a quasi-enveloped, single-stranded positive-sense RNA virus in the family Hepeviridae.[11] Hepeviridae contains several viral species that infect both humans and animals. In 2014, a new classification system for HEV was established.[12] Hepeviridae was divided into 2 genera, *Orthohepevirus* and *Piscihepevirus*. The *Orthohepevirus* includes all mammalian and avian isolates and is divided into 4 species: *Orthohepevirus A*, which includes isolates from humans, pigs, wild boar, deer, mongooses, rabbits, and camels; *Orthohepevirus B*, which includes isolates from chickens; *Orthohepevirus C*, which includes isolates from ferrets, rats, greater bandicoots, Asian musk shrews, and mink; and *Orthohepevirus D*, which includes isolates from bats. The *Piscihepevirus* genus only includes the fish isolate from trout (Cutthroat trout virus). At present, only viruses in *Orthohepevirus A* have been proven to infect humans and have a history of zoonosis,[11] although recent studies have shown that antibodies against *Orthohepevirus C* have been detected in humans in Germany and Vietnam.[13,14]

HEV in humans causes acute hepatitis E. Usually, this hepatitis is self-limiting, with full recovery in most cases.[11] However, the most serious form affects pregnant women during their third trimester of gestation. This infection causes fulminant liver failure with a mortality rate of almost 50% if liver transplantation is unavailable.[11]

HEV is transmitted via the fecal-oral route and in humans this is usually through contaminated food or water.[15] HEV infection in humans was originally suspected to be rare in developed countries.[11] More recent serosurveillance studies have demonstrated a high prevalence of HEV infection in the general population, which indicates the existence of an HEV endemic that has been underestimated.[11] These observations in developed countries suggest a cross-species transmission of zoonotic HEV from animal hosts to humans that depends on a variety of transmission routes other than the fecal-oral route.[11] This suspicion of zoonosis is further supported by a 2012 study finding a higher prevalence of *Orthohepevirus C* (Norway rat-associated HEV) antibodies in forestry workers compared with the general public in Germany.[13] Farmers, slaughterers, and veterinarians could be at a higher risk for zoonotic HEV infection as they work closely with potentially infected animals.[13]

Hepatitis E in Ferrets

HEV was first reported in ferrets in the Netherlands in 2012.[16] Since then, it has been reported in ferrets from the United States, Canada, Japan, and China.[17–20] Genetic analysis of the ferret HEV strains from different countries have found genetic similarity and clustering, but there are enough differences to suggest that the ferret HEV genome is genetically diverse.[17–20]

Surveillance studies of laboratory ferrets in Japan that were born in the United States found that 23.3% to 100%[17,21,22] of the ferrets had been exposed to HEV

(IgG in serum) and 60.3%[21]–100%[22] had HEV RNA in their feces or serum. In eastern China, 17.5% of laboratory ferrets had RNA in their fecal swabs.[20]

Although most of these surveillance studies have looked at natural infection in ferrets from breeding and research colonies, 1 study did look at natural infection in pet ferrets in Japan.[19] Samples from 10 hospitals in 5 prefectures (2009–2013) were tested. A total of 85 fecal samples and 10 serum samples were collected. Results found that 7.1% of the fecal samples were positive for HEV RNA and 10% of the serum samples were positive for IgM, and 20% were positive for IgG. These results suggested active ferret HEV transmission and prevalence among pet ferrets in Japan.[19] Genetically, the samples were most similar to strains from the United States and Canada, leading to the conclusion that ferret HEV has been introduced into Japan through importation from these countries.[19]

Experimentally, ferret HEV was successfully transmitted to other ferrets through the fecal-oral route and intravenous inoculation.[23] One study looking at natural infection in 8-week-old ferrets from US farms suspected that they were exposed to ferret HEV via the fecal-oral route after weaning at 6 weeks of age.[22] Another study looking at natural infection in ferrets born in the United States and imported to Japan detected ferret HEV RNA in both serum and fecal samples, suggesting that the ferret HEV infection induces viremia and virus shedding in feces, which may contaminate the environment.[21] The virus does not seem to be shed in the urine of infected ferrets.[22]

Ferret Hepatitis E Virus in Other Species

Rats, cynomolgus monkeys, and rabbits intravenously inoculated with ferret HEV did not develop infection.[20,23] This suggests that the reservoirs of ferret HEV in experimental animals is limited.[23]

Although ferret HEV infection has never been reported in humans, rat-associated HEV *Orthohepevirus C* antibodies have been detected in humans[13,14] and may have caused acute febrile illness with mild liver dysfunction in 1 patient in Vietnam.[14] Genetically, ferret HEV shares a high nucleotide sequence identity with rat HEV.[16]

Clinical Presentation

Both natural and experimental infections of HEV in ferrets indicate that this virus can cause liver damage in some ferrets.[19,21] Despite an increase in liver values, most ferrets do not show symptoms of liver disease, such as jaundice, diarrhea, fever, or lethargy.[21] One pet ferret in Japan had increased alanine aminotransferase (ALT), hepatomegaly, and anorexia.[19]

Two observational studies have found 3 patterns of natural infection in ferrets: subclinical infection, acute hepatitis, and persistent infection. All ferrets were positive for ferret HEV in their serum and feces.

- Subclinical infection: no significant increase of liver enzymes; diagnosed in 13/38 (34%) ferrets in a short-term study, 4/9 (44%) in a long-term study (74 days),[21] and 2/9 (22%) in a long-term study (20 weeks).[22]
- Acute hepatitis: an increase in the ALT value of greater than 100 IU/L that decreased as HEV RNA became undetectable in serum and feces; diagnosed in 25/38 (66%) ferrets in a short-term study,[21] 4/9 (44%) in a long-term study (74 days),[21] and 6/9 (67%) in a long-term study (20 weeks).[22]
- Persistent infection: increased ALT and constant positivity for ferret HEV RNA throughout the monitoring; diagnosed in 5/63 (8%) in a long-term study (74 and 153 days)[21] and 1/9 (11%) in a long-term study (20 weeks).[22]

Although the ferrets with different infection patterns had different levels of serum IgG and IgM, there were no clear differences between the viral strains, suggesting that the sequence does not contribute to the infection patterns.[22] The presence of subclinical infection with viral RNA in the serum and feces indicates that infected ferrets can shed the virus in their feces without showing clinical signs of disease or changes in their liver enzymes.

Based on the results of these studies, ferrets with HEV may have an increased ALT value and hepatomegaly. Other parameters were not investigated, such as changes in the red and white blood cell counts, changes in other liver-associated biochemistry values (ie, albumin, glucose, cholesterol, bile acids) and diagnostic imaging. Therefore, any ferret with an increased ALT and suspicion of acute or persistent hepatitis should have a full biochemistry profile, complete blood count, and diagnostic imaging, including radiographs and abdominal ultrasound.

Diagnostic Testing

Ferret HEV infection can be diagnosed with RNA detection of the virus in feces or serum. Exposure to the virus can be detected with serum IgG and IgM antibodies. At present, seroprevalence of this disease in pet ferrets has only been investigated in Japan.[19]

An observational study followed the natural infection in 9 juvenile ferrets for 16 to 20 weeks after importation from a breeding farm in the United States to a laboratory in Japan.[22] Diagnostic testing results differed depending on the pattern of infection.

- Subclinical infection (2/9): Ferrets had viral RNA detected in the feces 5 weeks after importation and in the serum 8 weeks after importation. Their IgM antibody levels peaked at 8 weeks and IgG at 12 weeks after importation. Both IgG and IgM levels were decreasing by the end of the study.
- Acute hepatitis (6/9): The serum RNA was positive 5 weeks after importation and remained detectable for a further 5 to 12 weeks, with all RNA detection decreasing to zero before the end of the study. Their IgG and IgM serum antibodies peaked at 5 to 8 weeks after importation. All IgM values were decreasing by the end of the study.
- Persistent infection (1/9): Viral RNA was first detected in the ferret's serum at 5 weeks after importation and was detected in the serum and feces at similar values for the entire 20-week study. The IgG and IgM antibodies remained increased at a high value for the entire 20-week study. The IgM levels decreased from 9 to 13 weeks but did not decrease further from 13 to 20 weeks after importation.

Based on these results, any ferret with a suspicion of HEV should have serum and fecal samples submitted for RNA viral detection and IgG and IgM serum antibodies measured. Detection in the feces and serum is likely to precede an increase in the IgG and IgM antibodies. If the virus remains detectable in the feces and serum at similar levels 5 to 12 weeks later, the ferret may have a persistent infection. In this case, the liver values, and IgG and IgM values, may remain increased indicating ongoing hepatitis and shedding of the virus.

UPDATES ON INFLUENZA

Influenza is an important zoonotic and anthroponotic disease that affects many species. The zoonotic spread of influenza from ferrets was first reported in the in 1930s, and more recently ferrets have been used as models for influenza infection.[24]

Readers are encouraged to refer to the 2013 article, "Selected Emerging Diseases in Ferrets," which discusses diagnostic testing and treatment options in ferrets.[24]

Since the 2013 article, there has been another case of suspected anthroponotic spread of influenza to a pet ferret in Taiwan.[25] An 8-year-old female spayed ferret presented for hyporexia, lethargy, hypothermia, coughing, and dyspnea. Diagnostic imaging revealed pulmonary consolidation and a bronchial pattern. The owner had experienced influenza-like symptoms 3 days before the ferret's signs. Despite fluid, antibiotic, and nebulization therapy, the ferret declined and was euthanized. PCR from the ferret's nasal swab was positive for influenza A(H1N1)pmd09, which caused the 2009 influenza pandemic that infected humans and ferrets in the United States.

Recently, ferrets have been experimentally infected with various types of influenza viruses that infect pets and humans. Although natural infection with these viruses has not yet been noted, the evidence of experimental infection in ferrets indicates there is anthroponotic and zoonotic potential. As veterinarians, we may be the first to see signs of another pandemic and could contract the disease from our patients.

A highly pathogenic H7N9 influenza virus with almost 40% mortality in humans caused 100% mortality in ferrets inoculated intranasally, compared with zero deaths in those inoculated with the H1N1 influenza virus that caused the 2009 pandemic.[26] These ferrets died due to hemorrhagic pneumonia and had high viral titers in their lungs. In other less-pathogenic types of influenza, the patient often dies of secondary pneumonia rather than the virus itself.

In addition to being susceptible to influenza viruses that infect humans, ferrets are also susceptible to those that infect dogs and cats. Ferrets intranasally inoculated with canine influenza H3N2 not only developed disease (15% weight loss, lethargy, sneezing, hyporexia), but the virus was spread to 50% of the cohoused naive ferrets.[27] Although the ferrets did not exhibit neurologic signs before euthanasia, necropsy found acute necrotizing bronchioalveolitis and nonsuppurative encephalitis. In the same study, those infected with human influenza H3N2 developed less severe clinical signs (8% weight loss, sneezing), but the virus was spread to 100% of the cohoused naive ferrets. A low pathogenic avian influenza H7N2, causing an outbreak of respiratory disease in a cat shelter, resulted in mild clinical signs in ferrets (5% weight loss, mild increase in body temperature) that were intranasally inoculated, but the virus was not spread to cohoused naive ferrets.[28] A veterinarian working in the cat shelter was infected by the cats, showing the zoonotic potential of this virus.

DISCLOSURE

The author has nothing to disclose.

REFERENCES

1. Chihab W, Alaoui AS, Amar M. *Chryseomonas luteola* identified as the source of serious infections in a Moroccan University Hospital. J Clin Microbiol 2004;42:1837–9.
2. Rahav G, Simhon A, Mattan Y, et al. Infections with *Chryseomonas luteola* (CDC group Ve-1) and *Flavimonas oryzihabitans* (CDC group Ve-2). Medicine 1995;74:83–8.
3. Altinok I, Balta F, Capkin E, et al. Disease of rainbow trout caused by *Pseudomonas luteola*. Aquaculture 2007;273:393–7.
4. Cantas L, Sørby JRT, Aleström P, et al. Culturable gut microbiota diversity in zebrafish. Zebrafish 2012;9:26–37.
5. Coignet S. Etude retrospective des infections a *Pseudomonas luteola* chez le furet. 2012. Available at: http://theses.vet-alfort.fr/telecharger.php?id=1893. Accessed October 4, 2019.

6. Martínez J, Martorell J, Abarca M, et al. Pyogranulomatous pleuropneumonia and mediastinitis in ferrets (Mustela putorius furo) associated with Pseudomonas luteola infection. J Comp Pathol 2012;146:4–10.

7. Schmidt L, Doss G, Hawkins S, et al. Cranial cervical abscessation and sialadenitis due to Pseudomonas luteola in two domestic ferrets (Mustela putorius furo). J Exot Pet Med 2019;31:120–6.

8. Baum B, Richter B, Reifinger M, et al. Pyogranulomatous panniculitis in ferrets (Mustela putorius furo) with intralesional demonstration of Pseudomonas luteola. J Comp Pathol 2015;152:114–8.

9. Fass RJ, Bamishan J. In vitro susceptibilities of nonfermentative gram-negative bacilli other than Pseudomonas aeruginosa to 32 antimicrobial agents. Rev Infect Dis 1980;2:841–53.

10. Furuhama K, Onodera T. The influence of cephem antibiotics on gentamicin nephrotoxicity in normal, acidotic, dehydrated, and unilaterally nephrectomized rats. Toxicol Appl Pharmacol 1986;86:430–6.

11. Nan Y, Wu C, Zhao Q, et al. Zoonotic hepatitis E virus: an ignored risk for public health. Front Microbiol 2017;8:2396.

12. Smith D, Simmonds P, Jameel S, et al, Members of the International Committee on the Taxonomy of Viruses Hepeviridae Study Group. Consensus proposals for classification of the family Hepeviridae. J Gen Virol 2015;96:1191–2.

13. Dremsek P, Wenzel JJ, Johne R, et al. Seroprevalence study in forestry workers from eastern Germany using novel genotype 3-and rat hepatitis E virus-specific immunoglobulin G ELISAs. Med Microbiol Immunol 2012;201:189–200.

14. Shimizu K, Hamaguchi S, Ngo CC, et al. Serological evidence of infection with rodent-borne hepatitis E virus HEV-C1 or antigenically related virus in humans. J Vet Med Sci 2016;78(11):1677–81.

15. Yugo DM, Cossaboom CM, Meng X-J. Naturally occurring animal models of human hepatitis E virus infection. ILAR J 2014;55:187–99.

16. Raj VS, Smits SL, Pas SD, et al. Novel hepatitis E virus in ferrets, the Netherlands. Emerg Infect Dis 2012;18:1369.

17. Yang T, Kataoka M, Ami Y, et al. Characterization of self-assembled virus-like particles of ferret hepatitis E virus generated by recombinant baculoviruses. J Gen Virol 2013;94:2647–56.

18. Li T-C, Yang T, Ami Y, et al. Complete genome of hepatitis E virus from laboratory ferrets. Emerg Infect Dis 2014;20:709.

19. Li T-C, Yonemitsu K, Terada Y, et al. Ferret hepatitis E virus infection in Japan. Jpn J Infect Dis 2015;68(1):60–2.

20. Wang L, Gong W, Fu H, et al. Hepatitis E virus detected from Chinese laboratory ferrets and farmed mink. Transbound Emerg Dis 2018;65:e219–23.

21. Li T-C, Yang T, Yoshizaki S, et al. Ferret hepatitis E virus infection induces acute hepatitis and persistent infection in ferrets. Vet Microbiol 2016;183:30–6.

22. Li T-C, Yoshizaki S, Kataoka M, et al. Genetic and physicochemical analyses of a novel ferret hepatitis E virus, and clinical signs of infection after birth. Infect Genet Evol 2017;51:153–9.

23. Li T-C, Yoshizaki S, Ami Y, et al. Monkeys and rats are not susceptible to ferret hepatitis E virus infection. Intervirology 2015;58:139–42.

24. Wyre NR, Michels D, Chen S. Selected emerging diseases in ferrets. Vet Clin North Am Exot Anim Pract 2013;16:469–93.

25. Lin H-T, Wang C-H, Wu W-L, et al. Natural A (H1N1) pdm09 influenza virus infection case in a pet ferret in Taiwan. Jpn J Vet Res 2014;62:181–5.

26. Yum J, Ku KB, Kim HS, et al. H7N9 influenza virus is more virulent in ferrets than 2009 pandemic H1N1 influenza virus. Viral Immunol 2015;28:590–9.
27. Lee Y-N, Lee D-H, Park J-K, et al. Experimental infection and natural contact exposure of ferrets with canine influenza virus (H3N2). J Gen Virol 2013;94:293–7.
28. Belser JA, Pulit-Penaloza JA, Sun X, et al. A novel A (H7N2) influenza virus isolated from a veterinarian caring for cats in a New York City animal shelter causes mild disease and transmits poorly in the ferret model. J Virol 2017;91 [pii:e00672-17].

Cystine Urolithiasis in Ferrets

Rebecca E. Pacheco, DVM

KEYWORDS

- Cystine urolithiasis • Cystinuria • Ferrets • Mustela putorius furo

KEY POINTS

- Urolithiasis in captive domestic ferrets previously has been predominantly struvite uroliths; however, more recent laboratory submissions show a shift to predominantly cystine uroliths.
- Genetic mutations for cystinuria have been identified in dogs, and it is suspected that underlying genetic mutations are partly responsible for the disease in ferrets.
- Surgery remains the only definitive treatment of cystine urolithiasis in ferrets, because dissolution protocols have not been explored thoroughly.
- Medical management with dietary and urinary manipulation should be considered for use in ferrets postoperatively, adapted from principles of cystine urolithiasis management in dogs.

INTRODUCTION

Urolithiasis in captive domestic ferrets has previously been well documented, with a predominance of struvite (magnesium ammonium phosphate) stones accounting for the historical majority of uroliths.[1,2] Recently, however, there has been a significant increase of cystine uroliths being reported and submitted to diagnostic laboratories in North America. Cystine urolithiasis is currently the most common urolith type recognized in North American ferrets.[3] Although the increased recognition and incidence of cystine stones in ferrets seem well accepted among specialty and general practitioners within the zoologic companion animal field, peer-reviewed literature investigating underlying genetic and physiologic causes, predisposing factors, true prevalence, and potential medical management and prevention options is extremely limited. The goal of this review is to summarize the anecdotal and limited peer-reviewed information available regarding cystine urolithiasis in ferrets for easy access to current knowledge for the practitioner.

Gulf Coast Veterinary Specialists, 8042 Katy Freeway, Houston, TX 77024, USA
E-mail address: rebecca.pacheco@gcvs.com

Vet Clin Exot Anim 23 (2020) 309–319
https://doi.org/10.1016/j.cvex.2020.01.015
1094-9194/20/© 2020 Elsevier Inc. All rights reserved.

UROLITH COMPOSITION IN DOMESTIC FERRETS

Urolithiasis is well established as a disease syndrome in ferrets, and ferret-specific urinary anatomy and physiology have been well described previously.[1] The most common type of urolith, until recent years, had predominantly been struvite. An article published in 2011 retrospectively reviewed urolith samples submitted to the Minnesota Urolith Center from 1981 to 2007 (n = 408), of which 272 (67%) were documented as struvite uroliths, and only 61 (15%) were cystine uroliths.[2] Shortly after that study, a review from 1992 to 2009 looked at 435 stone submissions, of which 277 (67%) were struvite stones, and only 70 (16%) were cystine. The third most common urolith composition in this review was calcium oxalate, comprising 50 (11%) of all submissions.[4] Within this review, during a time period from January 2010 and September 2012 (therefore not included in the study), an additional 69 uroliths were submitted to the laboratory. Evaluation of this subset of uroliths showed that 44 (64%) were cystine uroliths, 12 (17%) were struvite uroliths, 6 (9%) were calcium oxalate uroliths, 3 (4%) were ammonium nitrate uroliths, and the remaining 4 uroliths were of various other or mixed composition.[4]

The brief analysis of submissions from 2010 to 2012 signifies the first peer-reviewed notation comma not necessary where cystine urolithiasis represented the predominant urolith composition. A recent release of statistics (currently unpublished) from the Minnesota Urolith Center determined that during the time period from 2010 to 2017, the composition of ferret uroliths submitted (total n = 700) was 623 (89%) cystine, whereas only 46 (6.5%) were struvite (**Table 1** lists a summation of these data).[3] Further unpublished data currently in review evaluating submissions from multiple laboratories in North America from 2010 to 2018, including the data from the Minnesota Urolith Center, found that of approximately 1014 urolith submissions, 943 (93%) were composed of cystine.[5] An underlying cause for this shift has yet to be elucidated; however the Minnesota Urolith Center and University of Minnesota Canine Genetics Lab are currently redundant evaluating for genetic mutations that could be responsible for cystine urolithiasis in ferrets.

CYSTINE CHEMISTRY, METABOLISM, AND GENETICS

Cystine is a nonessential amino acid, derived from oxidation of the amino acid cysteine. Cysteine itself is derived from the essential amino acid methionine, which

Table 1
Overview of urolith composition over time by retrospective review

Years	Total Number of Uroliths Evaluated	Cystine	Struvite	Calcium Oxalate	Mixed/ Other
1981–2007 (Nwaokorie et al,[2] 2011)	408	61 (15%)	272 (67%)	43 (11%)	32 (8%)
1992–2009 (Nwaokorie et al,[4] 2013)	435	70 (16%)	277 (67%)	50 (11%)	40 (9%)
2010–2012 (Nwaokorie et al,[4] 2013)	69	44 (64%)	12 (17%)	6 (9%)	7 (10%)
2010–2017[a] (Minnesota Urolith Center,[3] 2018)	700	623 (89%)	46 (6.5%)	—	—

[a] This data set is not yet published as a retrospective study.
Data from Refs.[2–4]

is most commonly found in animal-based proteins; this becomes an important factor in management of human and canine cystinuria. Cystine is a sulfur-containing amino acid due to the addition of a disulfide link in the oxidation process, and provides the primary source of sulfur in protein synthesis. Sources of dietary cystine that are applicable to domestic ferrets include animal proteins such as beef, poultry, pork, lamb, dairy, and eggs. Other important sources include soy products, grains (barley, wheat, oats), and legumes (peas, beans, lentils).

In normal urinary metabolism, cystine is freely filtered in the glomerulus and is then reabsorbed from the urine in the proximal renal tubules. Therefore, a defect in renal tubule reabsorption of cystine is one contributing component of cystinuria that has been identified in dogs and humans.[6–8] Other contributing mechanisms of cystine urolith formation have yet to be identified in humans and dogs. Not all dogs with cystine crystalluria go on to develop cystine uroliths; thus it is thought there are other predisposing factors contributing to urolith formation. There is a paucity of data available assessing if ferrets develop cystinuria or cystine crystalluria prior to development of cystine urolithiasis; this may be because a majority of ferrets that present to clinics with urolithiasis present acutely obstructed without previous signs of urinary disease. Cystine crystals observed via urinalysis typically are visualized as flat, colorless, hexagonal crystals, often layered in sheets or clumped.[6] Cystine uroliths vary in gross appearance but generally appear as spherical or smooth polyhedronal in shape, vary in size from less than 1 mm to greater than 5 mm, and are commonly tan to yellow in color, although they can appear lighter (**Fig. 1**). Some cystine uroliths can have a rough outer texture, although most are smooth. Anecdotally, stones can range from a single stone to greater than 100 in ferrets; similar information has been reported for dogs.[6]

Genetic mutations altering renal cystine transporters have been identified in dogs, including one in relation to androgen-dependent cystinuria. Neutering has been considered a potential therapy to help reduce cystinuria in certain candidates with

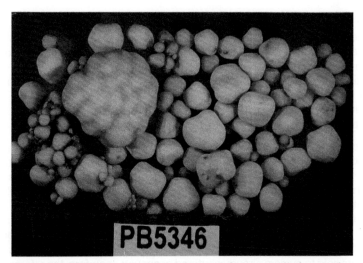

Fig. 1. Example of 100% cystine uroliths submitted from a male ferret. These uroliths demonstrate the smooth polyhedronal but overall spherical shape and yellow color common to most cystine uroliths. Note the variation in size. Each line on the ruler represents 1 mm. (*Courtesy of* Urolithiasis Laboratory, Houston, TX.)

this genetic mutation.[8,9] Genetic mutations identified affecting amino acid trans-porters in dogs include autosomal dominant mutations SLC3A1 and SLC7A9, and autosomal recessive mutation SLC3A1.[8,10] Genetic markers have yet to be identified in ferrets, and androgen-dependent cystine urolithiasis has not been evaluated to date.

EPIDEMIOLOGY OF CYSTINE UROLITHIASIS

There is little epidemiologic information available for cystine urolithiasis in ferrets. One retrospective review of a total of 69 cystine urolith submissions in ferrets revealed the following points regarding various factors evaluated based on information provided with submissions[4]:

Age

- Median age at time of presentation was 4 years, with most cases presenting be-tween the ages of 2.6 years and 5.6 years.
- The age group of 2-year-old to 4-year-old ferrets represented the largest propor-tion of cystine stone submissions (51%), followed by 4-year-old to 7-year-old fer-rets (21%).

These results show that cystine urolithiasis in ferrets appears most commonly in middle-aged individuals. The average reported lifespan of a domestic ferret ranges between 6 and 11 years, although in the author's experience it is rare to find an indi-vidual greater than 9 years old.[11,12] This is similar to dogs, where incidence of cystine uroliths is most common in the 2.3-year to 7.3-year range.[6] Cystine urolithiasis in dogs is known to be in part due to a genetic contribution, although the disease rarely man-ifests in juvenile animals as can be seen with some genetic diseases.[6] Thus, other instigating causes for urolith formation are thought to be necessary, since animals do not develop uroliths until well into life in most forms of cystinuria.[6] Similar mecha-nisms of urolith formation are likely in play for ferrets.

Sex Status

- Male ferrets were overrepresented, comprising 77% of cystine urolith cases. Male ferrets had 2.5-times the risk of developing cystine uroliths compared with female ferrets.
- Of all cystine uroliths, 93% were from neutered/spayed ferrets compared with 7% from intact animals.
- Neutered/spayed ferrets were approximately 3.1times more likely to develop cystine uroliths compared with intact animals.

Male ferrets are likely overrepresented, due in part to a longer lower urinary tract combined with a tightly angled pelvic urethral flexure, rigid os penis, and narrow ure-thral diameter that serve to predispose male ferrets to urinary blockage. Female ferrets have a shorter, wider, and less convoluted urethra and are able to pass smaller diam-eter uroliths without significant risk of obstruction. The role of androgen, a sex hor-mone found in higher levels in males than in females, is currently unknown in ferrets though is genetically linked to a particular type of cystinuria in dogs; in this form there also is a heavy predilection for males to be affected.[8] The majority of ferrets in North America are sold to owners already neutered or spayed, therefore, the reference study had a small number of intact cases to determine risk of urolith formation with regards to sex status. Therefore, it is not clear if overrepresentation of altered animals is truly due to an increased risk versus statistical overrepresentation or other factors.

Anatomical Location

- The lower urinary tract (bladder and urethra) was the source for 96% of submissions; the remaining 4% were voided; therefore, origin was considered undetermined.
- Of cystine stones found in the bladder and urethra, 84% were removed from the urethra and 16% were from the bladder.

These findings are consistent with the reported location of cystine urolithiasis in dogs, although there is a breed-related predisposition to nephroliths found in the Newfoundland, which is suspected to be related to the particular genetic cystinuria syndrome in that breed.[6] In the author's experience, renal mineral deposition has been noted on abdominal ultrasound of a subset of ferrets with cystine urolithiasis.

Seasonality

- Seasons did not seem to demonstrate a statistically significant effect on cystine urolith submissions.

In human medicine, several studies have shown that seasonality, in particular warm seasons, predisposes humans to the development of nephrolithiasis or urolithiasis.[13,14] To the author's knowledge, there has been no similar seasonal effect recognized in dogs or cats.

CLINICAL PRESENTATION AND PHYSICAL EXAMINATION FINDINGS

The presenting signs of cystine urolithiasis in ferrets can vary, although many ferrets present with signs of acute urinary obstruction. In these cases, patients typically present with a history of straining to urinate with no urine production, dribbling of urine, or scant production of blood-tinged urine. It is common for ferret owners to list the presenting complaint as straining to defecate, since it is easy to misinterpret the repeated action of attempting to urinate as attempts to defecate. Owners may notice that their ferret is restless and cannot get settled; alternatively, a patient may present lethargic to obtunded or even stuporous if significant acid-base alterations, renal derangements, or electrolyte abnormalities are present. Ferrets may vocalize or grunt during attempts to urinate, although this is not always present. Some ferrets may flatten their abdomens to the ground intermittently, whereas others may exhibit a hunched back. Many ferrets have a history of decreased to absent appetite and may have vomiting and/or diarrhea. The time frame for how long signs have been present prior to evaluation at the clinic is typically short, due to the rapid decline associated with full urinary obstruction. It is possible for a patient to have a more prolonged history of clinical signs with a less severe initial presentation if the ferret has not yet obstructed. In these cases, signs can include intermittent or mild stranguria, pollakiuria, hematuria, or urine dribbling. A ferret that has historically used a litter box may change habits and urinate inappropriately outside of the litter box. Changes in appetite, drinking habits, and energy levels may be noted by the owner. These signs may be present for days to weeks before a patient is presented to the clinic for evaluation.

In most cases of acute urinary obstruction, a large, round, and turgid bladder is palpable on examination. If the patient is able to pass a small amount of urine or has had the bladder drained prior to presentation, the bladder will be somewhat compressible. In rare instances, if a ferret has ruptured the bladder, the bladder may be small or nonpalpable, and an abdominal fluid wave or distended abdomen may be noted. Most obstructed ferrets exhibit mild to severe abdominal pain and resistance to bladder palpation. On examination, the prepuce may be erythematous and inflamed, and there may be tiny stones or fine grit visible at the distal end of the penis. Vital parameters can vary, with tachycardia noted in part from pain; however, arrhythmias, including bradyarrhythmias, can be auscultated with certain electrolyte abnormalities. The respiratory rate may be elevated as a compensatory mechanism if severe metabolic acidosis is present; however it may also be normal or even low in dull or obtunded animals.[15] Hypothermia may be present in azotemic animals, as is seen in dogs and cats.[16]

DIAGNOSTIC TESTING

In a ferret presenting acutely with signs of urinary obstruction, it is warranted to obtain a minimum database inclusive of a blood chemistry profile, complete blood cell count, and potentially venous blood gas and blood lactate levels. Depending on patient status on presentation, electrocardiogram for evaluation of cardiac arrhythmias, blood pressure, and urine can also be obtained. Urine for urinalysis and urine culture and sensitivity should be obtained if voided with clean catch at initial presentation and can also be collected during urethral catheterization, cystocentesis, or at the time of surgery if necessary.[17] Cystocentesis is not recommended in an animal with a turgid bladder due to the risk of intra-abdominal urine leakage or bladder rupture/tearing.

Once a patient is stabilized, diagnostic imaging is strongly recommended even if urolithiasis is obvious or has been confirmed previously. At a minimum, 2-view abdominal radiographs should be obtained, being sure to include the urethra at the level of the ischium (**Fig. 2**). A flexed pelvic view with pelvic limbs pulled forward is advised to better visualize uroliths that may be within the pelvic or penile urethra. Cystine stones are radiodense, although they are typically only of intermediate radiodensity.[6] Therefore, it can be difficult to visualize small uroliths, uroliths within the urethra, or urolithiasis where only a few are present. Contrast cystourethrogram can be helpful in cases of cystine uroliths that are less radiodense or to better visualize uroliths within the urethra. Abdominal ultrasound is helpful to visualize even small, more radiolucent cystoliths and can determine if nephroliths or ureteroliths are present.

The complete blood cell count erythrogram may reveal evidence of dehydration, although values can be within normal limits in cases of patients that remain eating and drinking. The leukogram may show leukocytosis; differentials include a

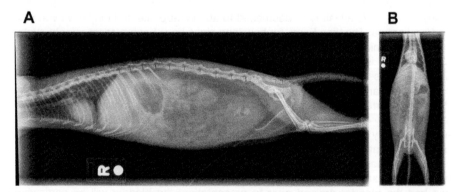

Fig. 2. (A) Right lateral and (B) ventrodorsal radiographs of a male ferret with confirmed cystine uroliths. Note the intermediate radiodensity of the uroliths as well as the presence of uroliths in the right kidney, bladder, and perineal urethra. A urinary catheter is placed in the penile urethra. (*Courtesy of* M. McNeil, DVM, Houston, TX. and S. Fronefield, DVM, DABVP (Avian), Houston, TX.)

physiologic stress response, urinary tract infection (UTI), sepsis, or a systemic inflammatory response in the event of vasculitis or peritonitis. Biochemistry values, in cases of complete urinary obstruction, nearly always show azotemia in the form of elevations in blood urea nitrogen (BUN) and possibly creatinine. These values at times can be severely elevated. In contrast to dogs and cats, ferret creatinine often is within normal limits even in ferrets with significant renal compromise. Therefore, an elevated BUN may be the only parameter elevated in an azotemic ferret, and even mild elevations in creatinine should be considered significant.[1] Other common biochemical and venous blood gas derangements include hyperkalemia, hyperphosphatemia, and hypocalcemia, which are secondary to alterations in normal renal function.[18] Venous blood gas often shows a metabolic acidosis with a lowered base excess.[18] If there is any concern for bladder rupture or leakage and ascites is present, abdominal fluid can be obtained for creatinine evaluation to compare the ratio of fluid creatinine with serum creatinine. In dogs and cats, a fluid to serum/plasma creatinine ratio greater than or equal to 2:1 confirms a diagnosis of uroabdomen.[19] Blood lactate is often elevated in conjunction with uremia and can be helpful in evaluating the degree of glomerular filtration rate compromise. Blood lactate can also be elevated if bladder wall compromise or necrosis is present. Normal lactate reference range reported for cats is 1 mmol/L to 2 mmol/L, and in a single study of urethral obstruction, showed average lactate levels of 2.2 mmol/L $\pm$ 1.3 mmol/L.[20] Normal lactate levels in ferrets have not been established.

Urinalysis in ferrets typically is less helpful than in dogs and cats, since normal urine specific gravity has not been determined in ferrets, and cystine crystals may not be seen in animals with cystine urolithiasis depending on urinary pH.[1,6] Based on information available in dogs, many cases of cystine urolithiasis show both proteinuria and hematuria of varying degrees.[6] Bacterial infection is uncommon with cystine urolithiasis in dogs, although leukocytes secondary to inflammation are not an uncommon finding.[6] Similar information based on comparison of struvite urolithiasis in cats and ferrets suggests that like cats, ferrets may exhibit a low frequency of urinary tract infection (UTI) associated with urolithiasis.[2] Urine culture and sensitivity remain prudent to rule out concurrent UTI, as other urinary factors may still predispose a patient to a UTI. A sterile urine sample can be collected for submission, and it is recommended to collect bladder mucosa and a urolith sample if surgery is performed.

Any uroliths retrieved during surgery should be submitted to a urolith laboratory for analysis. A thorough history, including signalment, diet, supplements and treats, diagnostic results, previous history of urinary disease, and any known familial relations and their history with urinary disease, should be included with submission or available on request.

TREATMENT

Ultimately, the only definitive treatment for a ferret patient with cystine cystolithiasis is via cystotomy and manual urolith removal. In unstable patients, alleviation of the obstruction via urinary catheterization is ideal, followed by medical management with an indwelling urinary catheter until the patient is more stable for anesthesia and surgery.[1] Fluid therapy, either intravenous or subcutaneous, prior to surgical intervention may also assist nephroliths or ureteroliths to be flushed into the bladder to reduce the risk of cystolithiasis recurrence immediately postoperatively.[21] In cases where an indwelling urinary catheter is unable to be placed, such as obstructive urethroliths or urethral stricture, decompressive cystocentesis can be considered to alleviate a critically full bladder.[1] This should always be performed with ultrasound guidance, and risks of bladder leakage or tearing leading to uroabdomen should be explained to the owner prior to performing this procedure.

Stable patients or patients found to have cystoliths without clinical signs will ultimately still need surgical intervention. No successful medical dissolution protocol has been described for ferrets yet; therefore, in a male ferret diagnosed with cystine urolithiasis, the stones pose a significant risk for urinary obstruction. Performing surgery while a patient is clinically stable instead of in an obstructive emergency is preferred. Increasing dietary water intake or diuresis with subcutaneous fluid therapy for several days prior to surgery, as well as initiating preventative medical management practices is reasonable prior to surgery in the stable patient.

Complications at the time of surgery are reported to include uroabdomen, peritonitis, cystic wall necrosis, complete obstruction of the urethra that is unable to be unobstructed, urethral tearing, and urethral necrosis. Other factors to consider going into surgery include the presence of ureteroliths or nephroliths. To date, there have been no published reports of laser lithotripsy used in ferrets with urolithiasis.

The most common surgical approach is a ventral midline incision in the body wall with a cranial to caudal, ventrally placed cystotomy incision. The cystotomy procedure can be performed in a ferret in similar fashion as in dogs and cats and has previously been well described by Miwa and Sladky.[22] During surgery, a urinary catheter should be fed retrograde and anterograde and flushed copiously to ensure urethral patency. A possible intraoperative complication encountered is uroliths that remain lodged within the lower urinary tract, commonly found at the pelvic flexure or proximal to the os penis.[1] These stones can simply be too large to successfully pass, may be partially embedded within the urethral mucosa, or may be lodged secondary to inflammation, stricture, or trauma to the urethra. In such cases, stones should be flushed retrograde and removed through the bladder. Retrograde hydropropulsion requires having an assistant with narrow fingers insert a lubricated finger into the rectum and apply gentle pressure ventrally on the urethra while the surgeon threads a catheter (3.5Fr or 5Fr red rubber catheter) into the distal tip of the urethra. The distal urethral opening should be gently pinched and closed around the catheter and the catheter filled with sterile saline with a 10 mL or greater size syringe, increasing pressure against the assistant's finger until the urethra is dilated. The assistant then releases pressure on the urethra as the surgeon continues to apply positive pressure to the syringe, thereby pulsing any stuck uroliths back toward the bladder. Uroliths can then be removed as they are flushed back into the bladder.

In cases of multiple urethral obstructions over time, complete urethral obstruction that cannot be alleviated with retrograde hydropropulsion, or urethral stricture leading to repeat urinary obstruction, additional intervention is necessary. Repeat cystotomy should be perfrmed, or, in selective cases, perineal urethrostomy can be performed to make a new, permanent urinary opening proximal to the site of obstruction.[1]

PREVENTION AND DIETARY MANAGEMENT

Cystine is relatively insoluble and is more insoluble in acidic urine than in alkaline urine. Therefore, modification of diet to achieve a urinary pH of 7.5 or greater has been implemented as a management technique for dogs with cystinuria and would likely function similarly in ferrets.[6] Historically, diets that derive their protein from cereal or plant sources tend to alkalinize the urine, but this presents a problem when considering cystine urolithiasis since alkaline urine can promote the formation of struvite uroliths.[23] Cystine is found in high levels in certain plant proteins such as legumes; consequently, plant proteins in the diet also may lead to higher levels of cystine in the urine.[6] Ferrets require high levels of protein (30%–35%) in their diet, even moreso than dogs or cats.[23] Therefore, maintaining captive ferrets on a diet based on high-quality animal protein sources while simultaneously increasing urinary pH is ideal.

Ideally, a diet for dissolution and/or prevention of cystine uroliths for ferrets would encompass the following factors:

- Increased alkalinity: Increases solubility of cystine to prevent urolith formation
- Low in methionine: Minimizes animal-based proteins such as muscle meat and dairy
- Low in cystine: Minimizes plant-based cystine sources such as legumes, grain, and soy
- Increased water content: Dilutes urine to reduce cystine concentration; consider feeding canned food or mixing food with water
- Low in sodium: Decreases cystine excretion into urine

Providing a diet that meets both the physiologic needs of a ferret as well as the necessary dissolution factors proves difficult. Prescription diets that promote alkalization exist for the dog, but the protein levels in these products vary between 10.9% and 13.4%, which are suboptimal to maintain a ferret long term.[24] Reducing both cystine and its precursor, methionine, eliminates many appropriate protein sources. Even with appropriate dietary management, cystine urolithiasis is commonly recurrent in dogs.[6,21]

Urine manipulation via other pathways may be a more successful focus until more is known about dietary protein manipulation. Potassium citrate, a urine alkylating agent, has been used successfully to increase urinary pH in dogs.[6,21,25] This medication has been used anecdotally in ferrets, although no peer-reviewed literature has been compiled to determine efficacy. If potassium citrate is implemented as part of a dietary management plan, regular monitoring of urine pH via dipstick at home is warranted to ensure efficacy of treatment. Optimal dosage for potassium citrate has not been determined for dogs or ferrets. Reported recommended starting doses for dogs are 150 mg/kg/d and 0.5 mEq/kg/d, which are then titrated to effect.[21,25]

Concentrated urine increases the saturation of cystine within the urine, promoting crystalluria and urolith formation. High moisture diets can dilute urine and aid in preventing cystine supersaturation. This can be achieved by offering multiple water stations, providing a ferret-appropriate canned food, or mixing water into a ferret's regular diet.[25] In humans, high dietary sodium causing natriuresis has been correlated to increased concentration of cystine in the urine. Consequently, in human medicine, low-sodium diets are advised to reduce the amount of cystine excreted into the urine and are also recommended in dogs as a management technique for cystinuria.[21,26,27] Commercially available ferret diets are typically well standardized to maintain similar levels of sodium; therefore, there are practical difficulties in finding a low-sodium, nutritionally appropriate ferret diet.[23]

Tiopronin is a medication used to effectively treat cystinuria in humans by complexing with cystine to form more soluble forms of tiopronin-cysteine. This helps to prevent crystallization and stone formation and promotes urinary excretion of cystine.[6] Tiopronin has also been used successfully in dogs, both to reduce recurrence of cystinuria and cystine urolithiasis as well as to assist in dissolving cystine stones already present.[28] Application of tiopronin in ferrets has not been evaluated.

There has been a purely anecdotal correlation between the increased incidence of cystine urolithiasis and the introduction of ferret diets in North America bolstered with legumes, with peas and lentils most commonly implicated. It is important to note that not all ferrets fed a grain-free diet go on to develop urolithiasis. In reviewing cases at a single hospital (Gulf Coast Veterinary Specialists, Houston, Texas), every ferret that presented with cystine urolithiasis was consuming a grain-free diet. At this facility, there were several multiferret households (4–15 individuals per household) that fed all ferrets exclusively grain-free diets. In these groups, only 1 to 2 individuals were presented for cystine urolithiasis. This anecdotal finding may support the theory of a genetic mutation playing a part in development of cystine urolithiasis; however, diet and the presence of legumes likely play a critical role in urolith development. Cystine uroliths have not been documented at a clinic in Hong Kong, where a majority of ferrets are fed diets without legume components (Nicole Wyre, DVM, DABVP Avian, Exotic Companion Mammal; personal correspondence, 2019). Similarly, in the United Kingdom, where ferrets more commonly are fed whole-prey or legume free diets, struvite remains the most common urolith, followed by calcium carbonate.[29]

After this correlation was noticed in the zoologic companion animal field, some diet manufacturers revised their ingredients to avoid legume ingredients. Many clinicians now recommend that owners feed their ferret a high-quality, ferret-specific diet that does not have legume ingredients. It is unclear if legume proteins truly contribute to cystine urolithiasis; however, there currently are many high quality commercial ferret diets that are exclusive of legumes to choose from.

DISCLOSURE

The author has nothing to disclose.

REFERENCES

1. Orcutt CJ. Ferret urogenital diseases. Vet Clin North Am Exot Anim Pract 2003; 6(1):113–38.
2. Nwaokorie EE, Osborne CA, Lulich JP, et al. Epidemiology of struvite uroliths in ferrets: 272 cases (1981-2007). J Am Vet Med Assoc 2011;239:1319–24.
3. Minnesota Urolith Center. Cystine rising: Ferreting out the cause. In: Minnesota Urolith Center image of the month. 2018. Available at: http://www.vetmed.umn. edu/sites/vetmed.umn.edu/files/ferret_cystine_rising.pdf. Accessed November 9, 2019.
4. Nwaokorie EE, Osborne CA, Lulich JP, et al. Epidemiological evaluation of cystine urolithiasis in domestic ferrets (Mustela putorius furo): 70 cases (1992–2009). J Am Vet Med Assoc 2013;242:1099–103.
5. Hanak EH, Di Girolamo N, DeSilva U, et al. Composition of ferret uroliths in North America and Europe: 1055 Cases (2010-2018). Abstract, presented at: Exotics Conference with AAZV, Saint Louis, MO, September 30, 2019.
6. Osborne CA, Sanderson SL, Lulich JP, et al. Canine cystine urolithiasis: cause, detection, treatment, and prevention. Vet Clin North Am Small Anim Pract 1999; 29(1):193–211.
7. Chillarón J, Font-Llitjós M, Palacín M, et al. Pathophysiology and treatment of cystinuria. Nat Rev Nephrol 2010;6(7):424–34.
8. Brons AK, Henthorn PS, Raj K, et al. SLC3A1 and SLC7A9 mutations in autosomal recessive or dominant canine cystinuria: a new classification system. J Vet Intern Med 2013;27(6):1400–8.
9. Henthorn PS, Liu J, Gidalevich T, et al. Canine cystinuria: polymorphism in the canine SLC3A1 gene and identification of a nonsense mutation in cystinuric Newfoundland dogs. Hum Genet 2000;107(4):295–303.
10. Harnevik L, Hoppe A, Söderkvist P. SLC7A9 cDNA cloning and mutational analysis of SLC3A1 and SLC7A9 in canine cystinuria. Mamm Genome 2006;17(7): 769–76.

11. Fox JG. Normal clinical and biologic parameters. In: Fox JG, Marini RP, editors. Biology and diseases of the ferret. 2nd edition. Baltimore (MD): Williams & Wilkins; 1998. p. 183–210.

12. Powers LV, Brown SA. Basic anatomy, physiology, and husbandry. In: Quesenberry KE, Carpenter JW, editors. Ferrets, rabbits, and rodents: clinical medicine and surgery. 3rd edition. St Louis (MO): Elsevier Saunders; 2012. p. 7.

13. Buttigieg J, Attard S, Carachi A, et al. Nephrolithiasis, stone composition, meteorology, and seasons in Malta: Is there any connection? Urol Ann 2016;8(3):325.

14. Fukuhara H, Ichiyanagi O, Kakizaki H, et al. Clinical relevance of seasonal changes in the prevalence of ureterolithiasis in the diagnosis of renal colic. Urolithiasis 2016;44(6):529–37.

15. Lee JL, Drobatz KJ. Historical and physical parameters as predictors of severe hyperkalemia in male cats with urethral obstruction. J Vet Emerg Crit Care 2006;16(2):104–11.

16. Kabatchnick E, Langston C, Olson B, et al. Hypothermia in uremic dogs and cats. J Vet Intern Med 2016;30(5):1648–54.

17. Pollock C. Emergency medicine of the ferret. Vet Clin North Am Exot Anim Pract 2007;10(2):463–500.

18. Freitas GC, Mori da Cunha MGMC, Gomes K, et al. Acid–base and biochemical stabilization and quality of recovery in male cats with urethral obstruction and anesthetized with propofol or a combination of ketamine and diazepam. Can J Vet Res 2012;76(3):201–8.

19. Stafford JR, Bartges JW. A clinical review of pathophysiology, diagnosis and treatment of uroabdomen in the dog and cat. J Vet Emerg Crit Care 2013; 23(2):216–29.

20. Lee JA, Drobatz KJ. Characterization of the clinical characteristics, electrolytes, acid-base and renal parameters in male cats with urethral obstruction. J Vet Emerg Crit Care 2003;13(4):227–33.

21. Lulich JP, Berent AC, Adams LG, et al. ACVIM Small animal consensus recommendations on the treatment and prevention of uroliths in dogs and cats. J Vet Intern Med 2016;30(5):1564–74.

22. Miwa Y, Sladky KK. Small mammals: common surgical procedures of rodents, ferrets, hedgehogs, and sugar gliders. Vet Clin North Am Exot Anim Pract 2016; 19(1):205–44.

23. Johnson-Delaney CA. Ferret nutrition. Vet Clin North Am Exot Anim Pract 2014; 17(3):449–70.

24. Veterinary team. Managing patients with feline lower urinary tract disease (FLUTD)/urolithiasis. In: Hill's Vet. 2012. Available at: https://www.hillsvet.com/products/product-algorithms. Accessed November 9, 2019.

25. Grauer GF. Feline Struvite & Calcium oxalate urolithiasis. In: Urology/renal medicine, Today's veterinary practice. 2014. Available at: https://todaysveterinarypractice.com/feline-struvite-calcium-oxalate-urolithiasis/. Accessed November 2, 2019.

26. Norman RW, Manette WA. Dietary restriction of sodium as a means of reducing urinary cystine. J Urol 1990;143(6):1193–5.

27. Dion M, Ankawi G, Chew B, et al. CUA guideline on the evaluation and medical management of the kidney stone patient - 2016 update. Can Urol Assoc J 2016; 10(11–12):347–58.

28. Hoppe A, Denneberg T. Cystinuria in the dog: clinical studies during 14 years of medical treatment. J Vet Intern Med 2001;15(4):361–7.

29. Rogers KD, Jones B, Roberts L, et al. Composition of uroliths in small domestic animals in the United Kingdom. Vet J 2011;188:228–30.

Update on Diseases in Chinchillas: 2013–2019

Anna Martel, DVM[a], Thomas Donnelly, BVSc, DACLAM,
DABVP (Small Mammals), DECZM[b],
Christoph Mans, Dr med vet, DACZM, DECZM[a],*

KEYWORDS

- *Chinchilla lanigera* • *Streptococcus equi* subsp *zooepidemicus*
- *Pseudomonas aeruginosa* • Urolithiasis • Cardiac disease • Penile disease
- *Rodentolepis nana*

KEY POINTS

- Penile disorders are common in chinchilla and, therefore, the glans penis and prepuce should be examined carefully during every physical examination.
- *Streptococcus equi* subsp *zooepidemicus* is an emerging pathogen in chinchillas and increasingly is diagnosed. Common clinical findings include subcutaneous abscesses and conjunctivitis.
- *Pseudomonas aeruginosa* is the most important pathogen in chinchillas and is the most common bacterial pathogen isolated in chinchillas with conjunctivitis.

NONINFECTIOUS DISEASES

Penile Disorders

Penile disorders are common in chinchillas. Conditions, such as penile fur rings, balanoposthitis, preputial abscesses, paraphimosis, and phimosis, have been described with recommendations for treatment[1] (**Fig. 1**). Diagnosis and management of phimosis and balanoposthitis recently have been reported.[2] Initially, the animal presented with lethargy and inappetence. Purulent discharge and phimosis were present on physical examination. Repeated mechanical breakdown of the adhesions between the prepuce and the glans penis was required to resolve the phimosis. Regular recheck examinations were performed to avoid recurrence of phimosis and balanoposthitis in this animal.[2]

[a] Department of Surgical Sciences, School of Veterinary Medicine, University of Wisconsin-Madison, 2015 Linden Drive, Madison, WI 53706, USA; [b] Exotic Pet Medicine Service, Alfort University Veterinary Teaching Hospital, Ecole Nationale Vétérinaire d'Alfort, 7 Avenue du Géneral de Gaulle, Maisons-Alfort Cedex 94704, France
* Corresponding author.
E-mail address: Christoph.mans@wisc.edu

Vet Clin Exot Anim 23 (2020) 321–335
https://doi.org/10.1016/j.cvex.2020.01.005
1094-9194/20/© 2020 Elsevier Inc. All rights reserved.
vetexotic.theclinics.com

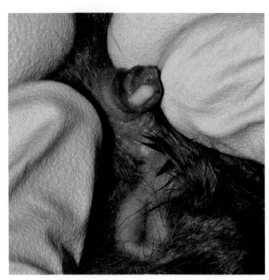

Fig. 1. Phimosis and balanoposthitis.

Urinary Tract Disorders

Urinalysis

Urine appearance can vary greatly in color and turbidity (**Fig. 2**). Urinalysis reference values recently have been reported.[3] Urine specific gravity in most chinchillas was greater than or equal to 1.050, although the range was 1.014 to greater than 1.060. Amorphous crystals were found by urinary sediment evaluation in 68% of samples (**Fig. 3**), whereas calcium carbonate crystals were not found in chinchilla urine because chinchillas do not excrete significant amount of calcium through the kidneys. Dipstick analysis revealed the presence of protein in the urine of healthy chinchillas. Dipstick urinary protein quantification did not correlate with gold standard quantitative protein analysis (biochemistry analyzer) and overestimated urinary protein. Urinary pH measured with urine dipstick was 8.5 in all chinchillas, but the upper limit of detection was 8.5. Ketonuria and decrease in urine pH are common findings in anorexic chinchillas (**Fig. 4**).[4,5] Therefore, urine dipstick monitoring of ketones and pH should be performed in any systemically diseased and anorexic chinchilla, because it represents a noninvasive and inexpensive way to diagnose and monitor chinchillas with catabolic metabolism.

Diagnostic imaging of the urinary tract

Ultrasonographic features of the chinchilla kidney have been described in a limited number of animals (n = 9). Compared with dogs and cats, chinchillas have a single papilla and wider renal pelvis. Chinchillas also appear to have a longer medullary area. The median (2.5%–97.5%) kidney length was 2 cm (1.8–2.2 cm) and kidney width was 1 cm (0.8–1.2 cm).[6] No difference in size between the left and right kidney was found and the right kidney was located more cranially.[6]

Urolithiasis

Urolithiasis is significantly more prevalent in male chinchillas compared with female chinchillas. In a retrospective study, 15 chinchillas diagnosed with urolithiasis were included and all were male with a median age of 30 months (range 11–132 months).[7] The most common presenting complaints included hematuria, pollakiuria, and stranguria, and a

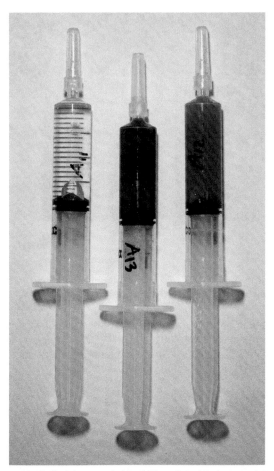

Fig. 2. Variations in gross appearance of chinchilla urine. (*Courtesy of* Grayson Doss, DVM, Dipl. ACZM, Madison, WI.)

majority of cases were painful on abdominal palpation or had palpable stones. If urolithiasis is suspected, radiographs are recommended, taking care to ensure the full length of the urethra is included in males (**Fig. 5**). A majority of stones reported in chinchillas were calcium carbonate.[7,8] Increased calcium in the diet has been anecdotally associated with increased urolithiasis in rabbits.[9] The risk factors of urolithiasis in chinchillas are unknown, however, it is unlikely that dietary calcium intake plays a role, because excess calcium is excreted in the feces and not the urine of chinchillas.[10] In addition to calcium carbonate uroliths, semen-matrix calculi also recently have been reported in a chinchilla.[11]

Uroliths located in the urinary bladder had a better prognosis compared with urethral stones, although both can occur alone or in conjunction. Urethral calculi require urinary catheterization and retropulsion of stones into the bladder, which can be challenging because many of these calculi are embedded in the mucosa and cannot be dislodged. Therefore, a majority (75%) of chinchillas diagnosed with urethral calculi were euthanized within 24 hours of diagnosis.[7] Cystotomy is recommended to treat cystic calculi; however, the owners should be informed of the high rate of recurrence. Recurrence rate in animals after surgical removal of the calculi was 50%. The median

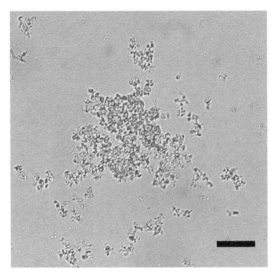

Fig. 3. Urine sediment: amorphous crystals are a common finding in healthy chinchillas. Bar, 50 μm. (*Courtesy of* Grayson Doss, DVM, Dipl. ACZM, Madison, WI.)

time to recurrence was 68 days (range 19–1440 days). Median survival time in chinchillas with calculi recurrence was 391 days (74–1074 days) and in animals without recurrence was 6 years (5–7 years). Close monitoring for recurrence and potential urinary obstruction should be performed postoperatively.[7]

Middle Ear Disease

Otitis media in chinchillas is not as prevalent as in guinea pigs but is increasingly reported in the literature.[12–15] Diagnosis is made by otoscopic examination and diagnostic imaging of the skull (**Figs. 6** and **7**). In addition to primary bacterial infections, frequently associated with *Pseudomonas aeruginosa*, neoplasms and polyps of the external ear also have been reported in chinchillas, resulting in secondary otitis media and otitis interna. An 8-year-old chinchilla presented with purulent, hemorrhagic discharge from

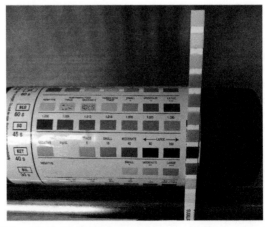

Fig. 4. Urine dipstick analysis. Note the large amounts of ketones present in the urine.

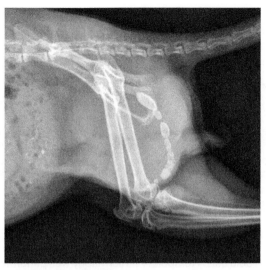

Fig. 5. Urethral calculi in a male chinchilla.

the left ear canal and vestibular disease. Based on computed tomography and biopsy, a leiomyosarcoma obstructing the ear canal causing secondary otitis media was diagnosed.[12] Inflammatory polyps of the ear canal have been reported in chinchillas. A 5-month-old female chinchilla with respiratory distress, head tilt, and suppurative otitis was diagnosed via magnetic resonance imaging with bilateral otitis media, exostosis of the left middle ear, and a polypoid mass. Video otoscopy was performed to flush the middle ear and remove the mass. Histology indicated an inflammatory polyp.[13] Inflammatory polyps are reported as a cause of otitis media in cats and dogs, but naturally occurring polyps have not been reported in rodents or rabbits. Another 5-month-old chinchilla that was presented for chronic nasal discharge and poor body condition was diagnosed with a cleft palate and bilateral otitis media by CT and necropsy. *Proteus mirabilis* and α-hemolytic *Streptococcus* species were cultured from the middle ears.[15]

Surgical management of chronic otitis media in a 6-year-old chinchilla has been reported. A modified total ear canal ablation and temporary fenestration of the caudodorsal and rostroventral chambers of the tympanic bulla were performed. The

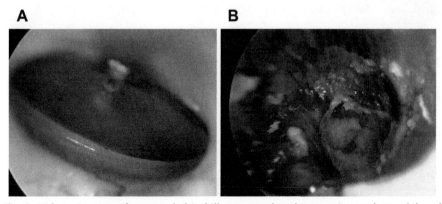

Fig. 6. Video otoscopy of a normal chinchilla ear canal and tympanic membrane (*A*) and from an animal with severe otitis media and perforated tympanic membrane (*B*).

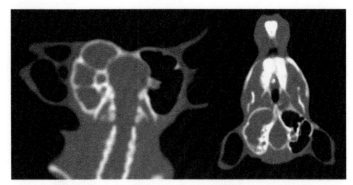

Fig. 7. Cross-sectional and coronal computed tomography sections of a chinchilla with severe right-sided otitis media.

temporary fenestration windows remained open for 5 weeks, allowing routine flushing and medicating with topical antibiotics. Multidrug-resistant *Pseudomonas* was cultured from the middle ear. A temporary tarsorrhaphy was performed due temporary facial nerve paralysis after surgery. Recheck computed tomography scan 2 months after surgery showed persistence of the otitis media.[14] Although the surgery successfully resolved the otitis externa, it was not possible to resolve the chronic otitis media. This is not surprising given the large size and multicambered anatomy of the tympanic bulla in chinchillas, in addition to the infection with multiresistant and biofilm-forming *Pseudomonas* species.

Ocular Disorders

Conjunctivitis and other ophthalmic disorders are commonly reported in pet chinchillas (**Fig. 8**). In a retrospective study, abnormalities of the lens were the most common finding followed by corneal abnormalities and conjunctivitis.[16] The prevalence of ophthalmic disorders in the population reported was 30/385, or 7.8%. Normal conjunctival bacterial isolates in healthy chinchillas are reported to be predominantly

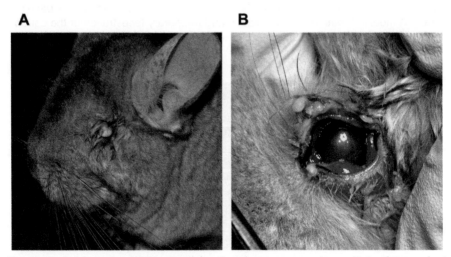

Fig. 8. Bacterial conjunctivitis caused by *Pseudomonas aeruginosa*. Note the purulent discharge (*A*) and severe chemosis (*B*).

gram-positive species (94%).[17] The most commonly isolated samples reported were *Streptococcus* species (27.5%), *Staphylococcus aureus* (23.5%), and coagulase-negative *Staphylococcus* (19.6%).[17]

In contrast, a majority of conjunctival bacterial isolates in 49 chinchillas diagnosed with conjunctivitis were gram-negative (62%) and the most common isolate was *P aeruginosa*, which was reported in 50% the cases, followed by *Staphylococcus* species (27%).[18] Chinchillas with an acute onset (1–3 days) of conjunctivitis were more likely to have gram-negative pathogens isolated and *P aeruginosa was isolated from all* animals with concurrent upper respiratory signs. Other parameters, however, such as reduced appetite or activity, severity of conjunctivitis, unilateral versus bilateral conjunctivitis, and presence of purulent discharge, were not significantly different between animals with gram-positive versus gram-negative isolates. Due to the high prevalence of *P aeruginosa,* aerobic bacterial culture and susceptibility testing should always be performed in chinchillas diagnosed with conjunctivitis. Empirical therapy with topical gentamicin or polymyxin B is recommended while awaiting culture results. A retrospective study showed that 89% of all bacterial isolates were susceptible to gentamicin, whereas susceptibility rates for ciprofloxacin and neomycin were 72% and 70%, respectively.[18] All *P aeruginosa* isolates were susceptible to polymyxin B[18]; therefore, commonly available ophthalmic antibiotic formulation containing polymyxin B and another antibiotics (eg, neomycin and bacitracin) should provide excellent empirical coverage. Systemic antimicrobial therapy should be considered, especially if other clinical signs (eg, respiratory signs) frequently associated with *Pseudomonas* species infections are present.

Cardiac Disease

Vertebral heart size (VHS) reference intervals have recently been reported in chinchillas and can be calculated based on radiographs (reference interval, 7.5–10.4) or computed tomography (reference interval, 7.1–9.4).[19] No difference between left and right thoracic radiographs or between male chinchillas and female chinchillas has been reported. The vertebral heart size for chinchillas is larger than reported values for other rodent species.

Echocardiographic measurements for healthy chinchillas under manual restraint, isoflurane anesthesia, and dexmedetomidine-ketamine anesthesia all have been reported.[20,21] Compared with animals examined under manual restraint alone, dexmedetomidine-ketamine anesthesia resulted in similar echocardiographic changes as reported with isoflurane anesthesia, including decreased fractional shortening and cardiac output.[20,21]

Although the prevalence of heart murmurs is high (23%) in chinchillas, reports on clinical management of cardiac disease in chinchillas are rare. Although many chinchillas have innocent (benign) murmurs, those with a murmur of grade 3 or higher were 29 times more likely to have echocardiographic abnormalities.[22] The clinical management of cardiac disease in chinchillas has not been reported in the literature. Therapy should be based on treatment recommendations in other similar species.

Diaphragmatic and Perineal Hernia

Two recent reports described hernias in chinchillas.[23,24] A 10-year-old neutered male chinchilla was presented with a 2-day history of anorexia, lethargy, and respiratory signs. Radiographs revealed pleural effusion and a soft tissue mass in the caudal thorax. Thoracic ultrasound was not able to identify the diaphragmatic hernia clearly. Necropsy revealed a true diaphragmatic hernia, with parts of the stomach and omentum having passed through an approximately 0.8 cm in diameter defect in the tendinous portion of the diaphragm.[23]

Perineal hernias have been reported in 2 adult intact male chinchillas that presented for a swelling in the perineal area.[24] Ultrasonography confirmed the tentative diagnosis of a perineal hernia in both cases. The hernia sac contained the urinary bladder in one case and fat in the other case. Unilateral perineal herniorrhaphies, including an internal obturator muscle flap transposition technique, were performed and both chinchillas recovered uneventfully.[24]

Fur Chewing

Fur chewing is an abnormal, repetitive, excessive grooming behavior reported in captive chinchillas.[4,25,26] The underlying etiology remains elusive; however, evidence supports stress as a cause of this compulsive behavior. The most severely affected fur-chewing female chinchillas demonstrated an elevated mean concentration of cortisol metabolites in the urine.[27] Typically, affected animals have normal fur on the head and distal extremities and shortened fur on the dorsum, from the lumbar area to the tail and laterally on the flanks (**Fig. 9**). Diagnostic testing should be performed to rule out underlying disease, including painful conditions, such as dental disease or otitis media. Husbandry changes to reduce stress, including dietary, and housing changes, should be considered.[4] Possible changes include reducing handling, light, and noise disturbances; separating animals; offering multiple sleeping and feeding areas; and offering enrichment items to redirect behavior. Fluoxetine has been suggested as a potential treatment.[4,25] In a recent study, however, fluoxetine 10 mg/kg orally every 24 hours) demonstrated limited success in reducing fur-chewing behavior.[25] Fur-chewing behavior in breeding female chinchillas were not associated with a decrease in reproductive performance, but there was a lower pup survival in 1 report.[28]

Neoplasia

Although neoplasia generally is considered uncommon in chinchillas, compared with guinea pigs and other rodents, it is increasingly reported in the literature. Since 2012, 11 new cases of neoplasia in chinchillas have been published, which include single

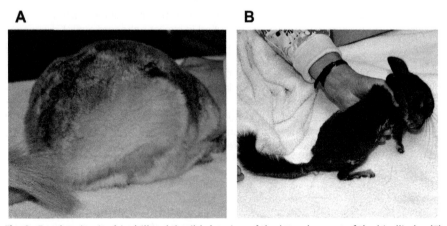

Fig. 9. Fur chewing in chinchillas. (A) mild chewing of the lateral aspect of the hindlimbs. (B) Generalized fur chewing affecting all body parts reachable by the animal. Only the head and tail are not affected.

cases of osteosarcoma,[29] mammary adenocarcinoma,[30] iridociliary adenocarcinoma,[31] uterine leiomyoma (**Fig. 10**),[32] uterine hemangioma,[32] vaginal leiomyoma,[33] aural leiomyosarcoma,[12] and gastric adenocarcinoma[34,35] and 3 cases of cutaneous squamous cell carcinoma.[36] The age and sex of 2 chinchillas were not described, but in the other 10 chinchillas (3 male and 6 female) the median an age was 12.5 years (range 5–17 years).

The 3 cases of cutaneous squamous cell carcinoma were diagnosed in animals older than 15 years and all had ulcerative skin masses ranging 2 cm to 5 cm in diameter and located on a limb. In all cases, self-mutilation of the tumor site was reported and all animals were euthanized within 2 months after initial diagnosis.[36]

INFECTIOUS DISEASES
Pseudomonas aeruginosa Infections

Pseudomonas aeruginosa is common isolated from diseased chinchillas; however, isolation of this organism from apparently healthy chinchillas also has been reported.[37–41] A recent study described the epidemiology of conjunctivitis cases in chinchillas, with the most commonly cultured species reported as *P aeruginosa* (50%).[18] Besides conjunctivitis, otitis media and upper respiratory disease are also common manifestation of pseudomonal infection in chinchillas.[14,42] Due to high rates of multidrug resistance in *Pseudomonas* species, culture and susceptibility testing are strongly recommended.[4,18] Empirical treatment is recommended while awaiting culture results, typically using fluoroquinolones, third-generation cephalosporins, or aminoglycosides.[1,4,18] Reported susceptibility rates of *P aeruginosa* isolated from chinchillas to potentiated sulfonamides, enrofloxacin, ciprofloxacin, gentamicin, amikacin, ceftazidime, and piperacillin were 8%, 36%, 63%, 89%, 100%, 100%, and 100%, respectively.[18] Due to the formation of biofilms, antimicrobial treatment alone may not be effective and surgical debridement as well as topical treatment should be considered, if feasible.

Giardia Infection

Giardia is not routinely isolated from fecal samples of wild chinchillas, but in captive chinchillas Giardia has a high prevalence in healthy and sick animals.[1] Because Giardia is highly prevalent in healthy pet chinchillas, concerns have been raised about zoonotic transmission.[43] Molecular analysis by multilocus genotyping of Giardia isolates from different host species has revealed at least 8 gene assemblages (A–H), which

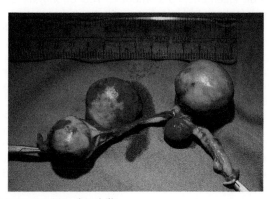

Fig. 10. Uterine leiomyoma in a chinchilla.

can aid in identifying chinchilla isolates as potentially zoonotic (assemblages A or B) or host-specific.[44]

A survey of Giardia in chinchillas from Europe found 61% of 326 chinchillas positive on coproantigen enzyme-linked immunosorbent assay (ELISA) assay.[45] ELISA-positive samples from 23 chinchillas were investigated by assemblage-specific polymerase chain reaction (PCR) and sequencing of fragments of 3 genes; 22 samples were positive for B assemblage and 1 sample was positive for D assemblage. In an earlier study in Belgium, Giardia cysts were detected in 66% of 80 pet chinchillas and in 22 isolates, molecular analysis revealed zoonotic assemblages A and B.[43] A study in China, sampling 140 pet chinchillas from 4 cities, found that 27% of the chinchillas that were positive for Giardia.[46] Molecular characterization of the 38 samples revealed assemblage A in 5 samples and assemblage B in 33 samples. Another study in Romania of farmed chinchillas tested 341 fecal samples and found 56% positive for Giardia infection.[47] Assemblages B (151/190), D (33/190), and E (6/190) were identified.

A case of direct zoonotic transmission of Giardia from a pet chinchilla to a child in the Netherlands recently was published.[48] The transmission from the chinchilla to the child was coprophagous after the 1-year-old child ingested pet chinchilla feces. Molecular analysis of fecal samples from both the child and the chinchilla classified the Giardia cysts into assemblage B. This was the first report of a true zoonotic transmission of giardiasis, supporting the zoonotic potential of assemblage B.

Mycobacterium genavense Infection

Mycobacterium genavense infection of the lungs and liver was reported in a 1-year old male neutered chinchilla that was presented for emaciation and progressive weight loss.[49] Radiographs demonstrated changes consistent with severe pneumonia and bullous emphysema in 1 lung lobe. Antibiotic treatment did not lead to improvement of clinical signs and the animal was euthanized within 6 weeks after initial presentation. Postmortem PCR and gene sequencing confirmed *M genavense*. Diagnosis with *M genavense* can be challenging.[50,51] Growth in vitro is poor and PCR testing is required for speciation.[52] Mycobacterium infections should be considered a differential diagnosis in chinchillas with progressive weight loss, poor body condition, and granulomatous inflammation.

Helminthic Infections

Captive chinchillas are reported to have a low prevalence of helminth infections. Previous reports include *Haemonchus contortus*, *Trichotrongylus colubriformis*, and *Ostertagia ostertagi* infections.[4,53] Infections with oxyurid species also have been reported. Recently, a case report identifying an oxyurid nematode infection in a chinchilla in Brazil was published.[53] An adult female chinchilla was presented with intense perianal pruritus. Clear, adhesive tape preparation of the anus recovered eggs demonstrating the characteristics of parasites in the superfamily Oxyuroidea. Further speciation was not possible. The animal was treated with fenbendazole and repeat testing was negative.

Cestode infections, including zoonotic *Rodentolepis nana*, a tapeworm parasite, previously known as *Hymenolepis nana*, also have been documented (**Fig. 11**)[4] Six of 13 pet chinchillas had ova of *R nana* on a fecal float in a survey performed in Italy.[54] Transmission is direct via the fecal-oral route and an intermediate host is not necessary. Therefore, superinfection due to coprophagy is possible and chinchillas can be infected with high numbers of this cestode. Clinical signs include anorexia, diarrhea, weight loss, and death. In mild infections, there may be no clinical

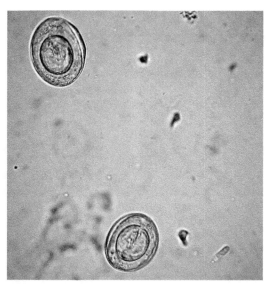

Fig. 11. *Rodentolepis nana* eggs from a fecal flotation. (*Courtesy of* Cathy Johnson-Delaney, DVM, Kirkland, WA.)

signs. Fecal flotation is recommended for diagnosis. Treatment with praziquantel at 5 mg/kg to 10 mg/kg orally or subcutaneously is recommended.[55]

Infections with *Taenia serialis*, *T pisiformis*, *T multiceps*, *Echinococcus granulosus*, and *E multilocularis* species also have been documented in chinchillas.[4] These cestode parasites use carnivores as definitive hosts, whereas rodents serve as intermediate hosts.[56] A case of disseminated *T crassiceps* was reported in an adult male chinchilla in a shelter in Switzerland. Initially, the animal demonstrated areas of subcutaneous fluctuant edema over the face and thoracic regions. This progressed and one mass was surgically excised. A diagnosis of *T crassiceps* infection was confirmed with PCR. Praziquantel was administered to the animal at 10 mg/kg, subcutaneously, every 10 days, for 3 doses, but it was not deemed an effective treatment because the subcutaneous swelling reoccurred after surgery. The chinchilla was euthanized 1.5 months after diagnosis due decline in condition. At necropsy, thousands of cysticerci were found in the subcutaneous tissues, thorax, larynx, pharynx, and retropharyngeal area. *T taeniaeformis* metacestodes also were found in the liver. The source of the infection was suspected to be foliage offered to the chinchilla for consumption collected from outside the shelter. The area where the material was collected was noted to have exposure to foxes and martens, which are definitive hosts for both *Taenia* species.

Streptococcus equi Subspecies *zooepidemicus* in Chinchillas

S equi subspecies *zooepidemicus* (*S zooepidemicus*) initially was diagnosed in farmed chinchillas around 2013 in Minnesota and California. Later reports included animals from Michigan, Nebraska and Colorado, and North Dakota. These reports usually described chinchilla with conjunctivitis and subcutaneous abscesses (**Fig. 12**); however, pyometra also has been anecdotally reported.[57] A conference paper in 2018 reported 2 6-month old female chinchillas in a Colorado laboratory animal facility with subcutaneous abscesses.[58] Both animals were euthanized and displayed evidence of sepsis on necropsy. Another 2 chinchillas from a shipment of 13 chinchillas were

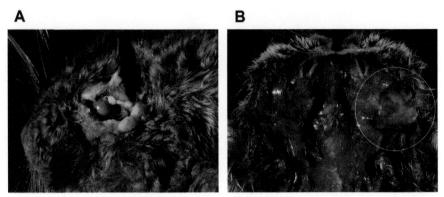

Fig. 12. *S equi* subsp *zooepidemicus* in chinchillas. (*A*) Conjunctivitis. (*B*) Subcutaneous cervical abscess. (*Courtesy of* Arno Wuenschmann, Dr. med. vet, DACVP, St. Paul, MN.)

positive for *S zooepidemicus* by oral swab. A 2019 case report described a 4-month-old, male pet chinchilla with a rapidly growing midcervical subcutaneous mass.[59] It was diagnosed as an *S zooepidemicus* abscess based on cytology and aerobic bacterial culture. The infection resolved after oral administration of trimethoprim-sulfamethoxazole.

S zooepidemicus is a mucosal commensal bacteria, especially in the horse, but it is unrestrained in its selection of hosts, causing opportunistic respiratory, wound, and genital infections in most species. It traditionally has been reported in guinea pigs as the cause of cervical lymphadenitis.[60] *S equi* remains viable in water for 4 weeks to 6 weeks but only for 1 to 3 days in feces or soil.[61] The prevalence of *S zooepidemicus* in chinchillas currently is unknown and, although it is an emerging pathogen in chinchillas, it does not appear to be a significant concern in pet chinchillas at this time.

Streptococcus *zooepidemicus* abscesses should drained and aerobic bacterial culture and susceptibility testing performed. While awaiting susceptibility testing, empirical antibiotic treatment with parenteral penicillin (the drug of choice in horses), parenteral ceftiofur or oral trimethoprim-sulfa should be considered. In farmed chinchillas, sulfadimethoxine administered in the drinking water has been used to treat outbreaks. Second-generation quinolones, such as enrofloxacin, are not ideal for treating infections caused by Streptococcus; therefore, other antibiotics should be considered first.[61] It currently is unknown if chinchillas treated with antimicrobials continue to carry the bacteria and remain a source of infection for other chinchillas. In horses, expression of clinical signs and degree of shedding depends on preexisting immunity to *S zooepidemicus*.[61]

DISCLOSURES

The authors have nothing to disclose.

REFERENCES

1. Mans C, Donnelly TM. Update on diseases of chinchillas. Vet Clin North Am Exot Anim Pract 2013;16(2):383–406.
2. Martel-Arquette A, Mans C. Management of Phimosis and Balanoposthitis in a pet chinchilla (Chinchilla lanigera). J Exot Pet Med 2016;25(1):60–4.
3. Doss GA, Mans C, Houseright RA, et al. Urinalysis in chinchillas (Chinchilla lanigera). J Am Vet Med Assoc 2016;248(8):901–7.

4. Mans C, Donnelly TM. Disease problems of chinchillas. In: Quesenberry KE, Carpenter JW, editors. Ferrets, rabbits, and rodents: clinical medicine and surgery. 3rd edition. St Louis (MO): W.B. Saunders; 2012. p. 311–25.

5. Mills R, Gilsdorf J. Middle-ear effusions following acute otitis media in the chinchilla animal model. J Laryngol Otol 1986;100(3):255–61.

6. Ferrari M, Carlos da Silva WA, Monteiro RV. Ultrasonographic features of the chinchilla (Chinchilla lanigera) kidney. J Exot Pet Med 2013;22(4):393–5.

7. Martel-Arquette A, Mans C. Urolithiasis in chinchillas: 15 cases (2007 to 2011). J Small Anim Pract 2016;57(5):260–4.

8. Osborne CA, Albasan H, Lulich JP, et al. Quantitative analysis of 4468 uroliths retrieved from farm animals, exotic species, and wildlife submitted to the Minnesota Urolith Center: 1981 to 2007. Vet Clin North Am Small Anim Pract 2009;39(1): 65–78.

9. Klaphake E, Paul-Murphy J. Disorders of the reproductive and urinary systems. In: Quesenberry KE, Carpenter JW, editors. Ferrets, rabbits, and rodents: clinical medicine and surgery. 3rd edition. St Louis (MO): W.B. Saunders; 2012. p. 217–31.

10. Hansen S, Wolf P, Kamphues J. Investigations on calcium metabolism, growth, attrition, and composition of the incisors with varying dietary calcium content and gnawing material in chinchillas (C. lanigera) (Thesis). Hannover (Germany): Institut fuer Tierernaehrung, Tieraerztliche Hochschule Hannover; 2012.

11. Higbie CT, DiGeronimo PM, Bennett RA, et al. Semen-matrix calculi in a juvenile chinchilla (Chinchilla lanigera). J Exot Pet Med 2019;28:69–75.

12. Bertram CA, Klopfleisch R, Erickson NA, et al. Leiomyosarcoma of the external ear canal as a cause of otitis externa, media, interna in a chinchilla (Chinchilla lanigera). J Exot Pet Med 2019;28:13–6.

13. Boncea AM, Măcinic M, Ifteme CV, et al. Inflammatory polyp in the middle ear of a chinchilla: a case report. J Exot Pet Med 2019;31:79–81.

14. Rockwell K, Wells A, Dearmin M. Total ear canal ablation and temporary bulla fenestration for treatment of otitis media in a chinchilla (Chinchilla laniger). J Exot Pet Med 2019;29:173–7.

15. Ozawa S, Mans C, Miller JL, et al. Cleft palate in a Chinchilla (Chinchilla lanigera). J Exot Pet Med 2019;28:93–7.

16. Müller K, Eule JC. Ophthalmic disorders observed in pet chinchillas (Chinchilla lanigera). J Exot Pet Med 2014;23(2):201–5.

17. Lima L, Montiani-Ferreira F, Tramontin M, et al. The chinchilla eye: morphologic observations, echobiometric findings and reference values for selected ophthalmic diagnostic tests. Vet Ophthalmol 2010;13(S):14–25.

18. Ozawa S, Mans C, Szabo Z, et al. Epidemiology of bacterial conjunctivitis in chinchillas (Chinchilla lanigera): 49 cases (2005 to 2015). J Small Anim Pract 2017; 58(4):238–45.

19. Doss GA, Mans C, Hoey S, et al. Vertebral heart size in chinchillas (Chinchilla lanigera) using radiography and CT. J Small Anim Pract 2017;58(12):714–9.

20. Linde A, Summerfield N, Johnston M, et al. Echocardiography in the chinchilla. J Vet Intern Med 2004;18(5):772–4.

21. Doss G, Mans C, Stepien R. Echocardiographic effects of dexmedeomidine-ketamine in chinchillas (Chinchilla lanigera). Lab Anim 2017;51(1):89–92.

22. Pignon C, Guzman DSM, Sinclair K, et al. Evaluation of heart murmurs in chinchillas (chinchilla lanigera): 59 cases (1996-2009). J Am Vet Med Assoc 2012; 241(10):1344–7.

23. Aymen J, Langlois I, Lanthier I. Diaphragmatic hernia in a pet chinchilla (Chinchilla lanigera). Can Vet J 2017;58(6):597–600.

24. Thöle M, Schuhmann B, Köstlinger S, et al. Treatment of unilateral perineal hernias in 2 male chinchillas (Chinchilla Lanigera). J Exot Pet Med 2018;27:43–9.

25. Galeano MG, Ruiz RD, de Cuneo MF, et al. Effectiveness of fluoxetine to control fur-chewing behaviour in the chinchilla (Chinchilla lanigera). Appl Anim Behav Sci 2013;146:112–7.

26. Franchi V, Aleuy OA, Tadich TA. Fur chewing and other abnormal repetitive behaviors in chinchillas (Chinchilla lanigera), under commercial fur-farming conditions. J Vet Behav Clin Appl Res 2016;11:60–4.

27. Ponzio MF, Monfort SL, Busso JM, et al. Adrenal activity and anxiety-like behavior in fur-chewing chinchillas (Chinchilla lanigera). Horm Behav 2012;61(5):758–62.

28. Galeano MG, Cantarelli VI, Ruiz RD, et al. Reproductive performance and weaning success in fur-chewing chinchillas (Chinchilla lanigera). Reprod Biol 2014; 14(3):213–7.

29. Hocker SE, Eshar D, Wouda RM. Rodent oncology: diseases, diagnostics, and therapeutics. Vet Clin North Am Exot Anim Pract 2017;20(1):111–34.

30. Konell AL, Gonçalves KA, de Sousa RS, et al. Mammary adenocarcinoma with pulmonary, hepatic and renal metastasis in a chinchilla (Chinchilla laniger). Acta Sci Vet 2018;46(S):310.

31. Ueda K, Ueda A, Ozaki K. Pleomorphic iridociliary adenocarcinoma with metastasis to the cervical lymph node in a chinchilla (Chinchilla lanigera). J Vet Med Sci 2018;81(2):193–6.

32. Bertram CA, Kershaw O, Klopfleisch R, et al. Uterine leiomyoma, fibroma, and hemangioma in 2 chinchillas *(Chinchilla laniger)*. J Exot Pet Med 2019; 28:23–9.

33. Bertram CA, Klopfleisch R, Müller K. Vaginal leiomyoma in a chinchilla (Chinchilla Laniger). J Small Anim Pract 2018;59(9):583.

34. Lucena RB, Rissi DR, Queiroz DMM, et al. Infiltrative gastric adenocarcinoma in a chinchilla (Chinchilla lanigera). J Vet Diagn Invest 2012;24(4):797–800.

35. Lucena RB, Giaretta PR, Tessele B, et al. Doenças de chinchilas [Diseases of chinchilla] (Chinchilla lanigera). Pesqui Vet Bras 2012;32(6):529–35.

36. Szabo Z, Reavill DR, Kiupel M. Squamous cell carcinoma in chinchillas: a review of three cases. J Exot Pet Med 2019;28:115–20.

37. Soldati G. Outbreak of Pseudomonas aeruginosa infection in chinchillas. Nuova Vet 1972;48:240–2.

38. Menchaca E, Moras E, Martin A, et al. Infectious diseases of the chinchilla IV. Gaceta veterinaria 1980;42:96–102.

39. Brem M. Investigations about the disease of the gastrointestinal tract in the chinchilla (Dr. med. vet. thesis). Munich (Germany): Medizinische Tierklinik, Ludwig Maximilians Universitaet; 1982.

40. Mathieu X, Duran J, Rivas M. Normal bacterial flora of the wild Chinchilla lanigera silvestre. Rev Latinoam Microbiol 1982;24(2):77–82.

41. Hirakawa Y, Sasaki H, Kawamoto E. Prevalence and analysis of Pseudomonas aeruginosa in chinchillas. BMC Vet Res 2010;6:52.

42. Wideman WL. Pseudomonas aeruginosa otitis media and interna in a chinchilla ranch. Can Vet J 2006;47(8):799–800.

43. Levecke B, Meulemans L, Dalemans T, et al. Mixed Giardia duodenalis assemblage A, B, C and E infections in pet chinchillas (Chinchilla lanigera) in Flanders (Belgium). Vet Parasitol 2011;177(1–2):166–70.

44. Ryan U, Zahedi A. Molecular epidemiology of giardiasis from a veterinary perspective. Adv Parasitol 2019;106:209–54.
45. Pantchev N, Broglia A, Paoletti B, et al. Occurrence and molecular typing of Giardia isolates in pet rabbits, chinchillas, guinea pigs and ferrets collected in Europe during 2006-2012. Vet Rec 2014;175(1):18.
46. Qi M, Yu F, Li S, et al. Multilocus genotyping of potentially zoonotic Giardia duodenalis in pet chinchillas (Chinchilla lanigera) in China. Vet Parasitol 2015; 208(304):113–7.
47. Gherman CM, Kalmár Z, Györke A, et al. Occurrence of Giardia duodenalis assemblages in farmed long-tailed chinchillas Chinchilla lanigera (Rodentia) from Romania. Parasit Vectors 2018;11(1):86.
48. Tůmová P, Mazánek L, Lecová L, et al. A natural zoonotic giardiasis: infection of a child via Giardia cysts in pet chinchilla droppings. Parasitol Int 2018;11:86.
49. Huynh M, Pingret JL, Nicolier A. Disseminated Mycobacterium genavense infection in a chinchilla (Chinchilla lanigera). J Comp Pathol 2014;151(1):122–5.
50. Ludwig E, Reischl U, Janik D, et al. Granulomatous pneumonia caused by mycobacterium genavense in a dwarf rabbit (Oryctolagus cuniculus). Vet Pathol 2009; 46(5):1000–2.
51. Dequéant B, Pascal Q, Bilbault H, et al. Identification of Mycobacterium genavense natural infection in a domestic ferret. J Vet Diagn Invest 2019;31(1):133–6.
52. Thomsen VO, Dragsted UB, Bauer J, et al. Disseminated infection with Mycobacterium genavense: a challenge to physicians and mycobacteriologists. J Clin Microbiol 1999;37(12):3901–5.
53. Cardia DFF, Camossi LG, Lux Hoppe EG, et al. An Oxyurid nematode identified in a pet chinchilla (Chinchilla lanigera). J Exot Pet Med 2016;25:311–3.
54. d'Ovidio D, Noviello E, Pepe P, et al. Survey of Hymenolepis spp. in pet rodents in Italy. Parasitol Res 2015;114(12):4381–4.
55. Mayer J, Mans C. Rodents. In: Carpenter JW, Marion CJ, editors. Exotic animal formulary. 4th edition. St Louis (MO): W.B. Saunders; 2018. p. 459–93.
56. Basso W, Rütten M, Deplazes P, et al. Generalized Taenia crassiceps cysticercosis in a chinchilla (Chinchilla lanigera). Vet Parasitol 2014;199(1–2):116–20.
57. Veterinary Information Network, Message Boards: Mammals Small and Exotic Folder. Three reports of chinchillas with Streptococcus equi subsp zooepidemicus infections (2015-2018). 2019. Available at: www.vin.com. Accessed September 1, 2019.
58. Mitchell C, Johnson L, Tousey S, et al. Diagnosis and surveillance of Streptococcus equi subspecies zooepidemicus infections in chinchillas (Chinchilla lanigera). J Am Assoc Lab Anim Sci 2018;57:551.
59. Berg CC, Doss GA, Mans C. Streptococcus equi subspecies zooepidemicus infection in a pet chinchilla (Chinchilla lanigera). J Exot Pet Med 2019;31:36–8.
60. Murphy JC, Ackerman JI, Marini RP, et al. Cervical lymphadenitis in guinea pigs: infection via intact ocular and nasal mucosa by Streptococcus zooepidemicus. Lab Anim Sci 1991;41(3):251–4.
61. Boyle AG, Timoney JF, Newton JR, et al. Streptococcus equi infections in horses: guidelines for treatment, control, and prevention of strangles—revised consensus statement. J Vet Intern Med 2018;32(2):633–47.

Update on Avian Bornavirus and Proventricular Dilatation Disease

Diagnostics, Pathology, Prevalence, and Control

Sharman M. Hoppes, DVM, DABVP-avian[a],*,
H.L. Shivaprasad, BVSc, MS, PhD, DACPVc, DACVP[b]

KEYWORDS

- Avian ganglioneuritis • Avian bornavirus • Proventricular dilatation disease
- Bornaviridae

KEY POINTS

- Avian bornavirus (ABV) is a causative agent of proventricular dilatation disease in birds.
- Birds intermittently shed the virus in their droppings, and seroconversion is unpredictable. This makes diagnosis challenging, requiring multiple negative polymerase chain reaction (PCR) and serology tests before determining that a bird is negative.
- Different genotypes of ABV may be more or less virulent depending on species of bird infected. Having exposure to one strain may not provide immunity to another strain.
- There is a large percentage of exposed birds that are serologically and/or ABV PCR positive yet clinically normal. It is unknown if these birds will ever develop disease.
- A clinically normal ABV-positive bird should not be euthanized.

INTRODUCTION

Avian bornavirus (ABV) is the only known etiological agent of proventricular dilatation disease (PDD). This infectious disease has been reported in more than 80 species of psittacine and nonpsittacine birds worldwide, both captive and in the wild.[1–12] PDD was first recognized in the early 1970s in macaws exported to Europe and North America from Bolivia[1] and has since then spread to Australia, Central and South America, Japan, the Middle East, and Africa. PDD is a progressive neurologic disease that is ultimately fatal once clinical signs develop. The predominant clinical feature of the disease in parrots is dilation of the proventriculus by accumulated food secondary to intestinal motility dysfunction (**Fig. 1**). The disease is also associated with significant

a Texas Avian and Exotic Hospital, 2700 West State Highway 114 Suite A, Building 2, Grapevine, TX 76051, USA; b University of California Animal Health and Food Safety Laboratory System-Tulare, University of California, Davis, 18760 Road 112, Tulare, CA 93274, USA
* Corresponding author.
E-mail address: shoppes@texasavian.com

Vet Clin Exot Anim 23 (2020) 337–351
https://doi.org/10.1016/j.cvex.2020.01.006
1094-9194/20/© 2020 Elsevier Inc. All rights reserved.

central nervous system damage.[1] PDD is really a misnomer, as many systems in the body can be affected by ABV and some cases lack proventricular dilation. Because of the wide array of clinical signs and the pathology present, this disease may be more appropriately termed "avian ganglioneuritis," as this better defines the disease process and takes the focus off the proventriculus.[12] It has also been suggested that PDD be renamed ABV disease or ABV syndrome, although no consensus on renaming the disease process has been obtained.[12]

CLINICAL SIGNS

Clinical signs include ataxia, difficulty perching, seizures, blindness, weight loss, crop stasis, regurgitation, proventricular and intestinal dilatation, maldigestion, and death. Affected birds may show neurologic and/or gastrointestinal signs. Feather damaging behavior (FDB) has been associated with PDD, but scientific evidence for causality has been lacking. A recent article by Fluck and colleagues[13] evaluated and compared viral RNA shedding and ABV antibody titers in clinically normal birds, birds with neurologic signs, and birds with FDB. Birds with neurologic signs had the highest titers and highest viral shedding, followed by birds with FDB having significantly lower values and clinically normal birds having the lowest values. There was no significant difference between antibody titers in the birds with feather destructive behavior and the clinically normal birds. This study provided no evidence to support PDD causing feather-damaging behavior, but further studies are necessary to rule out any link between PDD and FDB.[13] ABV has been detected in the skin (**Fig. 2**).

CAUSE

Recently ABVs have been reclassified. Currently there are 15 genetically diverse ABV genotypes comprising 6 distinct viral species identified. The 2 species known to cause PDD in parrots are psittaciform bornaviruses (PaBV) 1 and 2 and include PaBV genotypes 1 to 8. PaBV-2 and PaBV-4 are the most commonly reported genotypes in parrots.[14] Other known ABVs includes passeriform bornavirus-1 (canary bornavirus [CnBV] 1, 2, and 3) and (Munia finch bornavirus 1), passeriform bornavirus-2 (Estrildid finch bornavirus 1), and waterbird bornavirus 1 (aquatic bird bornavirus 1 [ABBV-1]).[14]

Readers are encouraged to refer to the 2013 Veterinary Clinics of North America chapter Avian Bornavirus and Proventricular Dilatation Disease: Diagnostics,

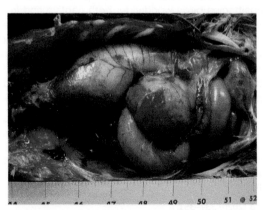

Fig. 1. Dilated proventriculus in an African Gray parrot (Psittacus erithacus) with PDD. (*Courtesy of* Gerry Dorrestein, DVM, PhD, Vessem, The Netherlands.)

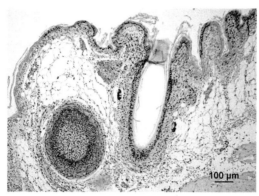

Fig. 2. IHC demonstrating ABV antigen mostly in the nucleus of cells in the epidermis, dermis, and feather follicles including the pulp of a cockatiel. IHC, immunohistochemistry.

Pathology, Prevalence, and Control for further information on cause and detailed descriptions of experiments that support the proposition that ABV is the sole cause of PDD in psittacines.

INCIDENCE

PaBV is widely distributed in captive and wild bird populations. The infection is common and widespread among captive psittacines in North America and Europe. Many healthy or subclinical carriers of several species have been documented. As many as 15% to 40% of normal healthy birds are positive for PaBV.[15] This investigator has detected PaBV RNA in 11 of 32 healthy appearing aviary birds (34%) (Sharman Hoppes, unpublished data, 2013). Nineteen of 59 healthy birds (32.2%) from an aviary with a history of PDD were found to be positive for ABV RNA in cloacal swabs.[16] A survey of laboratory samples submitted for other testing revealed PaBV in 271 of 791 samples (34%).[17] Herzog and colleagues[18] found 35 of 77 healthy birds from an aviary with a history of PDD positive for ABV antibodies. Payne and colleagues[6] have found a high infection rate in water fowl, and a large number of infected canaries have been reported in Germany.[19] A study involving 1442 live birds and 73 dead birds out of 215 aviaries in Spain, Germany, Italy, the United Kingdom, and Denmark revealed 22.8% of birds tested were positive for ABV infection. This study demonstrated that 100% of all dead birds with histopathological lesions confirmed PDD were positive for ABV. Only 19% of the dead birds dying from other causes were ABV positive. In addition, 67% of live birds with clinical signs of PDD were positive for ABV, and 19% of healthy birds were positive for ABV.[20] This study supports the high prevalence of ABV-infected parrots in captivity and that clinically healthy ABV-positive birds are common. It is likely most large collections of psittacine birds will have some individuals infected with PaBV.[21] The incidence of infected birds is much higher than the incidence of birds clinically ill. In fact, most PaBV-positive birds do not seem to exhibit clinical signs of disease. Until recently, it has been assumed that ABV was only in captive birds, but in 2014, Encinas-Nagel and colleagues[22] detected ABV-4 in free-ranging birds in Brazil. Few other tests have been performed in wild parrots, but ABV polymerase chain reaction (PCR) testing performed in wild macaws in Peru were negative (Sharman Hoppes, unpublished data from the Schubot Exotic Bird Health Center, 2013). In contrast, in free-ranging waterfowl, AVB-RNA shedding in asymptomatic birds ranged from 0% to 13%. In waterfowl cases selected based on histopathological lesions of PDD, the prevalence of ABV-RNA was 88.2%.[4–7]

TRANSMISSION

Transmission of ABV is not fully understood, but it is contagious. The spread of PaBV and PDD was documented by Kistler and colleagues,[23] who detailed the spread of disease through an aviary after introduction of an adult bird with fatal PDD. This study demonstrated that ABV infection precedes development of PDD. This outbreak suggests that the age at the time of infection affects the disease outcome. Chicks as young as 5 weeks of age on becoming anorexic developed central nervous system signs within 24 hours and died within 3 days, whereas older but unweaned chicks developed clinical disease within 2 to 4 weeks of exposure to PDD.[23]

Rubbenstroth and colleagues[24] performed a phylogenetic analysis of PaBV-2, PaBV-4, and ABBV-1 sequences obtained in a study of captive and free-ranging birds. They reported that within PaBV-2, PaBV-4, and ABBV-1, identical or genetically closely related bornavirus sequences were found in parallel in various avian species.

Because ABV is shed in droppings, the fecal-oral route of transmission is considered the most likely route of transmission.[1] Heatley and Villalobos also demonstrated that urine of ABV-positive birds was strongly positive with real-time PCR (RT-PCR).[25] PaBV RNA has been detected in the air of an infected aviary[1] and detected within lung tissue of infected birds (**Fig. 3**). Thus, it has been theorized that ABV may have a respiratory route of transmission.[1] Bornavirus has been detected in feather calami[26] and could be a source of airborne virus in feather dust.[1]

In spite of the above findings and the success of experimentally induced infections, a recent paper investigating different infection routes of PaBV in cockatiels revealed that transmission of PaBV by oral or intranasal routes was unsuccessful. Cockatiels were infected with PaBV-4 intranasally and orally. Clinical signs of disease were not observed during the 174-day observation period, and no PDD lesions were seen on necropsy. There was also no ABV-specific antigen in any of the birds.[27] A second

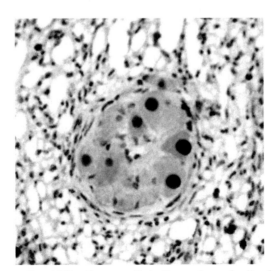

Fig. 3. IHC demonstrating ABV antigen mostly in the nucleus of cells of a ganglion in the lung of a cockatiel.

paper indicated that transmission of PaBV by direct contact is inefficient in immuno-competent, fully fledged birds.[28]

Vertical transmission of BDV has been observed in mammals but has proved difficult to confirm in birds. ABV was detected in 10 of 61 eggs from 2 confirmed PaBV-positive aviaries. The evaluated eggs were either nonviable or contained developing embryos. Two of those embryos also had PaBV RNA detected in their brain tissue.[29] Lierz and colleagues[30] also found similar evidence ofPaBV in eggs. Kerski and colleagues[31] obtained eggs, embryos, and hatchlings from 4 pairs of sun conjures (*Aratinga solstitialis*) naturally infected with PaBV-2. PaBV RNA was detected in embryos and a 2-week-old hatchling. Vertical transmission was not confirmed, however, because unless the eggs are incubator hatched and hand raised in isolation, infection may develop after hatch.

PaBV is not an environmentally stable virus. It is easily destroyed with soap or diluted bleach and is inactivated by ultraviolet light and desiccation.[32] This suggests that the virus loses its viability soon after being shed further reducing risk of transmission.

At this time, transmission of PaBV is not fully understood. In spite of the high prevalence of ABV-positive healthy birds, anecdotally, many birds that have been housed for years with ABV-positive birds remain negative.[1] Host factors such as species, age, and immunosuppression may play a factor. ABV genotype may also play a role. Some have proposed that there may be a need for presence of mucosal or skin lesions for infection to occur.[33]

INCUBATION PERIOD

The large number of asymptomatic infected birds makes determining an incubation period difficult. Asymptomatic ABV infections have been identified both in experimentally and naturally infected birds. Many healthy appearing psittacines can harbor the infection for prolonged periods.[1] The factors that trigger the development of clinical signs are unknown. Experimentally, disease varies with species, age, and immune competency.[28] The age that the bird is infected may determine incubation period. Young birds seem to have a more rapid onset and course of disease than older birds.[23] The ABV genotype may also affect the incubation period and course of disease.[34]

Clinical observation suggests the incubation period of PaBV can be as short as weeks to as long as decades.[1] In many cases, birds have developed disease years after exposure to another bird indicating the disease can lay dormant for extended periods of time.[1] Although a direct relationship between genotype and virulence has not been proved, a recent study indicates differences in pathogenicity between ABV isolates with PaBV-2–infected cockatiels showing earlier and more severe clinical signs compared with PaBV-4–infected birds.[34]

PATHOGENESIS

The Pathogenesis of ABV is a complicated and controversial topic. For a more complete review, Tizard and colleagues[35] and Rossi and colleagues[15] are recommended readings.

DIAGNOSIS

In the classical form of the disease, decreased motility or blockage of the proventriculus results in dilation of the proventriculus. Subsequently, birds begin to regurgitate ingested foods, pass undigested food, and ultimately die of starvation (**Fig. 4**). Birds

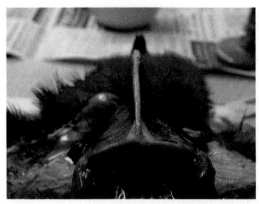

Fig. 4. Severe atrophy of pectoral muscles in a Hahns macaw (Aranobilis) due to PDD. (*Courtesy of* Dr. Gerry Dorrestein, DVM, PhD, Vessem, The Netherlands.)

may exhibit neurologic signs such as difficulty perching, an inability to fly, or blindness, in addition to or instead of gastrointestinal signs. PDD should be considered in the differential diagnosis of any bird exhibiting neurologic signs, blindness, gastrointestinal signs, or signs of cardiac disease.[36,37] Survey films, contrast radiography, and flouroscopy can be used to further support the clinician's suspicions. The proventriculus is often severely dilated, filling the left side of the coelomic cavity (**Fig. 5**). The ventriculus and intestines may also be dilated. Contrast studies often reveal prolonged transit times throughout the gastrointestinal tract. Serum chemistry and hematology are often normal although there may be an elevated creatine phosphokinase, mild anemia, heterophilia, and/or hyperproteinemia. Some birds may present with gram-negative or clostridial enteritis.

It is important to know that there are other diseases that can mimic the clinical signs of PDD. These include intestinal parasites, tumors, granulomas, papillomas, or foreign bodies of the gastrointestinal tract. In small birds *macrorhabdus ornithogaster* can

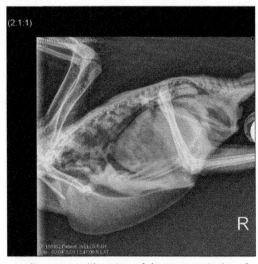

Fig. 5. Radiograph revealing severe dilatation of the proventriculus of a PaBV PDD–affected parrot.

cause similar signs. Heavy metal poisoning, especially lead, can mimic both the gastrointestinal and central nervous system signs.

Definitive diagnosis is confirmed with histopathology. Characteristic myenteric ganglioneuritis lesions may be seen in the crop, proventriculus, ventriculus, or adrenal gland. Crop biopsies are reported to be diagnostic of PDD in only about 30% to 35% of cases.[38] Failure to observe lesions in the crop does not rule out disease. Diagnosis of PDD often occurs at necropsy. Histologic examination should be performed on the crop, proventriculus, ventriculus, duodenum, adrenal gland, heart, kidney, spleen, and brain.[38–40]

Polymerase Chain Reaction

With the discovery of PaBV as the causative agent for PPD, diagnostic testing has focused on reverse transcriptase–PCR for the detection of ABV RNA in affected birds. Most agree that urine, feces, and cloacal swabs are the samples most likely to contain virus. Shedding, however, is intermittent, which can lead to a false-negative test result.[1,25] Many healthy infected birds shed ABV infrequently and conversely many confirmed cases of PDD have been reportedly PaBV negative with multiple tests. Some birds, especially those with clinical disease, may shed the virus on a continuous basis. Because of all these variations, the testing of a single dropping or cloacal swab from a single bird is of limited usefulness. deKloet and colleagues[26] have suggested that RT-PCR performed on a feather sample is a reliable testing procedure. However, others have had limited success using the RT-PCR assay on feather calami, and the opinion among most other researchers at the 2014 ABV research forum was that the feather PCR was not an adequate sample for accurate testing. Similarly, Dalhausen and Orosz have suggested that the use of RT PCR on whole blood of birds is a sensitive diagnostic test,[17] but other studies have not supported this.[33] Although RT-PCR is the most commonly performed test for ABV, at this time there is no standardized method of testing among laboratories offering this service. Reported rates of ABV-positive birds among commercial laboratories and university settings range from 3% to 33%. This may be due to intermittent shedding or because the known ABV genotypes vary in sequence identity so some assays may not detect all genotypes.

Immunohistochemistry

Ouyang and colleagues[38] used immunohistochemistry (IHC) to detect the presence of ABV in 24 stored avian brain samples from birds diagnosed with PDD. Raghav and colleagues[41] performed IHC using antinucleoprotein antibodies on birds with PDD and consistently detected antigen in brain, spinal cord, adrenal, pancreas, and kidney. Antigen was also detected in the anterior gastrointestinal tract as well as heart, testes, ovary, and thyroid.

Serology

The assessment of PaBV infection and the diagnosis of PDD are difficult, because although PaBV infection is common, the development of clinical PDD is rare. Thus, tests that simply detect the presence of PaBV may not be useful for the antemortem diagnosis of PDD. This is further complicated by some PaBV-infected birds not developing a detectable antibody response, although, conversely, there does seem to be a positive correlation between the level of antibodies produced and the development of disease.[16] Although following the natural course of infection in parrots Heffels-Redmann and colleagues[42] found that birds with a high PaBV load in their crop and cloaca combined with the presence of high levels of antibodies had the highest risk of developing disease. Birds that are positive on PaBV PCR and negative on serology have been documented as have birds that are intermittently positive on serology.[1,12,42] Some birds have suddenly seroconverted immediately before the onset of clinical disease. This confirmed the investigators' experience that antibodies or prior ABV infection does not protect against disease.[34] Western blot and the indirect fluorescent antibody assays have been used the most.[15,18]

One of the major difficulties in developing a serologic assay is determining the nature of the standard of comparison. There is poor correlation between the presence of antibodies, fecal shedding of ABV, and clinical disease. Widespread persistent asymptomatic infection without clinical disease is a consistent feature of bornavirus infections. This may be due to the noncytopathic effect of bornaviruses and their ability to escape recognition from the immune system. Even clinically affected birds may or may not have detectable antibodies or fecal PCR positivity.

Antiganglioside Antibodies

Some researchers have proposed serologic testing for antiganglioside (anti-GSL) antibodies, markers of immune-mediated disease, stating that it seems more accurate in detecting clinically affected birds.[43] Rossi and colleagues[43] suggest that bornavirus infection results in the production of anti-GSL antibodies. They suggest that immunization of birds with gangliosides resulted in lesions consistent with PDD. Leal de Araujo and colleagues[44] have repeated their studies in both chickens and Quaker parrots and both failed to generate any lesions resembling PDD. Further studies are needed to determine if anti-GSL antibodies will be diagnostic for PDD.

Recommended Diagnostics and Interpretation

In a clinical setting, the following tests are recommended[1,45]:

- A choanal and cloacal RT-PCR with a serologic assay offers the best combination to determine infection, recognizing that one negative test on all does not rule out infection.

Interpretation of tests

- Birds positive for both PCR and serology should be considered positive and housed separate from negative birds.
- Birds positive for PCR only should be retested in 4 to 6 weeks. They should be housed separate from other birds until deemed negative (3 negative tests). If they seroconvert or test positive on additional tests they should be considered positive.
- Birds positive only on serology should be considered positive and housed separately from negative birds.
- Some birds are infected and will not test positive on any test, and infection is found at necropsy (Sharman Hoppes, personal experience, 2013).

As previously discussed, positive ABV PCR and serology results in a healthy bird do not predict that a bird will ever become clinically ill with PDD.

TREATMENT PROTOCOLS

At this time, there is no cure and few treatment options. Based on the observed inflammatory histopathologic lesions, nonsteroidal antiinflammatory drugs (NSAIDs) are widely used. The effectiveness of treatment may depend on the time of onset of treatment and the stage of the disease when initiated. Most clinicians believe the preferential and selective COX -2 inhibitors improve and extend the quality of life of PDD birds.

Cyclooxygenase-2 Inhibitors

Celecoxib was the first of this class of medication to be used. Dalhausen and colleagues[46] administered celecoxib at 10 mg/kg orally once daily for 6 to 12 weeks to birds with clinically diagnosed PDD. They reported that birds had marked clinical improvement, but unfortunately, there were no control groups for comparison, so the significance of this report is unclear. Based on this initial data with increasing dosages recommended over the years, it is currently the recommended treatment. The current dosage for celecoxib (Celebrex, Pfizer Inc, Mission KS, USA) for PDD birds is 15 to 30 mg/kg PO q12 h. For severe central nervous system involvement, 30 to 40 mg/kg PO q12 h is recommended.[15,47]

Although meloxicam has been used widely by practitioners for the treatment of PDD, preliminary studies performed at the authors' facility did not demonstrate efficacy of treatment with meloxicam in cockatiels experimentally challenged with ABV strain M24.[48] This study found that birds treated with meloxicam that were challenged with ABV-M24 did not survive. In contrast, birds challenged with ABV-M24 that did not receive meloxicam and the control birds that did receive meloxicam all survived to the study endpoint.[48] In spite of this study in cockatiels, anecdotally most practitioners report beneficial effects in PDD birds using oral and injectable meloxicam. Anecdotal dosages of meloxicam (Metacam, BoehringerIngelheimVetmedica Inc., St Joesph, MO, USA) for treatment of PDD birds is 0.5 to 1 mg/kg IM or PO q12 to 24 h.

Robenacoxib (Onsior, Novartis Animal Health, North Ryde, NSW) has also been used by some practitioners with equivocal results for the treatment of PDD. Robenacoxib has been used at dosages of 2 to 10 mg/kg IM weekly for 4 weeks and then monthly.[15,47]

Cyclosporine

Cyclosporine is a calcineurin inhibitor and immunosuppressant that selectively suppresses T-cell function. In preliminary studies, the authors found that in ABV-challenged cockatiels, there was no significant difference in the development of lesions between control groups and groups treated with cyclosporine. However, on necropsy, the treated birds had more organs that were RT-PCR positive for ABV.[49] Anecdotally, cyclosporine has been successful in treating some PDD birds that were unresponsive to NSAIDs alone. Cyclosporine at 10 mg/kg PO BID was used along with a cyclooxygenase-2 (COX-2) inhibitor in birds who presented with end-stage PDD who were not responding to COX-2 inhibitors alone. In many of these birds, the addition of cyclosporine seemed to reduce the clinical signs and prolonged their life. Because cyclosporine is an immunosuppressive drug, the birds were on antibiotics and antifungals prophylactically (IME and personal communication AdyGanz). Gancz and colleagues described long-term survival and clinical remission in an African Gray parrot using cyclosporine A treatment.[50]

Ribavirin

Ribavirin (Virazole, Valeant Pharmaceuticals International, Bridgewater, NJ, USA) is a ribonucleic analogue that stops viral RNA synthesis and readily kills ABV in tissue culture. Mammalian Borna disease virus shows a high degree of sensitivity to ribavirin, but preliminary studies on ABV-infected birds found no measurable effect on viral shedding.[51] Preliminary pharmacokinetic data on birds show that it is rapidly excreted and that doses appropriate for mammals are insufficient to reach and maintain therapeutic levels in birds.[52] Reuter and colleagues demonstrated a synergistic effect with ribavirin and interferon (IFN) alpha against PaBV in avian cells, suggesting that a combination of ribavirin with type 1 IFNs may be more effective in vivo. In this study, replication of the virus resumed after treatment cessation.[52] Studies on the use of higher and more frequent dosing with ribavirin with and without IFNs are needed.

Favipiravir (T-705)

Tokunaga and colleagues performed a study looking at favipiravir (T-705) (Toyama Chemical Company, Ltd. Tokyo, Japan), an antiviral similar to ribavirin. Favipiraivr was found to be a potent inhibitor of both BoDV-1 and PaBV-4. T-705 suppressed BoDV-1 and PABV-4 replication in a dose-and time-dependent manner during the 4-week observation period. At 28 days of treatment, T-705 reduced PaBV-4 RNA to an almost undetectable level, whereas PaBV-4 RNA was still detected in ribavirin-treated cells. Furthermore, they did not detect a significant increase in the amount of PaBV-4 RNA by 14 days posttreatment.[53] Further studies are needed to determine if T-705 could be used to treat persistent bornavirus infection in various animals in vivo.

Gabapentin

Gabapentin (Neurontine, Pfizer, New York, NY, USA) is a gamma-amino butyric acid agonist. It relieves neuropathic pain in mammals and birds. Although there are no controlled studies in birds, anecdotally there are positive clinical responses. A dose of 10 to 25 mg/kg PO q12 h is recommended for central or peripheral nervous system signs such as seizures or ataxia. Gabapentin 50 mg/kg PO has been used in birds that self-mutilate.[15,47]

Adjunctive Therapies

Adjunctive therapies for birds with PDD include gastrointestinal prokinetic agents such as cisapride (Propulsid; Janssen Pharmceutica, Inc., Titusville, NJ) and metoclopramide (Reglan; Schwarz Pharma, Seymour, IN) to improve gastrointestinal tract transit. Antibiotics or antifungals may be necessary for secondary infections. Essential fatty acids in flax seed oil at 0.1 mL/kg PO daily or Vet Omega (Avian Studios North Salt lake, UT, USA) at 0.22 to 0.44 mL/kg PO daily have been recommended to reduce inflammation. Anecdotally, stress has been deemed a factor in development of clinical signs. Owners should avoid overcrowding of birds, practice good hygiene, and provide nutritionally adequate diets. Reproductive stress may also exacerbate clinical signs. Leuprolide acetate (Leupron depot, AbbVie, Chicago IL) or the deslorelin implant (Suprelorin, Virbac Animal Health, Fort Worth, TX, USA) have been used to reduce reproductive hormones.

Vaccination

Because ABV disease is T-cell mediated, theoretically, a vaccination could exacerbate disease. Nonetheless, several studies looking at vaccination options have been performed. Two recent reports of the use of viral vector vaccines against parrot bornaviruses (PaBVs) used a prime boost strategy and showed that vaccinated cockatiels had a reduced viral load and reduced shedding as well as a delayed course of infection.[54,55]

Olbert and colleagues established a vaccination strategy using recombinant Newcastle disease virus (NDV) and modified vaccinia virus Ankara (MVA) that were engineered to express the phosphoprotein and nucleoprotein genes of 2 ABVs, PaBV-4 and CnBV-2. The vaccine established self-limiting infections and induced a bornavirus-specific humoral immune response in cockatiels (Nymphicushollandicus) and common canaries (Serinuscanaria forma domestica). Infected birds were challenged with a homologous bornavirus. Immunized birds had significantly reduced shedding of bornavirus RNA and reduced viral loads in tissue. However, the birds still developed clinical signs of PDD.[54]

Runge and colleagues revealed that prime-boost vaccination of cockatiels with NDV and modified vaccinia virus Ankara vectors expressing the nucleoprotein and phospho-protein genes of PaBV-4 substantially blocked bornavirus replication following paren-teral challenge infection with 103.5 ffu of heterologous PaBV-2. In this study only 2 of 6 vaccinated birds developed mild PDD-associated lesions, whereas the unvaccinated birds were not protected from PBV-2 infection or the inflammatory lesions.[55]

Hameed and colleagues demonstrated that vaccination with killed PaBV with recom-binant PaBV-4 nucleoprotein N in alum was protective against disease in cockatiels chal-lenged with a virulent bornavirus isolate (PaBV-2).[49] After challenge, both vaccinated and unvaccinated birds developed gross and histologic lesions of PDD. Vaccinated birds remained largely free of disease, despite persistence of virus in multiple organs. Similar results occurred when vaccinated with recombinant N in alum. There was no evidence that vaccination before or postchallenge made infection more severe.[49]

These results suggest that vaccination can protect against disease and does not exacerbate infection but does not reduce viral persistence. These studies supported that ABV may be immune mediated so Hameed and colleagues performed an additional study using cyclosporine A in unvaccinated birds beginning day 1 before challenge. This treatment also conferred protection from clinical disease but not infec-tion.[49] Results reflect the complex pathogenesis of PDD.

CONTROL

There is no available vaccine and should this disease prove immunologically medi-ated, it is possible that no effective vaccine will be produced. Infection with one geno-type does not seem to confer protection for a different genotype. In the absence of effective treatments and effective vaccines, control must be sought by other methods. Fortunately, ABV is not an environmentally stable virus. It is easily destroyed with soap or diluted bleach and is inactivated by ultraviolet light and desiccation. The control of ABV in aviaries and homes, therefore, requires a multimodal approach.

- Good hygiene and housing birds outdoors when temperature permits.
- Avoid overcrowding and provide good nutrition.
- Isolation of all new, sick, or PaBV-positive birds, separation of birds from a flock when they are PaBV positive.
- Existing birds and newly presenting birds should be tested using both serology and PCR, and birds should be separated based on the results of this testing. There should be at least 3 negative tests at 4- to 6-week intervals before consid-ering a bird negative.
- With the likelihood of vertical transmission, chicks from infected birds should be incubator hatched, hand raised, kept separate from other noninfected birds, and monitored for development of disease.
- Because of the intermittent shedding and inconclusive serology results, testing and separating birds may require years to obtain PaBV-negative aviaries.
- Healthy birds that test positive with either PCR or serology testing should not be euthanized.

SUMMARY

Previously, observations on PDD cases suggested sporadic infections and a relative lack of ABV outbreaks. Now, it is known that ABV infection is common and widespread throughout captive psittacine birds. Healthy and subclinical carriers of multiple species are documented. Considerable research has been performed on ABV and PDD, but there are still many unanswered questions. Continued studies are needed to determine mode of transmission and development of more efficient tests that accurately diagnose clinical PDD. Improved treatment protocols, including further work on antivirals and development of a vaccine, are needed. Presently, NSAIDs, treatment of secondary infections, reducing stress, providing a nutritionally adequate diet, and good sanitation are the only tools for improving both the quality and longevity of life of PaBV-/PPD-affected birds. Implementing appropriate therapy early in the course of disease seems most effective. In severely ill birds, therapy may be less effective.

ACKNOWLEDGMENTS

The authors would like to acknowledge Dr. Ian Tizard's co-authorship in the 2013 chapter Avian Bornavirus and Proventricular Dilatation Disease: Diagnostics, Pathology, Prevalence, and Control and thank him for his expert advice and help in editing the current article.

DISCLOSURE

The authors have nothing to disclose.

REFERENCES

1. Hoppes S, Gray PL, Payne S, et al. The isolation, pathogenesis, diagnosis, transmission, and control of avian bornavirus and proventricular dilatation disease. Vet Clin North Am ExotAnimPract 2010;13(3):495–508.
2. Perpiñan D, Fernandez-Bellon H, Lopez C, et al. Lymphocytic myenteric, subepicardial and pulmonary ganglioneuritis in four nonpsittacine birds. J Avian Med Surg 2007;21:210–4.
3. Daoust PY, Julian RJ, Yason CV, et al. Proventricular impaction associated with nonsuppurative encephalomyelitis and ganglioneuritis in 2 Canada geese. J Wildl Dis 1991;27:513–7.
4. Smith D, Berkvens C, Kummrow M, et al. Identification of avian bornavirus in the brains of Canada geese (Brantacanadensis) and trumpeter swans (Cygnus buccinator) with non-suppurative encephalitis. Proc Wildlife Disease Assoc. Puerto Iguazu, May 30–June 4, 2010.
5. Delnatte P, Ojkic D, DeLay J, et al. Pathology and diagnosis of avian bornavirus infection in wild Canada geese (Brantacanadensis), trumpeter swans (Cygnus buccinator) and mute swans (Cygnus olor) in Canada: a retrospective study. AvianPathol 2013;42(2):114–28.
6. Payne S, Covaleda L, Jianhua G, et al. Detection and characterization of a distinct bornavirus lineage from healthy canada geese (Brantacanadensis). J Virol 2011;85:12053–6.
7. Payne SL, Guo J, Tizard I. Bornaviruses. In: Hambrick J, Gammon LT, editors. North American Waterfowl. In Ducks: habitat, behavior and diseases. New York: Nova Scientific Publishers; 2012. p. 1–20.
8. Payne SL, Delnatte P, Guo J, et al. Birds and bornaviruses. AnimHealth ResRep 2012;13(2):145–56.
9. Weissenbock H, Sekulin K, Bakonyi T, et al. Novel avian bornavirus in a nonpsittacine species (canary; Serinuscanaria) with enteric ganglioneuritis and encephalitis. J Virol 2009;83(113):67–71.

10. Shivaprasad HL. Proventricular dilatation disease in a Peregrine falcon (Falco peregrinus).ProcAnnuConfAssoc Avian Vet, Monterrey, CA, 2005;107–8.
11. Berg M, Johansson M, Montell H, et al. Wild birds as a possible natural reservoir of Borna disease virus. Epidemiol Infect 2001;127:173–8.
12. Avian Bornavirus Research Forum. Association of Avian Vet Conference. New Orleans (LA), August 2–6, 2014.
13. Fluck A, Enderlein D, Piepenbring A, et al. Correlation of avian bornavirus-specific antibodies and viral ribonucleic acid shedding with neurological signs and feather-damaging behaviour in psittacine birds. Vet Rec 2019. https://doi.org/10.1136/vr.104860.
14. Kuhn JH, Durrwald R, Bao Y, et al. Taxonomic reorganization of the family borna-viridae. Arch Virol 2015;160:621–32.
15. Rossi G, Dahlhausen R, Orosz S. Avian ganglioneuritis in clinical practice. Vet Clin North Am ExotAnimPract 2018;21:33–67.
16. Lierz M, Hafez HM, Honkavouri KS, et al. Anatomical distribution of avian borna-virus in parrots, its occurrence in clinically healthy birds and ABV- antibody detection. AvianPathol 2009;38:491–6.
17. Dahlhausen RD, Orosz SE. Avian borna virus infection rates in domestic psitta-cine birds. ProcAnnuConfAssoc Avian Vet. San Diego (CA), August 1–5, 2010. p. 49.
18. Herzog S, Enderlein D, Heffels-Redmann U, et al. Indirect immunofluorescence assay for *intra vitam* diagnostic of avian Borna virus infection in psittacine birds. J ClinMicrobiol 2010;48(6):2282–4.
19. Rubbenstroth D, Rinder M, Stein M, et al. Avianbornaviruses are widely distrib-uted in canary birds (Serinuscanaria f. domestica). Vet Microbiol 2013;165: 287–95.
20. HeffelsRedmann U, Enderlean D, Herzog S, et al. Occurrence of avian bornavirus infection in captive psittacines in various European Countries and its association with proventricular dilatation disease. AvianPathol 2011;40(4):419–26.
21. de Kloet SR, Dorrestein GM. Presence of avian bornavirus RNA and anti-avian bornavirus antibodies in apparently healthy macaws. Avian Dis 2009;53:568–73.
22. Encinas-Nagel N, Enderlein D, Piepenbring A, et al. Avian Bornavirus in free-ranging psittacine birds, Brazil. Emerg Infect Dis 2014;20(12):2103–6.
23. Kistler AL, Smith JM, Greninger AL, et al. Analysis of naturally occurring avian bornavirus infection and transmission during an outbreak of proventricular dilata-tion disease among captive psittacine birds. J Virol 2010;84:2176–9.
24. Rubbenstroth D, Schmidt V, Rinder M, et al. Phylogenetic analysis supports hor-izontal transmission as a driving force of the spread of Avian Bornaviruses. PLoS One 2016. https://doi.org/10.1371/journal.pone.0160936.
25. Heatley JJ, Villalobos AR. Avian bornavirus in the urine of infected birds. Vet Med Res Rep 2012;3:19–23.
26. de Kloet AH, Kerski A, de Kloet SR. Diagnosis of avian bornavirus infection in Psittaciformes by serum antibody detection and reverse transcription polymerase chain reaction assay using feather calami. J Vet Diagn Invest 2011;23:421–9.
27. Heckmann J, Enderlein D, Piepenbring AK, et al. Investigation of different infec-tion routes of parrot bornavirus in cockatiels. Avian Dis 2017;61:90–5.
28. Rubbenstroth D, Brosinski K, Rinder M, et al. No contact transmission of avian bor-navirus in experimentally infected cockatiels (Nymphicushollandicus) and domes-tic canaries (Serinuscanaria forma domestica). Vet Microbiol 2014;172:146–56.
29. Monaco E, Hoppes S, Guo J, et al. The detection of avian bornavirus within psit-tacine eggs. J Avian Med Surg 2012;26:144–8.

30. Lierz M, Piepenbring A, Herden C, et al. Vertical transmission of avian bornavirus in psittacines. Emerg Infect Dis 2011;17:2390–1.

31. Kerski A, de Kloet AH, de Kloet SR. Vertical transmission of Avian Bornavirus in Psittaciformes: avian bornavirus RNA and anti-avian bornavirus antibodies in eggs, embryos, and hatchlings obtained from infected sun conures (aratingasolstitialis). Avian Dis 2012;56:471–8.

32. Kranz JB, Escandon P, Musser JMB. Environmental stability of avian Bornavirus:pH and drying. ProcExoticsCon. San Antonio (TX), August 29–September 2, 2015. p. 89.

33. Leal de Araujo J, Rech R, Heatley J, et al. From nerves to brain to gastrointestinal tract: A time-based study of parrot bornavirus2 (PaBV-2) pathogenesis in cockatiels (Nymphicushollandicus). PLoS One 2017. https://doi.org/10.1371/journal.pone.0187797.

34. Mirhosseini N, Gray PL, Hoppes S, et al. Proventricular dilatation disease in cockatiels (Nymphicushollandicus) following infection with a genotype 2 avian bornavirus. JAvian Med Surg 2011;25:199–204.

35. Tizard I, Shivaprasad HL, Guo J, et al. The pathogenesis of proventricular dilatation disease. AnimHealth Res Rev 2017;17(2):110–26.

36. Weissenbock H, Bakonyi T, Sekulin K, et al. Avian bornaviruses in psittacine birds from Europe and Australia with proventricular dilatation disease. Emerg Infect Dis 2009;15:1453–9.

37. CazayouxVice CA. Myocarditis as a component of psittacineproventricular dilatation syndrome in a Patagonian conure. Avian Dis 1992;36(4):1117–9.

38. Ouyang N, Storts R, Tian Y, et al. Histopathology and the detection of avian bornavirus in the nervous system of birds diagnosed with proventricular dilatation disease. AvianPathol 2009;38:393–401.

39. Lierz M, Piepenbring A, Heffels-Redmann U, et al. Experimental infection of cockatiels with different avian bornavirus genotypes. ProcAnnuConfAssoc Avian Vet, Louisville, KY, 2012;9–10.

40. Rossi G, Galosi L, Dahlhausen B, et al. Unusual and severe lesions of proventricular dilatation disease in lories. In: Proceedings of the 3rd ICARE, International Conference on Avian Herpetological and Exotic Mammal Medicine. Venice (Italy), March 25–29, 2017. p. 663.

41. Raghav R, Taylor M, DeLay J, et al. Avian bornavirus is present in many tissues of psittacine birds with histopathologic evidence of proventricular dilatation disease. J Vet Diagn Invest 2010;22:495–508.

42. Heffels-Redmann U, Enderlein D, Herzog S, et al. Follow-up investigations on different courses of natural avian bornavirus infections in Psittacines. Avian Dis 2012;56:153–9.

43. Rossi G, Ceccherelli R, Crosta L, et al. Anti-ganglioside auto-antibodies in ganglia of PDD affected parrots. ProcEurAssn Avian Vets, Madrid (Spain), April 26-30, 2011; 177–8.

44. Leal de Araujo J, Tizard I, Guo J, et al. Are anti-ganglioside antibodies associated with proventricular dilatation disease in birds? PeerJ 2017. https://doi.org/10.7717/peerj.3144.2017.

45. Lierz M. Avian bornavirus and proventricular dilation disease. In: Speer B, editor. Current therapy in avian medicine and surgery. St Louis (MO): Elsevier; 2016. p. 28–46.

46. Dahlhausen R, Aldred S, Colaizzi E. Resolution of clinical proventricular dilatation disease by cyclooxygenase 2 inhibition. ProcAnnuConfAssoc Avian Vet, Monterrey, CA, 2002;9–12.

47. Clubb SL. Clinical management of psittacine birds affected with proventricular dilatation disease. ProcAnnuConfAssoc Avian Vet. San Antonio (TX), August 29–September 2, 2015. p. 85–90.
48. Hoppes S, Heatley J, Guo J, et al. Meloxicam treatment in cockatiels (Nymphicushollandicus) infected with avian bornavirus. J Exot Pet Med 2013;22:275–9.
49. Hameed S, Guo J, Tizard I, et al. Studies on immunity and immunopathogenesis of parrot bornaviral disease in cockatiels. Virology 2018;515:81–91.
50. Gancz A, Elbaz D, Farnoushi Y, et al. Clinical recovery from proventricular dilatation disease following treatment with cyclosporine A in an African gray parrot (Psitticuserithacus). 17. DVG- TagunguberVogelkrankheiten, Munich, Germany, 2012.
51. Musser J, Heatley J, Koinis A, et al. Ribavirin inhibits parrot bornavirus 4 replication in cell culture. PLoS One 2015. https://doi.org/10.1371/journal.pone.0134080.
52. Reuter A, Horie M, Höper D, et al. Synergistic antiviral activity of ribavirin and interferon-a against parrot bornaviruses in avian cells. J Gen Virol 2016;97:2096–103.
53. Tokunaga T, Yamamoto Y, Sakai M, et al. Antiviral activity of favipiravir (T-705) against mammalian and avian bornaviruses. Antiviral Res 2017;143:237–45.
54. Olbert M, Römer-Oberdörfer A, Herden C, et al. Viral vector vaccines expressing nucleoprotein and phosphoprotein genes of avian bornaviruses ameliorate homologous challenge infections in cockatiels and common canaries. Sci Rep 2016;6:36840.
55. Runge S, Olbert M, Herden C, et al. Viral vector vaccines protect cockatiels from inflammatory lesions after heterologous parrot bornavirus 2 challenge infection. Vaccine 2017;35(4):557–63.

Selected Emerging Infectious Diseases of Squamata: An Update

La'Toya V. Latney, DVM, DECZM, Dip ABVP (Reptile/Amphibian)[a],*,
James F.X. Wellehan, DVM, MS, PhD, DACZM, DACVM[b]

KEYWORDS

- Reptile • *Cryptosporidium* • Bacterial • Fungal • Viral • Emerging disease

KEY POINTS

- Advances in *Cryptosporidium* treatment suggest that the use of paramomycin in squamates can help ameliorate shedding but will not eradicate infection.
- *Paranannizziopsis*, *Nannizziopsis*, and *Ophidiomyces* cause primary fatal fungal infections in captive and wild squamates.
- Diverse paramyxoviruses infect squamates, lack species specificity, and may readily cross species barriers.
- While sunshine viruses and bornaviruses are now known to impact snakes, nidoviruses have emerged to cause fatal infections in boa and colubrid species.
- Divergent reptarenaviruses cause inclusion body disease in boid snakes with variable disease progression based on affected species.

PARASITIC DISEASES

Cryptosporidium

Cryptosporidium, a genus of coccidian parasites known to infect many vertebrate orders, remains a significant concern for squamates. In clinical practice, polymerase chain reaction (PCR)-based methods are the most sensitive and specific to identify the presence of the organism in clinical or subclinical cases.[1,2] There are 2 acceptable methods for identification of PCR products, sequencing and probe hybridization. Other methods should not be relied upon for making clinical decisions. Most available testing utilizes pan-*Cryptosporidium* primers that will amplify any species, and the species identification is done by sequencing. Probe hybridization is most commonly

[a] Avian and Exotic Medicine & Surgery, The Animal Medical Center, 610 East 62nd Street, New York, NY 10065, USA; [b] Zoological Medicine Service, University of Florida College of Veterinary Medicine, PO Box 100126, 2015 Southwest 16th Avenue, Gainesville, FL 32608-0125, USA
* Corresponding author.
E-mail address: latoya.latney@amcny.org

Vet Clin Exot Anim 23 (2020) 353–371
https://doi.org/10.1016/j.cvex.2020.01.009
1094-9194/20/© 2020 Elsevier Inc. All rights reserved.
vetexotic.theclinics.com

utilized in TaqMan quantitative PCR (qPCR) and involves a probe that binds to a specific sequence. It is crucial that a probe hybridization qPCR is properly validated and shown not to cross-react against other species that may be present. For example, *Cryptosporidium serpentis* and *C muris* are closely related, but the first is a significant snake pathogen, and the other is a commonly seen pass-through from prey that is clinically irrelevant. *Cryptosporidium* species require sequence identification for reliable identification; morphology is unreliable for species identification.[3] Proper species identification is necessary to make clinical decisions.

Cryptosporidium spp. divide into clades that correlate more with site of infection (gastric vs intestinal) than host species. Oocysts can be detected on fecal or gastric lavage samples with acid-fast staining, with fecal samples better for intestinal species and gastric washes better for gastric species. However, the sensitivity and specificity of acid-fast staining is generally poor.[4] In squamates, the most common clinically significant species with gastric tropism is *C serpentis*. Clinical disease caused by *C serpentis* presents as hypertrophic gastritis, regurgitation, and a midbody swelling.

Intestinal cryptosporidiosis can cause chronic wasting secondary to enteritis. *Cryptosporidium varanii* (sometimes incorrectly called *C saurophilum*[5]) is the most common. *C avium* also causes intestinal disease in squamates, but extraintestinal infections have been documented, including cystitis and cloacal infections in green iguanas (*Iguana iguana*).[6] This organism was first identified in cockatiel feces (*Nymphicus hollandicus*), where it was initially called avian genotype V.[7] As seen in iguanas, *C avium* also infects the urinary tract and cloaca in birds.[8] An unnamed third intestinal *Cryptosporidium* species was first identified in a fecal sample from a viper boa (*Candoia asper*).[9] It was later found in 57 of 223 wild Japanese grass snakes (*Rhabdophis tigris*) associated with mucosal edema, goblet cell loss, and scattered necrosis in the small intestine.[10]

Cryptosporidium species that infect prey items commonly pass through in feces of squamates without clinical signs or histologic evidence of infection. *C muris* (formerly considered a *C parvum* genotype) and *C tyzzeri*, both utilizing mouse hosts, are commonly seen when healthy snake feces are tested[11] An unnamed rat genotype has been reported from the feces of a boa constrictor.[12] *C baileyi* has been reported in farmed snakes in China and was considered to be a pass-through pathogen from avian prey.[8] A previous experimental study provided evidence that *C parvum* oocysts were not infectious to reptiles.[13]

Reports of treatment successes remain scarce. One clinical trial evaluated paromomycin in bearded dragons (*Pogona vitticeps*) gavaged with feces from a positive animal.[14] However, the species of *Cryptosporidium* was not identified, and coinfection with *Isospora* was noted.[14] Oral treatment with paromomycin began 7 weeks after infection in the treatment group using 100 mg/kg every 24 hours for 7 days, then twice a week for 6 weeks, and then 360 mg/kg every 48 hours for 10 days. Fecal and histologic evaluations were performed. *Cryptosporidium* species were only detected in the intestinal lumens in the nontreated lizards. Renal gout was noted in some patients. Once the treatment frequency was decreased to 100 mg/kg twice a week, a reoccurrence of shedding by a large proportion of the animals was noted, indicating that infection was not cleared. It is expected that different *Cryptosporidium* species will have different drug susceptibilities.

Captive green iguanas infected with an unidentified *Cryptosporidium* species were treated with halofuginone and hyperimmune bovine colostrum in 1 treatment group, and a combination of sulfadiazine and trimethoprim, spiramycin, metronidazole, and hyperimmune bovine colostrum was used in the other treatment group.[15] Fecal shedding and clinical response were not seen for 18 monthly follow rechecks. PCR testing was not done. Older reports of bovine hyperimmune serum have been provided in previous reviews, but efficacy for treating *Cryptosporidium* species that do not infect cattle are highly questionable.[16]

A more recent treatment success has been reported in a king cobra (*Ophiophagus hannah*) infected with *C serpentis*.[17] A course of paromomycin, inserted in feeder rats, was initiated at 360 mg/kg orally, twice weekly for 6 weeks. Feces collected at the end of treatment were negative for *Cryptosporidium* on PCR, as were feces collected 3 weeks, 6 months, 12 months, and 18 months later.[17]

Transmission prevention and environmental decontamination remain pivotal in decreasing the disease burden for all genotypes. Routine disinfectants are typically ineffective; 2.5% glutaraldehyde exposure for over 10 hours may inactivate spores, but the presence of organic materials prevents this.[18] Previous studies looking at desiccation may have considerably underestimated parasite viability, and desiccation cannot be considered a reliable approach.[19] Freezing is also not an effective method of disinfection.[20] Currently, moist heat (56–70°C for 20 minutes) appears to be the most effective way to clean the environment.[21]

BACTERIAL DISEASE
Austwickia Chelonae

A chelonae (phylum Actinobacteria, formerly *Dermatophilus chelonae*) was first reported in squamates in a king cobra with granulomatous disease.[22] It has recently been reported as causing high mortality in crocodile lizards (*Shinisaurus crocodilurus*).[23] *Austwickia* has a potent diptheria-like biotoxin.[24]

Devriesea Agamarum

D agamarum (phylum Actinobacteria) is associated with severe hyperkeratotic dermatitis, cheilitis, and potential septicemia in *Uromastyx* and other agamid species.[25–27] Part of the oral microbiota in a variety of species, it has emerged as a primary pathogen of captive *Uromastyx*, *Crotaphytus*, *Physignathus*, *Agama* spp, and the critically endangered Lesser Antilles iguana (*Iguana delicatissima*)[28] with increased virulence in other agamid, iguanid, and euphlebarid species.

Experimental transmission studies demonstrated that dermal inoculation of *D agamarum* induces dermatitis as early as 5 to 9 days after exposure.[29] Distinctive dermal crusts are noted on the lips and other dermal sites in affected species.[29] Asymptomatic *P vitticeps* have been identified as reservoirs.[30,31]

Initial debridement and intramuscular administration of ceftiofur at 5 mg/kg every 24 hours for an average of 18 days in *P vitticeps* and 12 days in *Uromastyx* sp was an effective treatment.[30] Enrofloxacin did not eliminate the bacteria.[30] *D agamarum* was inhibited by ceftazidime, erythromycin, and tetracycline in clinically affected *Uromastyx sp*. The highest resistance was found to enrofloxacin, penicillin, and gentamicin.[30] Ceftazidime, 10 mg/kg intramuscularly every 72 hours for 15 days, proved clinically effective for treating *Uromastyx* species.[26]

D agamarum is resistant in the environment and can remain infective for over 5 months in humid sand and distilled water and for 57 days in dermal crusts from affected animals.[32] Sodium hypochlorite (0.05%–0.5%), chlorhexidine (0.05%–0.5%), boric acid (0.01%), and ethanol (70%) disinfect hard surfaces with a minimum 5 minutes of contact time.[32]

FUNGAL DISEASE

As Earth experiences the sith mass extinction event in the geologic record, fungal pathogens are emerging in response to climate change.[33] Reptiles and amphibians are 2 taxa that have and are consistently predicted to experience the greatest losses first.[34-36] Bohm and colleagues[35] have shown that regardless of location, squamates that are range-restricted habitat specialists living in areas highly accessible to people are likely to become extinct first.

Fungi in the order Onyenales contain some of the most serious fungal pathogens of vertebrates, including *Blastomyces, Histoplasma, Coccidioides, Microsporum, Trichophyton, Lacazia, Paracoccidioides, Nannizziopsis, Paranannizziopsis,* and *Ophidomyces*[37-39].

This fungal order has reduced numbers of plant cell wall–degrading enzymes and increased numbers of keratinases, which are adaptations for living on animal hosts. Fungi within this order are a dangerous group of primary fungal pathogens in squamates. Nannizziopsis spp (family *Nannizziopsiasceae)* infect lizards, crocodilians, turtles, and mammals; *Paranannizziopsis* spp (family *Nannizziopsiasceae)* infect squamates and sphenodontids; and, to date, *Ophidomyces ophiodiicola* (family *Onygenaceae*) only infects snakes[40].

Nannizziposis and Paranannizziopsis

Many squamates are affected by *Nannizziopsis* and *Paranannizziopsis*; a species review is available.[41-43] *Nannizziopsis guarroi* has been reported in inland bearded dragons, central bearded dragons, green iguanas, and a European green lizard (*Lacerta viridis*).[44] *Nannizziopsis chlamydospora, N draconii,* and *N barbata* cause dermatomycosis in bearded dragons.[37,45,46] *N. dermatitidis* has been reported in chameleons (three species), leopard geckos,[47] and day geckos (*Phelsuma* sp). *P crustacea, P californiensis,* and *P longispora* (formerly *C longisporum*) cause necrotic dermatitis in tentacled snakes in zoologic institutions.[37,38,48,49] *P crustacea* was isolated from snakes in Ontario, Canada, and *P californiensis* from snakes in California.[38,49] More recently, *Nannizziopsis crocodili* has been reported in fresh water crocodiles.[50] *Paranannizziopsis australasiensis* has been reported in tuatara,[51] and *P tardicrescens* in Wagler vipers, tentacled snakes, and a rhinoceros snake.[52]

Ophidiomyces

To date, many free-ranging species in the eastern and midwestern United States have been infected with *O ophiodiicola*, (also known as snake fungal Disease or SFD). Wild European snakes are afflicted by a genetically distinct clade,[53] and disease has been noted in captive snakes.[38,54] In 2018, 2 snakes imported from Asia to Europe had localized and systemic *O ophiodiicola* infections[55] (**Table 1**).

Prevalence

Although most prevalence studies of *Ophidiomyces* are in wild snakes, as the veil between captive and wild snake disease shears, the practitioner needs to be aware of this disease. It is not uncommon to see *O ophiodiicola* in captive snakes; the authors have witnessed the disease in captive native and non-native species. A study in Virginia found that 40% of 30 free-ranging snakes had lesions suggestive of *Ophidiomyces*, including pustules, dry thickened and crusty scales, dysecdysis, and ocular opacity.[56] Most lesions were detected in April (73% lesions), with fewer in May (0%) and June (25%). Affected species included northern water snakes, brown water snakes, eastern racers and rainbow snakes.[56] Studies in Georgia in eastern indigo snakes (*Drymarchon couperi*) report 43.9% prevalence,[74] and in Illinois in eastern massasauga report 18% and 24% prevalence for 2013 and 2014, respectively.[66] Allender and colleagues[67] have reported the significant disease impact in wild eastern

Table 1			
Serpentes affected by *Ophidiomyces ophiodiicola*			
Region	**Colubrids**	**Viperids**	**Boids**
United States	Eastern racer (*Coluber constrictor*)[56] Black racer (*C constrictor priapus*)[56] Rat snake (*Pantherophis obsoletus*)[58] Ribbon snake (*Thamnophis proximus*)[58] Rainbow snake (*Farancia erytrogramma*)[56] Salt marsh snake (*Nerodia clarkii compressicauda*)[56] Ring-necked snakes (*Diadophis punctatus*)[59,60] Brown water snake (*Nerodia taxispilota*)[56] Plains garter snake (*Thamnophis radix*)[57,61] Milk snake (*Lampropeltis triangulum*)[62] Mud snake (*Farancia abacura*)[63] Northern water snake (*Nerodia sipedon*)[56]	Eastern massasauga (*Sistrurus catenatus*)[64–68] Pygmy rattlesnake (*Sistrurus miliarius*)[58,69,70] Timber rattlesnake (*Crotalus horridus*)[71,72] Copperheads (*Agkistrodon contortrix*)[59] Cottonmouth (*Agkistrodon piscivorus*)[59,73]	
Europe, captive	Brown tree snakes (*Boiga irregularis*)[37,55] Water snakes (*Nerodia clarkii*)[37,55] Milk snakes (*Lampropeltis* sp)[37,55] Corn snakes (*Pantherophis guttatus*)[37,55] Broad-headed snake (*Hoplocephalus bungaroides*)[37,55] Garter snake (*Thamnophis sirtalis*)[37,54]	Eastern diamondback rattlesnake (*Crotalus adamanteus*)[38,54]	Ball pythons (*Python regius*)[38,54] Rock pythons (*Python sebae*)[38,54] Green anacondas (*Eunectes murinus murinus*)[38,54]
Europe, wild-genetically distinct clade	British grass snakes (*Natrix natrix*)[53] Dice snake (*Natrix tessellata*)[53] Smooth snake (*Coronella austriaca*)[53]		Adder (*Vipera berus*)[53]
Asian, captive imported to Europe	Bocourt water snakes (*Subsessor bocourti*)[55] Pueblan milk snake (*Lampropeltis triangulum campbelli*)[55]		

Data from Refs.[37,38,53–56,58–73]

massasauga, in a call for changing the species' conservation status to threatened because of population declines caused by *Ophidiomyces*.

Clinical presentation, diagnosis, and treatment

Clinical signs include severe necrogranulomatous dermatitis, cellulitis, stomatitis, osteolysis, and panophthalmitis. Earlier reports of the disease suggested crotalids only contracted localized disease along the snout and labial pits; however, systemic dissemination in captive viperids[75] and free-ranging colubrids[61,63] have since been reported. The authors have diagnosed several captive pet species with clinical signs like those reported in free-ranging snakes (**Figs. 1 and 2**).

The fungus grows in cold environments (22°C) and is inhibited at 35°C; therefore, samples should be kept cool (refrigeration or −80°C freezer). PCR detection using nylon swabs is highly sensitive and specific, yet sampling technique is imperative, as false negatives can be common. PCR detection has been reported 3 days after infection; however, on average, clinical signs develop 6 to 7 weeks after exposure.[41] Molecular testing for confirmation and speciation is needed, although a fungal stain performed on tape impression may help guide treatment decisions and disinfection protocols pending PCR confirmation (**Table 2**).

VIRAL DISEASES
Mononegavirales

The order Mononegavirales contains RNA viruses with unsegmented negative sense genomes. Some of the most significant viral pathogens of vertebrates may be found in this order, including Ebola virus, rabies, and canine distemper. All mononegavirales have 5 core genes with a standard gene order. The largest gene, the polymerase, is most conserved, and can be aligned across diverse families in the genome to study evolution and relationships in the order. They are enveloped viruses, making them more susceptible to commonly used disinfectants.

Paramyxoviridae

Historically, Paramyxoviridae was divided into 2 subfamilies, Pneumovirinae and Para-myxovirinae, but Pneumoviridae was elevated to its own family status in 2015.[79] The

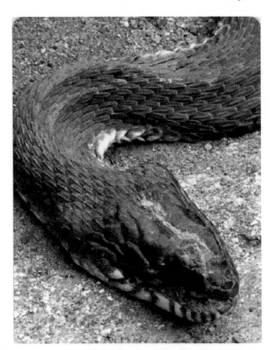

Fig. 1. Wild northern water snake (*Nerodia sipedon*) found in a state park in Philadelphia, Pennsylvania (LL) with severe facial disfiguration, necrodermatitis and osteolysis caused by *Ophidiomyces ophiodiicola*.

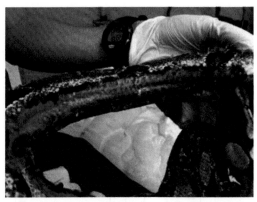

Fig. 2. Captive ball python (*Python regius*) presented with severe full thickness necrodermatitis of the gastropeges caused by *Ophidiomyces ophiodiicola* after being exposed to outdoor leaves as a form of enrichment for an indoor enclosure.

genus known to impact squamates is Ferlavirus. Ferlaviruses have 4 known genogroups: A, B, C, and tortoise.[80] Animals present with severe respiratory, neurologic, and immunosuppressive disease. Disease is not limited to snakes and is seen across the Toxicofera; reports include disease in caiman lizards (*Dracaena guianensis*)[81] and bearded dragons.[82] Serologic evidence is present in a wide variety of squamates.[83]

Since the last review of reptile paramyxoviridae,[16] new reports of ferlaviruses have surfaced globally. A seroprevalence study in 150 captive viperids in 9 different collections in Costa Rica revealed antibodies to a genogroup B strain in 26.6% and antibodies to a genogroup A strain in 30%.[84] Only 3 snakes tested positive by PCR and sequencing, and these snakes had no detectable ferlavirus antibodies in their serum.[84] Although it is unknown whether seropositive snakes had truly cleared the infection or were just not shedding virus at detectable levels when sampled, this study serves to illustrate the differences between measurement of humoral immune response and measurement of viral presence.

Ferlaviruses have been found by reverse transcriptase PCR (RT-PCR) and sequencing in snakes of more than 25 species, more than 15 genera, and 4 different families (Viperidae, Colubridae, Boidae, and Pythonidae).[85–87] All paramyxoviruses in snakes and other reptiles are associated with high mortality rates. Many reports have shown that ferlaviruses may cross species barriers readily.[85]

In 1 recent study evaluating the clinical progression of experimentally infected corn snakes, significant differences in pathogenicity were demonstrated between ferlavirus genotypes A, B, and C.[80] Genotype A induced moderate disease noted as a low amount of mucus secretion in the oral cavity on day 49 in 2 out of 12 challenged corn snakes. No animals died or were euthanized. Fifty percent of corn snakes infected with a genotype B isolate displayed severe clinical signs including abnormal respiratory sounds, purulent tracheal discharge, abnormal position, and apathy by day 16. One snake died. Corn snakes challenged with a genotype C isolate demonstrated mild clinical signs including minimal mucus secretion in the oral cavity in 3 snakes. Another report on the same snakes found that those challenged with genotype B had the highest white cell counts, but because of severe clinical signs, the animals died or were euthanized at day 36.[88] In the group challenged with genogroup A, antibodies started to rise at day 36. Snakes challenged with genogroup C showed an earlier rise in antibody titer, at 28 days. Cellular immune response, which is the more important for intracellular pathogens, was not assayed. *Salmonella* sp (all

Table 2
Summary of *Ophidiomyces ophidiicola* diagnostic options, treatments and disinfection agents

	Features	Diagnosis		References
		Definitive		
Microscopy (tape impression)	• Fungal hyphae: 5 μm (2–6 um) • Irregular septation • Refractile walls • Right angle branching • Terminal chains: 6–8 μm oval spores	No, if features are seen, begin disinfection and treatment pending PCR confirmation		Paré and Sigler,[41] 2016
PCR	Detects *Ophidiomyces* DNA	Yes, highly sensitive and specific		Hileman et al,[68] 2018
Note on Sampling	• Temperature sensitive (inhibited at 35°C) • False negatives common • Nylon swabs	• 5 swabs resulted in a 72% reduction in false negatives for diseased animals with clinical signs • 12% reduction for diseased animals without clinical signs		Hileman et al,[68] 2018

	Dose	Treatment		
		Species, Outcome		
Terbinafine	Nebulization: 2 mg/mL at 20–30 min, maintained therapeutic blood levels for 12 h	Cottonmouths		Kane et al,[76] 2017
Terbinafine	Subcutaneous implants: 26.4 mg lasted 5 wk at therapeutic blood levels	Cottonmouths		Kane et al,[76] 2017
Voriconazole	Single subcutaneous dose: 5 mg/kg Subcutaneous osmotic pump: 1.02–1.6 mg/kg/h Subcutaneous osmotic pump: 12.1–17.5 mg/kg/h	Cottonmouths, 4 died, 3 lived Eastern massasaugas (N = 2), not efficacious Timber rattlesnake (N = 1), maintained levels		Lindemann et al,[77] 2017 Lindemann et al,[77] 2017 Lindemann et al,[77] 2017
Itraconazole	Intracloacal: 10 mg/kg Oral: 10 mg/kg every 24 every 7 d for 3 wk	Cottonmouths, not efficacious Bocourt water snakes and a Pueblan milk snake, clinical resolution with cotherapy (enilconazole)		Lindemann et al,[77] 2017 Picquet et al,[55] 2018
Enilconazole	Topical: 2 mg/mL every 4 d for 1 mo	Bocourt water snakes and a Pueblan milk snake, clinical resolution with cotherapy (itraconazole)		Picquet et al,[55] 2018
Treatment notes	Adjunctive treatments include surgical debridement, fluid therapy, antibiotics, and increased environmental temperature			

	Disinfection		
Contact Time	Effective Agents	Noneffective Agents	
2, 5, 10 min	3% and 10% bleach Benzalkonium chloride 0.16% 70% Ethanol		Rzadkowska et al,[78] 2016
10 min	Lysol power bathroom cleaner Lysol all-purpose cleaner CLR 409 NPD quaternary ammonium 0.4% 70% ethanol		Rzadkowska et al,[78] 2016
Any concentration or contact time		Nolvasan 2% Simple Green Spectracide Immunox (propiconazole) in high and low formulations – did not inactive spores	Rzadkowska et al,[78] 2016

Data from Refs.[41,55,68,76–79]

groups), *Citrobacter freundii* (groups B and C), and *Klebsiella* (group C) were isolated from the lungs of clinical snakes. The authors concluded that viral strains differed in pathogenicity, and that primary lung damage and suppression of the host immune response significantly influences further disease processes.

Sunviridae

In 2012, a novel virus was found during an investigation of an outbreak of neurorespiratory disease in a collection of Australian pythons. Hindbrain white matter spongiosis and gliosis, with extension to the surrounding gray matter and neuronal necrosis were noted in severe cases. Sixty-three percent of infected snakes also had mild bronchointerstitial pneumonia.[89] Phylogenetic analyses supported the clustering of this virus within the order Mononegavirales, near the subfamily Paramyxovirinae.[89] When the subfamilies Paramyxoviridae and Pneumoviridae were reclassified as distinct mononegaviral families, this virus (sunshine virus) was recognized as the first member of a novel family, Sunviridae.[90] Findings from naturally infected animals from 2 collections showed that PCR testing of brain, kidney, lung, and liver (in order of preference) were suitable tissues.[89] Vertical transmission was demonstrated from PCR-positive dam and sire carpet pythons.[91] Sunshine virus was detected in extraembryonic membranes (allantois and amnion) and embryonic tissues but not on the surface of each egg (21 viable, 3 nonviable). The nonviable embryos were PCR positive for sunshine virus. Recently, a novel sunvirus with 69% homology to sunshine virus was discovered in an outbreak of respiratory disease in sidewinders (*Crotalus cerastes*) in a North American zoo.[92] A qPCR assay found greater numbers of virus present in tracheal washes than in blood or buffy coats.

Bornaviridae

The family Bornaviridae are neurotropic viruses in the order Mononegavirales. Borna disease virus causes encephalitis in mammals, and other bornaviruses cause ganglioneuritis in birds. Bornaviruses were found when sequencing RNA from the venom gland of a Gaboon viper (*Bitis gabonicus*).[93] A bornaviral genome was also found in a museum specimen of an African garter snake.[94] Unfortunately, there were no clinical data from either case. Through next-generation sequencing, a novel bornavirus was found in pythons (*Morelia spilota* and *Antaresia* sp) from Australia with progressive caudal paresis, flaccid paralysis, delayed righting reflex, and incoordination.[95] The virus (carpet python bornavirus) was divergent at the level of a novel genus and classified as the first member of a novel genus, *Carbovirus*, while previously known bornaviruses were classified as *Orthobornavirus*.[90] Twenty-seven snakes were PCR positive for carboviruses, 12 of which had neurologic signs. On necropsy, 4 affected snakes had nonsuppurative encephalitis, as did 2 of the 15 PCR-positive snakes without neurologic signs.[95]

Bornaviruses are atypical RNA viruses that replicate in the nucleus, where they are more likely to be reverse transcribed and incorporated into host genomes. It has been demonstrated that partial viruses incorporated into host genomes are protective against related viruses. The closest relatives of carboviruses are viral genes that were only incorporated into mammal genomes approximately 70 million years ago, just prior to the end-Cretaceous extinction event that killed the big dinosaurs. This may have protected the mammals from carboviral infection and provided a selective advantage in the recovery from this extinction event.[95]

Nidovirales

The Nidovirales are an order of large, enveloped viruses with nonsegmented positive-sense RNA genomes; members infecting vertebrates include the families Coronaviridae, Arteriviridae, and Tobaniviridae.

Tobaniviridae

In 2014, novel divergent nidoviral pathogens in the family Tobaniviridae were characterized in ball pythons in the United States and Indian pythons in Germany. Affected snakes suffered from a severe proliferative pneumonia, stomatitis, tracheitis, and esophagitis.[96–98] These nidoviruses are now classified within the subfamily Serpentovirinae.[99,100] The highest viral load was found in respiratory tissues, particularly the lungs.[101] Experimental challenge with ball python nidovirus 1 found that disease transmission is likely through oral secretions and feces. The virus causes mucinous chronic inflammation and proliferative interstitial pneumonia; choanal and oral/esophageal swabs are good samples for antemortem diagnosis.[100] This virus appears to be the most clinically significant disease of ball pythons.

There is considerable diversity of tobaniviruses now being characterized from snakes. A serpentovirus has been reported to cause respiratory disease in green tree pythons.[102] A study of 201 snake oral swabs submitted in Europe found a serpentovirus PCR prevalence of 27.4% in pythons and 2.4% in boas.[101] In a study of antemortem swabs from 639 snakes from 62 species from 12 US collections, 54 new tobanivirus genotypes were identified.[100] The overall serpentovirus prevalence was 26%. Two major clades were identified. The first clade contained python-only sequences, including the previous ball python isolate and new isolates including those recovered from python species in the genera *Morelia*, *Python*, *Aspidites*, and *Antaresia*. Clinical disease was consistently observed for all virus genotypes detected in this clade. Longitudinal sampling of pythons in a single collection over 28 months revealed that serpentovirus infection is persistent, and viral clearance was not observed.[100] A 75% mortality rate was observed in pythons.

The second clade contained sequences from boas (genera *Corallus* and *Chilabothrus*), a colubrid (genus *Lampropeltis*), reticulated pythons (genus *Malayopython*) and sequences from colubrid and homalopsid snakes in China.[103] Within this second clade, clinical disease was not detected in boas, colubrids, or reticulated pythons.

The authors also detailed quarantine measures that may have reduced transmission (85% infection rate in quarantine vs 5% in the main collection), which included designated individuals or days for managing quarantined snakes, separate air flow and ventilation, shower-out procedures, quarantine-specific clothes, shoes, and equipment, 1-way flow of bedding and feeder rodents, disposable glove changes between racks and hand sanitizer disinfection of gloves between breed rotations in racks, and disinfection of all surfaces and instruments following use.[100]

Although there has been an investigative bias toward snakes, other reptiles also have tobaniviruses. A novel serpentovirus in wild shingle-back lizards (*Tiliqua rugosa*) with respiratory disease was documented in 2016.[104] Additionally, a novel serpentovirus has been implicated in a mortality event in endangered Bellinger River snapping turtles (*Myuchelys georgesi*).[105]

Arenaviridae

The family Arenaviridae are viruses with bipartite genomes in the order Bunyavirales. There are 3 genera, *Mammarenavirus*, *Reptarenavirus*, and *Hartmanivirus*, of which the first infects mammals and the latter 2 infect snakes.

Reptarenaviruses, the causative agents of inclusion body disease (BIBD) in henophid snakes, were characterized using high-throughput sequencing in 2012.[106] Two viruses that caused disease in annulated tree boas (*Corallus annulatus*) (California Academy of Sciences [CAS] virus) and 2 species of boa constrictors (Golden Gate virus [GGV]) were completely sequenced. A third partially characterized virus was isolated from a moribund boa (Collierville virus). The *Reptarenavirus* glycoprotein gene originates from a lateral gene transfer from filoviruses.[107,108] Additional divergent viruses were isolated in Europe.[107,109–112] In 123 infected snakes sampled in the United States, many were infected by more than 1 virus strain, and there was significant recombination between viruses, likely caused by mixing of geographically diverse species of infected snakes in captivity[107]. Reptarenaviruses infect not only henophids, but also asymptomatic colubrids.[113] As of April 2019, the International Committee on Taxonomy of Viruses listed 5 species in the genus Reptarenavirus: Golden reptarenavirus (GoGV), Rotterdam reptarenavirus (ROUTV and UHV), California reptarenavirus (CASV), ordinary reptarenavirus (TSMV-2), and G reptarenavirus (UGV1–3) (ICTV). Giessen reptarenavirus appears to be the most common in boa constrictors in the United STates.

Challenge studies showed that ball pythons infected with GoGV displayed severe neurologic signs within 2 months.[114] Viral replication was detected only in the central nervous system. Pronounced inflammation was observed. In contrast, GoGV-infected boa constrictors remained free of clinical signs for 2 years, despite high viral loads and the accumulation of large intracellular inclusions in multiple tissues, including the brain, without associated inflammation. Infected ball pythons remained RT-PCR negative on blood samples, whereas blood PCR detection in infected boas was consistent.[114] Another study looking at RT-PCR prevalence in esophageal swab versus blood samples in 30 snakes in Germany found that several animals with negative blood samples had positive esophageal swabs, including both pythons and boas.[112] Further study on shedding at different sites by different species is needed.

Transmission of the virus is thought to be primarily via contact with infected animals or contaminated materials. Most Bunyavirales are vectored by arthropods, and it has been hypothesized that reptarenaviruses may be transmitted by snake mites.[115] Reptarenaviruses can survive in arthropod cell lines.[111] Although cell culture studies initially found that *R reptarenavirus* only replicated in mouse cell cultures at lower temperatures,[116] experimental infection of mice with *R reptarenavirus* resulted in increasing virus titers detected by RT-qPCR along with minimal pathology.[117] Rodents are the primary reservoir hosts for mammarenaviruses. Reptarenaviruses may also be vertically transmitted.[118] It is strongly recommended that animals with BIBD/reptarenavirus infection not be bred.

Hartmanivirus contains 4 viruses that infect snakes: old schoolhouse virus, Dante Muikkunen virus, Veterinary Pathology Zurich virus, and Haartman Institute snake virus-1 (HISV-1).[119] *Reptarenavirus* and *Mammarenavirus* are more closely related to each other than to *Hartmanivirus*. Unlike reptarenaviruses, HISV-1 does not produce intracellular inclusion bodies. Hepojoki and colleagues[119] found HISV-1 to be slightly cytopathic for cultured boid cells, but histology and immunohistology showed no evidence of pathology. In a collection of 71 animals, 60% were found to be positive.

Further comments

The Association of Reptile and Amphibian Veterinarians' Infectious Disease Committee complies a quarterly list of reptile infectious disease publications in peer-reviewed literature, entitled "Infectious Diseases of Reptiles and Amphibians: Peer-Reviewed Publications." The lists are published in the Journal of Herpetological Medicine & Surgery and serve as a valuable resource for practitioners.

DISCLOSURE

The authors have nothing to disclose.

REFERENCES

1. Richter B, Nedorost N, Maderner A, et al. Detection of *Cryptosporidium* species in feces or gastric contents from snakes and lizards as determined by polymerase chain reaction analysis and partial sequencing of the 18S ribosomal RNA gene. J Vet Diagn Invest 2011;23(3):430–5.
2. da Silva DC, Paiva PR, Nakamura AA, et al. The detection of *Cryptosporidium serpentis* in snake fecal samples by real-time PCR. Vet Parasitol 2014; 204(3–4):134–8.
3. Fall A, Thompson RA, Hobbs RP, et al. Morphology is not a reliable tool for delineating species within *Cryptosporidium*. J Parasitol 2009;89(2):399–402.
4. Graczyk TK, Cranfield MR, Fayer R. A comparative assessment of direct fluorescence antibody, modified acid-fast stain, and sucrose flotation techniques for detection of *Cryptosporidium serpentis* oocysts in snake fecal specimens. J Zoo Wildl Med 1995;1:396–402.
5. Pavlasek I, Ryan U. *Cryptosporidium varanii* takes precedence over C. saurophilum. Exp Parasitol 2008;118(3):434–7.
6. Kik MJ, van Asten AJ, Lenstra JA, et al. Cloaca prolapse and cystitis in green iguana (Iguana iguana) caused by a novel *Cryptosporidium* species. Vet Parasitol 2011;175(1):165–7.
7. Abe N, Makino I. Multilocus genotypic analysis of *Cryptosporidium* isolates from cockatiels, Japan. Parasitol Res 2010;106(6):1491–7.
8. Xiao X, Qi R, Han HJ, et al. Molecular identification and phylogenetic analysis of *Cryptosporidium, Hepatozoon* and *Spirometra* in snakes from central China. Int J Parasitol Parasites Wildl 2019;10:274–9.
9. Curtiss JB, Leone AM, Wellehan JFX, et al. Renal and cloacal cryptosporidiosis (*Cryptosporidium avian* genotype V) in a major Mitchell's Cockatoo Lophochroa leadbeateri. J Zoo Wildl Med 2015;46(4):934–7.
10. Kuroki T, Izumiyama S, Yagita K, et al. Occurrence of Cryptosporidium sp. In snakes in Japan. Parasitol Res 2008;103(4):801–5.
11. Osman M, El Safadi D, Benamrouz-Vanneste S, et al. Prevalence, transmission, and host specificity of *Cryptosporidium* spp. in various animal groups from two French zoos. Parasitol Res 2017;116(12):3419–22.
12. Xiao L, Ryan UM, Graczyk TK, et al. Genetic diversity of *Cryptosporidium* spp. In captive reptiles. Appl Environ Microbiol 2004;70(2):891–9.
13. Graczyk TK, Cranfield MR. Experimental transmission of *Cryptosporidium oocyst* isolates from mammals, birds and reptiles to captive snakes. Vet Res 1998;29(2):187–96.
14. Grosset C, Villeneuve A, Brieger A, et al. Cryptosporidiosis in juvenile bearded dragons (*Pogona vitticeps*): effects of treatment with paromomycin. J Herpetol Med Surg 2011;21(1):10–5.
15. Gałęcki R, Sokół R. Treatment of cryptosporidiosis in captive green iguanas (Iguana iguana). Vet Parasitol 2018;252:17–21.
16. Latney L, Wellehan J. Selected emerging infectious diseases of squamata. Vet Clin North Am Exot Anim Pract 2013;16(2):319–38.
17. Rivas AE, Boyer DM, Torregrosa K, et al. Treatment of *Cryptosporidium serpentis* infection in a king cobra (Ophiophagus hannah) with paromomycin. J Zoo Wildl Med 2018;49(4):1061–3.
18. Wilson J, Margolin AB. Efficacy of glutaraldehyde disinfectant against *Cryptosporidium parvum* in the presence of various organic soils. J AOAC Int 2003; 86(1):96–100.

19. Robertson LJ, Casaert S, Valdez-Nava Y, et al. Drying of *Cryptosporidium* oocysts and *Giardia* cysts to slides abrogates use of vital dyes for viability staining. J Microbiol Methods 2014;96:68–9.

20. Duhain GL, Minnaar A, Buys EM. Effect of chlorine, blanching, freezing, and microwave heating on *Cryptosporidium parvum* viability inoculated on green peppers. J Food Prot 2012;75(5):936–41.

21. Shahiduzzaman M, Dyachenko V, Keidel J, et al. Combination of cell culture and quantitative PCR (cc-qPCR) to assess disinfectants efficacy on *Cryptosporidium* oocysts under standardized conditions. Vet Parasitol 2010;167(1):43–9.

22. Wellehan JF, Turenne C, Heard DJ, et al. Dermatophilus chelonae in a king cobra (Ophiophagus hannah). J Zoo Wildl Med 2004;35(4):553–6.

23. Jiang H, Zhang X, Li L, et al. Identification of *Austwickia chelonae* as cause of cutaneous granuloma in endangered crocodile lizards using metataxonomics. PeerJ 2019;7:e6574.

24. Mansfield MJ, Sugiman-Marangos SN, Melnyk RA, et al. Identification of a diphtheria toxin-like gene family beyond the Corynebacterium genus. FEBS Lett 2018;592(16):2693–705.

25. Martel A, Pasmans F, Hellebuyck T, et al. Devriesea agamarum gen. nov., sp. nov., a novel actinobacterium associated with dermatitis and septicaemia in agamid lizards. Int J Syst Evol Microbiol 2008;58(9):2206–9.

26. Lukac M, Horvatek-Tomic D, Prukner-Radovcic E, et al. Findings of *Devriesea agamarum* associated infections in spiny-tailed lizards (Uromastyx sp.) in Croatia. J Zoo Wildl Med 2013;44(2):430–4.

27. Rossier C, Hoby S, Wenker C, et al. Devriesea in a Plumed basilisk (Basiliscus pulmfrons) and Chinese water dragons (Physignathus cocincinus) in a zoological collection. J Zoo Wildl Med 2016;47(1):280–5.

28. Hellebuyck T, Questel K, Pasmans F, et al. A virulent clone of *Devriesea agamarum* affects endangered Lesser Antillean iguanas (Iguana delicatissima). Sci Rep 2017;7(1):12491–7.

29. Hellebuyck T, Martel A, Chiers K, et al. *Devriesea agamarum* causes dermatitis in bearded dragons (Pogona vitticeps). Vet Microbiol 2009;134(3):267–71.

30. Hellebuyck T, Pasmans F, Haesebrouck F, et al. Designing a successful antimicrobial treatment against *Devriesea agamarum* infections in lizards. Vet Microbiol 2009;139(1):189–92.

31. Devloo R, Martel A, Hellebuyck T, et al. Bearded dragons (Pogona vitticeps) asymptomatically infected with *Devriesea agamarum* are a source of persistent clinical infection in captive colonies of dab lizards (Uromastyx sp.). Vet Microbiol 2011;150:297–301.

32. Hellebuyck T, Pasmans F, Blooi M, et al. Prolonged environmental persistence requires efficient disinfection procedures to control *Devriesea agamarum* associated disease in lizards. Lett Appl Microbiol 2011;52(1):28–32.

33. Fisher MC, Henk DA, Briggs CJ, et al. Emerging fungal threats to animal, plant and ecosystem health. Nature 2012;484(7393):186–94.

34. Alroy J. Current extinction rates of reptiles and amphibians. Proc Natl Acad Sci U S A 2015;112(42):13003–8.

35. Böhm M, Williams R, Bramhall HR, et al. Correlates of extinction risk in squamate reptiles: the relative importance of biology, geography, threat and range size. Glob Ecol Biogeogr 2016;25(4):391–405.

36. Ripple WJ, Wolf C, Newsome TM, et al. Extinction risk is most acute for the world's largest and smallest vertebrates. Proc Natl Acad Sci 2017;114(40): 10678–83.

37. Stchigel AM, Sutton DA, Cano-Lira JF, et al. Phylogeny of chrysosporia infecting reptiles: proposal of the new family Nannizziopsiaceae and five new species. Persoonia 2013;31:86–100.
38. Sigler L, Hambleton S, Paré JA. Molecular characterization of reptile pathogens currently known as members of the *Chrysosporium* anamorph of Nannizziopsis vriesii complex and relationship with some human-associated isolates. J Clin Microbiol 2013;51(10):3338–57.
39. Sigler L, Hambleton S, Paré JA. Molecular characterization of reptile pathogens currently known as members of the chrysosporium anamorph of nannizziopsis vriesii complex and relationship with some human-associated isolates. JCM 2013;51(10):3338–57.
40. Wellehan JF, Divers SJ. Mycology. In: Mader DR, Divers SJ, Stahl SJ, editors. Reptile and amphibian medicine and surgery. 3rd edition. St Louis (MO): WB Saunders; 2019. p. 270–80.
41. Paré JA, Sigler L. An overview of reptile fungal pathogens in the genera *Nannizziopsis, Paranannizziopsis*, and *Ophidiomyces*. J Herpetol Med Surg 2016; 26(1–2):46–53.
42. Schneider J, Heydel T, Klasen L, et al. Characterization of *Nannizziopsis guarroi* with genomic and proteomic analysis in three lizard species. Med Mycol 2018; 56(5):610–20.
43. Le Donne V, Crossland N, Brandão J, et al. *Nannizziopsis guarroi* infection in 2 inland bearded dragons (Pogona vitticeps): clinical, cytologic, histologic, and ultrastructural aspects. Vet Clin Pathol 2016;45(2):368–75.
44. Rhim H, Han JI. *Nannizziopsis chlamydospora* associated necrotizing dermatomycosis in a bearded dragon (Pogona vitticeps). J Exot Pet Med 2019;31:1–2.
45. Abarca ML, Martorell J, Castella G, et al. Dermatomycosis in a pet inland bearded dragon (Pogona vitticeps) caused by a *Chrysosporium* species related to Nannizziopsis vriesii. Vet Dermatol 2009;20:295–9.
46. Schmidt-Ukaj S, Loncaric I, Spergser J, et al. Dermatomycosis in three central bearded dragons (Pogona vitticeps) associated with *Nannizziopsis chlamydospora*. J Vet Diagn Invest 2016;28(3):319–22.
47. Paré JA, Sigler L, Hunter DB, et al. Cutaneous mycoses in chameleons caused by the *Chrysosporium* anamorph of *Nannizziopsis vriesii* (Apinis) Currah. J Zoo Wildl Med 1997;28(4):443–53.
48. Bertelsen MF, Crawshaw GJ, Sigler L, et al. Fatal cutaneous mycosis in tentacled snakes (Erpeton tentaculatum caused by the *Chrysosporium* anamorph of *Nannizziopsis vriesii*. J Zoo Wildl Med 2005;36(1):82–7.
49. Nichols DK. Case 4, skin-snake. In: AFIP WSC Conference, 23. 2009. Available at: http://www.askjpc.org/wsco/wsc_showcase2. php?id=204. Accessed October 1, 2019.
50. Hill AG, Sandy JR, Begg A. Mycotic dermatitis in juvenile freshwater crocodiles (Crocodylus johnstoni) caused by *Nannizziopsis crocodili*. J Zoo Wildl Med 2019;50(1):225–30.
51. Humphrey S, Alexander S, Ha HJ. Detection of *Paranannizziopsis australasiensis* in tuatara (Sphenodon punctatus) using fungal culture and a generic fungal PCR. N Z Vet J 2016;64(5):298–300.
52. Rainwater KL, Wiederhold NP, Sutton DA, et al. Novel *Paranannizziopsis* species in a Wagler's viper (Tropidolaemus wagleri), tentacled snakes (Erpeton tentaculatum), and a rhinoceros snake (Rhynchophis boulengeri) in a zoological collection. Med Mycol 2018;57(7):825–32.

53. Franklinos LH, Lorch JM, Bohuski E, et al. Emerging fungal pathogen *Ophidiomyces ophiodiicola* in wild European snakes. Sci Rep 2017;7(1):3844.

54. Ohkura M, Fitak RR, Wisecaver JH, et al. Genome sequence of *Ophidiomyces ophiodiicola*, an emerging fungal pathogen of snakes. Genome Announc 2017; 5(30):e00677-17.

55. Picquet P, Heckers KO, Kolesnik E, et al. Detection of *Ophidiomyces ophiodiicola* in two captive bocourt water snakes (subsessor bocourti) and one captive pueblan milk snake (lampropeltis triangulum campbelli). J Zoo Wildl Med 2018; 49(1):219–22.

56. Guthrie AL, Knowles S, Ballmann AE, et al. Detection of snake fungal disease due to *Ophidiomyces ophiodiicola* in Virginia, USA. J Wildl Dis 2015;52(1): 143–9.

57. Ohkura M, Worley JJ, Hughes-Hallett JE, et al. *Ophidiomyces ophiodiicola* on a captive black racer (Coluber constrictor) and a garter snake (Thamnophis sirtalis) in Pennsylvania. J Zoo Wildl Med 2016;47(1):341–6.

58. Cheatwood JL, Jacobson ER, May PG, et al. An outbreak of fungal dermatitis and stomatitis in a free-ranging population of pigmy rattlesnakes (Sistrurus miliarius barbouri) in Florida. J Wildl Dis 2003;39(2):329–37.

59. Paré JA. Update on fungal infections in reptiles. In: Mader DR, Divers SJ, editors. Current therapy in reptile medicine and surgery. 1st edition. St. Louis: Saunders; 2014. p. 53–6.

60. Sleeman JM. Snake fungal disease in the United States National Wildlife Health Center Wildlife Health Bulletin 2013–02. United States Geological Survey, Madison, WI. Available at: http://www.nwhc.usgs.gov/publications/wildlife_health_bulletins/WHB_2013-02_Snake_Fungal_Disease.pdf. Accessed October 1, 2019.

61. Dolinski AC, Allender MC, Hsiao V, et al. Systemic *Ophidiomyces ophiodiicola* infection in a free-ranging plains garter snake (Thamnophis radix). J Herpetol Med Surg 2014;24(1):7–10.

62. Ravesi MJ, Tetzlaff SJ, Allender MC, et al. Detection of snake fungal disease from a Lampropeltis triangulum (eastern milksnake) in northern Michigan. Northeast Naturalist 2016;23(3):18–21.

63. Last LA, Fenton H, Gonyor-McGuire J, et al. Snake fungal disease caused by *Ophidiomyces ophiodiicola* in a free-ranging mud snake (Farancia abacura). J Vet Diagn Invest 2016;28(6):709–13.

64. Allender MC, Hileman E, Moore J, et al. Ophidiomyces detection in the eastern massasauga in Michigan. Report prepared for the US fish and wildlife service, East Lansing Field Office, Michigan. 2014. Available at: https://www.researchgate. net/profile/Sasha_Tetzlaff/publication/280134467_Ophidiomyces_detection_in_the_ Eastern_Massasauga_in_Michigan/links/55ac3da308aea3d08685ebde.pdf. Accessed October 1, 2019.

65. Allender MC, Junge RE, Baker-Wylie S, et al. Plasma electrophoretic profiles in the eastern massasauga (Sistrurus catenatus) and influences of age, sex, year, location, and snake fungal disease. J Zoo Wildl Med 2015;46(4):767–73.

66. Allender MC, Phillips CA, Baker SJ, et al. Hematology in an eastern massasauga (Sistrurus catenatus) population and the emergence of *Ophidiomyces* in Illinois, USA. J Wildl Dis 2016;52(2):258–69.

67. Allender MC, Hileman ET, Moore J, et al. Detection of *Ophidiomyces*, the causative agent of snake fungal disease, in the eastern massasauga (Sistrurus catenatus) in Michigan, USA, 2014. J Wildl Dis 2016;52(3):694–8.

68. Hileman ET, Allender MC, Bradke DR, et al. Estimation of *Ophidiomyces* prevalence to evaluate snake fungal disease risk. J Wildl Manag 2018;82(1):173–81.

69. Lind CM, McCoy CM, Farrell TM. Tracking outcomes of snake fungal disease in free-ranging pygmy rattlesnakes (Sistrurus miliarius). J Wildl Dis 2018;54(2):352–6.

70. Lind CM, Clark A, Smiley-Walters SA, et al. Interactive effects of food supplementation and snake fungal disease on pregnant pygmy rattlesnakes and their offspring. J Herpetol 2019;53(4):282–8.

71. McBride MP, Wojick KB, Georoff TA, et al. Ophidiomyces ophiodiicola dermatitis in eight free-ranging timber rattlesnakes (Crotalus horridus) from Massachusetts. J Zoo Wildl Med 2015;46(1):86–94.

72. Nordberg EJ, Cobb VA. Body temperatures and winter activity in overwintering timber rattlesnakes (Crotalus Horridus) In Tennessee, USA. Herpetol Conserv Biol 2017;12(3):606–15.

73. Allender MC, Raudabaugh DB, Gleason FH, et al. The natural history, ecology, and epidemiology of *Ophidiomyces ophiodiicola* and its potential impact on free-ranging snake populations. Fungal Ecol 2015;17:187–96.

74. Chandler HC, Allender MC, Stegenga BS, et al. Ophidiomycosis prevalence in Georgia's Eastern Indigo Snake (Drymarchon couperi) populations. PLoS One 2019;14(6):e0218351.

75. Robertson J, Chinnadurai SK, Woodburn DB, et al. Disseminated *Ophidiomyces ophiodiicola* infection in a captive eastern massasauga (Sistrurus catenatus catenatus). J Zoo Wildl Med 2016;47(1):337–40.

76. Kane LP, Allender MC, Archer G, et al. Pharmacokinetics of nebulized and subcutaneously implanted terbinafine in cottonmouths (Agkistrodon piscivorus). J Vet Pharmacol Ther 2017;40(5):575–9.

77. Lindemann DM, Allender MC, Rzadkowska M, et al. Pharmacokinetics, efficacy, and safety of voriconazole and itraconazole in healthy cottonmouths (Agkistrodon piscivorus) and massasauga rattlesnakes (Sistrurus catenatus) with snake fungal disease. J Zoo Wildl Med 2017;48(3):757–66.

78. Rzadkowska M, Allender MC, O'Dell M, et al. Evaluation of common disinfectants effective against *Ophidiomyces ophiodiicola*, the causative agent of snake fungal disease. J Wildl Dis 2016;52(3):759–62.

79. ICTV. Virus taxonomy: 2017 release. Available at: https://talk.ictvonline.org/taxonomy/. Accessed October 30, 2019.

80. Pees M, Schmidt V, Papp T, et al. Three genetically distinct ferlaviruses have varying effects on infected corn snakes (Pantherophis guttatus). PLoS One 2019;14(6):e0217164.

81. Jacobson ER, Origgi F, Pessier AP, et al. Paramyxovirus infection in caiman lizards (Draecena guianensis). J Vet Diagn Invest 2001;13(2):143–51.

82. Abbas MD, Ball I, Ruckova Z, et al. Virological screening of bearded dragons (Pogona vitticeps) and the first detection of paramyxoviruses in this species. J Herpetol Med Surg 2012;22(3):86–90.

83. Marschang RE, Papp T, Frost JW. Comparison of paramyxovirus isolates from snakes, lizards and a tortoise. Virus Res 2009;144:272–9, pmid:19501125.

84. Solis C, Arguedas R, Baldi M, et al. Seroprevalence and molecular characterization of ferlavirus in captive vipers of Costa Rica. J Zoo Wildl Med 2017;48(2):420–30.

85. Marschang RE. Viruses infecting reptiles. Viruses 2011;3(11):2087–126.

86. Papp T, Pees M, Schmidt V, et al. RT-PCR diagnosis followed by sequence characterization of paramyxoviruses in clinical samples from snakes reveals concurrent infections within populations and/or individuals. Vet Microbiol 2010; 144(3–4):466–72.

87. Jacobson ER. Viruses and viral diseases of reptiles. In: Jacobson ER, editor. Diseases and pathology of reptiles. Boca Raton (FL): Taylor and Francis; 2007. p. 395–460.

88. Neul A, Schrödl W, Marschang RE, et al. Immunologic responses in corn snakes (Pantherophis guttatus) after experimentally induced infection with ferlaviruses. Am J Vet Res 2017;78(4):482–94.

89. Hyndman TH, Marschang RE, Wellehan JF Jr, et al. Isolation and molecular identification of sunshine virus, a novel paramyxovirus found in Australian snakes. Infect Genet Evol 2012;12(7):1436–46.

90. Amarasinghe GK, Arechiga Ceballos NG, Banyard AC, et al. Taxonomy of the Mononegavirales: update 2018. Arch Virol 2018;163(8):2283–94.

91. Hyndman TH, Johnson RS. Evidence for the vertical transmission of Sunshine virus. Vet Microbiol 2015;175(2–4):179–84.

92. Wellehan J, Rivera S, Ossiboff R, et al. Identification of a novel sunshine virus in sidewinders (Crotalus cerastes) with pneumonia in North America. Proceedings of the 9th World Congress of Herpetology. Dunedin, New Zealand, January 5-10, 2020.

93. Francischetti IM, My-Pham V, Harrison J, et al. Bitis gabonica (Gaboon viper) snake venom gland: toward a catalog for the full-length transcripts (cDNA) and proteins. Gene 2004;337:55–69.

94. Stenglein MD, Leavitt EB, Abramovitch MA, et al. Genome sequence of a bornavirus recovered from an African garter snake (Elapsoidea loveridgei). Genome Announc 2014;2(5) [pii:e00779-14].

95. Hyndman TH, Shilton CM, Stenglein MD, et al. Divergent bornaviruses from Australian carpet pythons with neurological disease date the origin of extant Bornaviridae prior to the end-Cretaceous extinction. PLoS Pathog 2018;14(2):e1006881.

96. Stenglein MD, Jacobson ER, Wozniak EJ, et al. Ball python nidovirus: a candidate etiologic agent for severe respiratory disease in Python regius. mBio 2014;5(5):e01484-14.

97. Uccellini L, Ossiboff RJ, De Matos RE, et al. Identification of a novel nidovirus in an outbreak of fatal respiratory disease in ball pythons (Python regius). Virol J 2014;11(1):144.

98. Bodewes R, Lempp C, Schürch AC, et al. Novel divergent nidovirus in a python with pneumonia. J Gen Virol 2014;95(11):2480–5.

99. Ziebuhr J, Baric RS, Baker S, et al. Reorganization of the family Coronaviridae into two families, Coronaviridae (including the current subfamily Coronavirinae and the new subfamily Letovirinae) and the new family Tobaniviridae (accommodating the current subfamily Torovirinae and three other subfamilies), revision of the genus rank structure and introduction of a new subgenus rank. In: International Committee on Taxonomy of Viruses. University of Otago, New Zealand, 2018.

100. Hoon-Hanks LL, Ossiboff RJ, Bartolini P, et al. Longitudinal and cross-sectional sampling of serpentovirus (nidovirus) infection in captive snakes reveals high prevalence, persistent infection, and increased mortality in pythons and divergent serpentovirus infection in boas and colubrids. Front Vet Sci 2019;338(6):1–17.

101. Marschang RE, Kolesnik E. Detection of nidoviruses in live pythons and boas. Tierarztliche Praxis Ausgabe K Kleintiere/heimtiere 2017;45(1):22–6.

102. Dervas E, Hepojoki J, Laimbacher A, et al. Nidovirus-associated proliferative pneumonia in the green tree python (Morelia viridis). J Virol 2017;91(21): e00718-17.
103. Shi M, Lin X-D, Chen X, et al. The evolutionary history of vertebrate RNA viruses. Nature 2018;556:197–202.
104. O'Dea MA, Jackson B, Jackson C, et al. Discovery and partial genomic characterisation of a novel nidovirus associated with respiratory disease in wild shingleback lizards (Tiliqua rugosa). PLoS One 2016;11(11):e0165209.
105. Zhang J, Finlaison DS, Frost MJ, et al. Identification of a novel nidovirus as a potential cause of large scale mortalities in the endangered Bellinger River snapping turtle (Myuchelys georgesi). PLoS One 2018;13(10):e0205209.
106. Stenglein MD, Sanders C, Kistler AL, et al. Identification, characterization, and in vitro culture of highly divergent arenaviruses from boa constrictors and annulated tree boas: candidate etiological agents for snake inclusion body disease. mBio 2012;3. e00180–00112.
107. Stenglein MD, Jacobson ER, Chang LW, et al. Widespread recombination, reassortment, and transmission of unbalanced compound viral genotypes in natural arenavirus infections. PLoS Pathog 2015;11(5):e1004900.
108. Koellhoffer JF, Dai Z, Malashkevich VN, et al. Structural characterization of the glycoprotein GP2 core domain from the CAS virus, a novel arenavirus-like species. J Mol Biol 2013;426:1452–68.
109. Bodewes R, Kik MJ, Raj VS, et al. Detection of novel divergent arenaviruses in boid snakes with inclusion body disease in The Netherlands. J Gen Virol 2013; 94(6):1206–10.
110. Hetzel U, Sironen T, Laurinmäki P, et al. Isolation, identification, and characterization of novel arenaviruses, the etiological agents of boid inclusion body disease. J Virol 2013;87(20):10918–35.
111. Hepojoki J, Salmenperä P, Sironen T, et al. Arenavirus coinfections are common in snakes with boid inclusion body disease. J Virol 2015;89(16):8657–60.
112. Aqrawi T, Stöhr AC, Knauf-Witzens T, et al. Identification of snake arenaviruses in live boas and pythons in a zoo in Germany. Tierärztl Prax Aus K Kleintiere Heimtiere 2015;43:239–47.
113. Hyndman TH, Marschang RE, Bruce M, et al. Reptarenaviruses in apparently healthy snakes in an Australian zoological collection. Aus Vet J 2019;97(4): 93–102.
114. Stenglein MD, Guzman DS, Garcia VE, et al. Differential disease susceptibilities in experimentally reptarenavirus-infected boa constrictors and ball pythons. J Virol 2017;91(15):e00451-17.
115. Chang L, Jacobson ER. Inclusion body disease, A worldwide infectious disease of boid snakes: a review. J Exot Pet Med 2010;19(3):216–25.
116. Hepojoki J, Kipar A, Korzyukov Y, et al. Replication of Boid inclusion body disease-associated arenaviruses is temperature sensitive in both boid and mammalian cells. J Virol 2015;89:1119–28.
117. Abba Y, Hassim H, Hamzah H, et al. Pathological vicissitudes and oxidative stress enzyme responses in mice experimentally infected with reptarenavirus (isolate UPM/MY01). Microb Pathog 2017;104:17–27.
118. Keller S, Hetzel U, Sironen T, et al. Co-infecting reptarenaviruses can be vertically transmitted in boa constrictor. PLoS Pathog 2017;13(1):e1006179.
119. Hepojoki J, Hepojoki S, Smura T, et al. Characterization of Haartman Institute snake virus-1 (HISV-1) and HISV-like viruses—the representatives of genus Hartmanivirus, family Arenaviridae. PLoS Pathog 2018;14(11):e1007415.

Updates on Thyroid Disease in Rabbits and Guinea Pigs

Peter M. DiGeronimo, VMD, MSc[a,b,*], João Brandão, LMV, MS, DECZM (Avian)[c]

KEYWORDS

- *Cavia porcellus* • Guinea pig • Hyperthyroidism • *Oryctolagus cuniculus* • Rabbit
- Thyroxine

KEY POINTS

- Hyperthyroidism is not uncommon in guinea pigs and may be underdiagnosed, albeit rare, in rabbits.
- Prevalence of thyroid disease in guinea pigs and rabbits is likely to increase because of the availability of clinical veterinary literature in English.
- In guinea pigs, disease may be more common in older animals, with no clear sex or breed predilections.
- Clinical signs of hyperthyroidism in guinea pigs may include weight loss, palpable cervical mass, behavioral changes, poor coat quality, polyuria and/or polydipsia, tachycardia, and tachypnea.
- Diagnosis is supported by clinical signs and elevated circulating thyroxine concentrations.

INTRODUCTION

Some of the earliest reports of naturally occurring primary thyroid disease in guinea pigs in the English-language veterinary literature were in the 1970s.[1,2] Since then, few clinically relevant papers were published prior to a review of guinea pig thyroid disease by Mayer and colleagues[3] in 2010. The authors observed that at the time of publication there had been few reports of spontaneous hyperthyroidism in guinea pigs in the English literature, although the disease had been commonly reported in the German literature. They speculated that guinea pig thyroid disease is likely under-reported given the difficulty to arrive at a definitive diagnosis and given that evidence of the disease was largely anecdotal for the English-speaking community. This was substantiated by a retrospective study of thyroid gland neoplasms in guinea pigs that has since been published in the peer-reviewed literature.[4] Subsequent reviews on the topic have thoroughly summarized the clinical literature.[5–7] Additionally, several

[a] Adventure Aquarium, 1 Riverside Drive, Camden, NJ 08103, USA; [b] Animal & Bird Health Care Center, 1785 Springdale Road, Cherry Hill, NJ 08003, USA; [c] Department of Veterinary Clinical Sciences, College of Veterinary Medicine, Oklahoma State University, 2065 W. Farm Road, Stillwater, OK 74078, USA
* Corresponding author.
E-mail address: pmdigeronimo@gmail.com

Vet Clin Exot Anim 23 (2020) 373–381
https://doi.org/10.1016/j.cvex.2020.01.007
1094-9194/20/© 2020 Elsevier Inc. All rights reserved.
vetexotic.theclinics.com

papers have been published in English, including a case series[8] and case report[9] of confirmed hyperthyroidism in guinea pigs and a retrospective study on hyperthyroidism in guinea pigs in Germany.[10] This article will review the most recent advancements in the understanding of guinea pig thyroid disease in light of these publications. For more comprehensive reviews on the etiology, diagnosis, and treatment of rodent endocrine disease, readers are directed to previous publications.[5–7]

PATHOLOGY

Hyperthyroidism was diagnosed in 1.3% of guinea pigs (4 of 309 cases) presented to a veterinary referral hospital in Austria over a 30-month period.[8] This supports previous speculations that hyperthyroidism is a rare, likely underdiagnosed disease in guinea pigs. In a retrospective study of guinea pig case submissions to a veterinary pathology service over 10 years, thyroid neoplasms comprised 3.6% of cases (19 out of 526 submissions).[4] Thyroid tumors were the fifth most common neoplasia after lipomas, trichoepitheliomas, lymphoid neoplasms, and mammary gland neoplasms.[4] Among the thyroid neoplasias, 12 of these (63%) were adenomas, and 7 (37%) were carcinomas.[4] Only grossly enlarged glands were included in the study, and thus prevalence may be greater in cases of thyroid disease without gross enlargement of the glands. In a retrospective study of tumors and tumor-like lesions of the cervix and uterus of guinea pigs, 1 out of 83 animals (1.2%) examined had a concurrent thyroid adenoma along with a nonmetastatic malignant mixed Müllerian uterine tumor, integumentary sarcoma, and a bronchial adenoma.[11] One single case report also described a case of a thyroid adenoma in an approximately 5-year-old male guinea pig with an ectopic thyroid carcinoma at the base of heart.[12]

SIGNALMENT

Previous reviews suggested anecdotally that female guinea pigs may be more predisposed to hyperthyroidism than male guinea pigs.[3] In the previously mentioned retrospective study of 19 cases of thyroid neoplasms, 10 were from female guinea pigs, 7 from male guinea pigs, and 2 from animals of unknown sex.[4] Of 40 cases of guinea pigs with elevated total thyroxine measured using a canine chemiluminescence immunoassay ($TT_4 > 66.9$ nmol/L [>5.2 µg/dL]), 21 were intact female guinea pigs, 11 intact male guinea pigs, 7 castrated male guinea pigs, and 1 of unknown sex.[10] Hyperthyroidism has also been documented in a neutered female guinea pig.[8] Diagnosis of hyperthyroidism may be positively associated with age. The median age of animals with elevated TT_4 was 5 years (range 2–8 years).[10] The age of animals with confirmed thyroid neoplasia ranged from 2.5 to 6 years, with a median of 4.3 years.[4] At the time of writing, genetic or breed predispositions have not been published.

CLINICAL SIGNS

Much of the current understanding of the systemic effects of thyroid disease has been derived from experimentally induced hyperthyroidism and hypothyroidism in rabbit and guinea pig models. Unfortunately, many of these studies are not necessarily clinically relevant to the veterinary practitioner.[13–15] Experimentally induced hyperthyroidism was documented to cause weight loss, alopecia, loss of nails, radiographically evident osteoporosis, and dental lesions similar to those caused by hypovitaminosis C (scurvy).[16]

Of 19 cases of guinea pigs with grossly enlarged thyroid glands and confirmed thyroid neoplasia, the most common antemortem clinical signs were a palpable ventral cervical mass ($n = 10$) and weight loss ($n = 9$).[4] These same clinical signs were observed in other reports of confirmed hyperthyroidism in guinea pigs, with findings of weight loss in 95% of the cases and a palpable cervical mass in 45% of the cases.[8–10] Note, however, that these signs are not specific to hyperthyroidism, as other common guinea pig diseases such as dental disease and cervical lymphadenopathy may present similarly. Other clinical signs documented in hyperthyroid guinea pigs include behavioral changes (eg, hyperactivity, restlessness, difficulty rousing from sleep, and sleeping in lateral recumbency),[8,10] polyuria and/or polydipsia, hair loss or poor coat quality, diarrhea, heart murmur, tachycardia, bounding pulses, and tachypnea.[8,10] Changes in appetite seem to be inconsistent across cases, and increased, decreased, or static food intake may be reported or observed.[10]

Accurate measurement of arterial blood pressure of guinea pigs is challenging in clinical settings. Experimental models have shown hyperthyroid guinea pigs to be tachycardic and hypertensive relative to controls.[13] This may also be true in cases of naturally occurring hyperthyroidism. This may be mediated by increased conversion of prorenin to renin due to thyroxine-induced prorenin converting enzyme mk9 in the liver[17] and by the potentiation of β-adrenoceptors in the heart.[18]

Comorbidities may be present either coincidentally or secondary to hyperthyroidism.[3] Some of those reported include ovarian cysts, ocular disease, acariasis, dental, or gastrointestinal disease,[10] as well as hepatopathies, nephropathies, and cardiomyopathies that may be more urgent medical concerns.[4] Of animals that died with thyroid neoplasia, pulmonary congestion and myocardial degeneration were the most common comorbidities found at necropsy.[4]

DIAGNOSIS

Hyperthyroidism should be included on a differential diagnosis list based on signalment, history, and physical examination findings. Diagnosis is supported by elevated circulating TT_4 measured by competitive chemiluminescent immunoassay[8] or radioimmunoassay (RIA) and/or free thyroxine (FT_4) measured by equilibrium dialysis.[9] Circulating FT_4 concentrations may be more sensitive indicators of hyperthyroidism, as these are less likely to be affected by concurrent illness.

Several reference intervals for serum TT_4, FT_4, total triiodothyronine (TT_3), and free triiodothyronine (FT_3) stratified by age, sex, and reproductive status using several methodologies are available for guinea pigs[19–22] and have been thoroughly summarized elsewhere.[5,6] Note that the presence or absence of a palpable cervical mass and the size of that mass, when present, have been shown to be independent of circulating TT_4 concentrations.[10] Therefore, absence of a cervical mass does not rule out hyperthyroidism, and presence or size of a cervical mass does not indicate severity of disease.

Circulating TT_4 concentrations in euthyroid guinea pigs were documented to increase by at least 2.6 times 3 to 4 hours following intramuscular administration of recombinant human thyroid-stimulating hormone (rhTSH).[23] Therefore a rhTSH test is feasible in guinea pigs, although the cost and availability of rhTSH may be prohibitive.

Osseous metaplasia was observed in 8 out of 19 cases of thyroid neoplasia in adenomas and carcinomas and may be present radiographically even if a cervical mass is not palpated.[4] There may be indications for ultrasonography, computed tomography, MRI, and nuclear scintigraphy, although these modalities may be less practical or unavailable and have been discussed previously.[3,6,24]

Diagnostic imaging, specifically nuclear medicine, has historically been used for the diagnosis of hyperthyroidism and ectopic thyroid tissue. This imaging modality takes advantage of the physiologic iodine/iodide cycle by using a radioactive isotope with high affinity to the thyroid gland. The uptake of the isotope by the thyroid gland is either quantified or compared with another organ. Normal ratios for guinea pigs have not been well established, but this modality has been used for the diagnosis of hyperthyroidism in 1 guinea pig.[25]

TREATMENT

Treatment options for hyperthyroidism include radioactive iodine, oral or transdermal thyreostatic agents (methimazole/thiamazole, or carbimazole), and surgical thyroidectomy.

According to 1 study, treatment times with thyreostatic drugs ranged from 1 week to 10 months, with 11% of cases showing complete resolution, and 11% showing no response to treatment.[10] In some animals, hyperthyroidism was refractory to medical management determined by serial TT_4 monitoring and observation of persistent or worsening clinical signs.[10] Although 41% of the animals in this retrospective were reported to have died, no information was available on clinical response to treatment prior to death, time to death, or cause of death,[10] precluding prognostication of thyreostatic treatment. However, clinical response has been documented in animals treated with methimazole at dosages extrapolated from feline practice.[8,9] In a published case series, 2 animals treated medically survived for 18 and 28 months, respectively, with dosages adjusted according to changes in clinical signs and circulating TT_4 concentrations.[8] Another animal responded well to methimazole treatment for 4 months prior to treatment with radioactive iodine, after which it survived for an additional 7 months.[8]

Surgical thyroidectomy has been described in the laboratory animal literature[26] and has been applied clinically. According to 1 retrospective study, 3 of 6 hyperthyroid guinea pigs treated with surgical thyroidectomy showed moderate resolution of clinical signs of hyperthyroidism, and 1 of 6 showed complete resolution of clinical signs, surviving for 18 months postoperatively.[10] The remaining 2 guinea pigs showed no signs of improvement, with 1 dying postoperatively.[10] A study looking at the removal of normal thyroid glands in euthyroid guinea pigs found that 42% of the guinea pigs had thyroid regeneration 2 to 3 months postoperatively.[26] In another retrospective study of hyperthyroid guinea pigs, 3 of 7 thyroidectomized guinea pigs died within days of surgery.[4] Although direct cause of death is a matter of speculation, iatrogenic hypoparathyroidism was ruled out by histologic examination of surgically excised tissues.[4] Other publications report perianesthetic deaths.[2,8]

There is still much to learn regarding the treatment of hyperthyroidism in guinea pigs. In the absence of controlled clinical trials for the various treatment options with long-term follow-up, clinicians must use their judgment on the appropriate intervention for each patient. Little evidence has been presented to change previously published discussions of the advantages and disadvantages of the various treatment modalities.[3,5–7] The choice to pursue medical or surgical intervention may be based on the presence of comorbidities, surgical or anesthetic risk, client compliance, relative cost, or failure to respond to the first line of treatment chosen. In any case, thorough patient evaluation and serial monitoring of clinical signs and blood thyroxine concentrations are recommended.

RABBITS

Thyroid disease has not been historically reported in domestic rabbits, likely because of low prevalence, lack of published clinical cases, and the difficulty of diagnosis.[27]

Similar to guinea pig thyroid disease, diagnosis of potentially affected rabbits may be confounded by nonspecific clinical signs, lack of recognition on the part of clinicians, and paucity of available validated diagnostic assays or clinically applicable reference intervals for blood thyroid hormone concentrations.[27]

Hyperthyroidism has been suggested in 2 spayed female rabbits (8 and 5 years old) that presented for paradoxic hyperexia with weight loss. A grade 3 heart murmur was also noted in 1 of the cases, while dermatologic changes (generalized alopecia) were noted on the other case. Based on echocardiography (bilateral atrial dilation [severe dilation of the left atrium and moderate dilation of the right atrium] and mild atrial fibrillation without signs of congestion) and skin histopathology findings, presumptive clinical suspicion of hyperthyroidism was made.[28] Outside of these 2 cases, understanding of manifestations of functional thyroid disorders in rabbits is derived from experimental models. Rabbits with experimentally induced hyperthyroidism had higher resting heart rates and arterial blood pressure than controls.[13] Experimentally induced hypothyroidism in rabbits induced uterine hyperplasia and inflammation.[29] It is unknown whether hypothyroidism is a spontaneously occurring condition in the domestic rabbit population.

The diagnosis of hyperthyroidism in 2 rabbits was supported by nuclear scintigraphy, although circulating thyroid hormone concentrations were not demonstratively elevated.[27] In 1 case, fT4 (by equilibrium dialysis) and TT4 (by radioimmunoassay) were 28 pmol/L and 46 nmol/L, respectively, while in the second case, fT4 and TT4 (both by radioimmunoassay) were 50 pmol/L and 36 nmol/L, respectively. Thyroid scintigraphy with intravenous technetium 99^{mc} pertechnetate was performed and revealed a significantly elevated thyroid-to-salivary gland ratio.[28,30]

Reference intervals for circulating thyroid concentrations in apparently healthy, euthyroid rabbits are presented in **Table 1**.[31,32] One study used serum from venous blood samples and found that FT_4 measured by equilibrium dialysis provided a narrower interval than both TT_4 and FT_4 by RIA and may be of the most diagnostic value.[31] A more recent investigation compared TT_4 and fT_4 plasma concentrations between healthy rabbits and those affected by disease.[32] The investigators used heparinized plasma from arterial blood samples and measured thyroxine concentrations by chemiluminescence immunoassay.[32] As for other species, practitioners should consider the method of thyroxine measurement when choosing reference intervals with which to compare and evaluate their clinical results. Ideally, laboratory specific reference ranges should also be established.

Table 1
Reference intervals for thyroid hormones by radioimmunoassay (RIA), chemiluminescence immunoassay (CIA), and equilibrium dialysis (EqD) in healthy domestic rabbits (*Oryctolagus cuniculus*)

Thyroid Hormone	Assay	Mean ± Standard Deviation	Range	Sample Size
Total T3	RIA	0.46 ± 0.13 nmol/L	0.3–0.7 nmol/L	n = 36
Free T3	RIA	6.8 ± 2.4 pmol/L	1.7–12.4 pmol/L	n = 42
Total T4	RIA	35.7 ± 9.6 nmol/L	18–59 nmol/L	n = 43
	CIA	20.8 ± 7.1 nmol/L	7.7–37.3 nmol/L	n = 56
Free T4	RIA	50.7 ± 16.1 pmol/L	21–80 pmol/L	n = 48
	EqD	22.9 ± 7.0 pmol/L	9–40 pmol/L	n = 48
	CIA	13.3 ± 2.7 pmol/L	8.2–18 pmol/L	n = 28

Data from Brandão J, Rick M, Tully TN. Measure of serum free and total thyroxine and triiodothyronine concentrations in rabbits. ExoticsCon 2016 Proceedings: Portland, OR, August 27 – September 1, 2016. P. 485-486 and Thöle M, Brezina T, Fehr M, Schmicke M. Presumptive nonthyroidal illness syndrome in pet rabbits (*Oryctolagus cuniculus*). *Journal of Exotic Pet Medicine*. 2019;31:100-103.

Prior to these studies, reference intervals could only be gleaned from experimental literature that reported the mean circulating TT_4 of euthyroid rabbits to be 2.94 plus or minus 0.59 µg/dL as measured by RIA.[33] Whether these concentrations are affected by signalment or season remains open to speculation. In 1 free-ranging population of rabbits (Oryctolagus cuniculus), circulating TT_4 concentrations were found to vary seasonally in sexually intact male rabbits signaled by photoperiod and ambient temperatures, with significantly higher concentrations coinciding with the breeding season.[34] The breeding seasonality of this population was observed not to be consistent across free-ranging rabbit populations,[34] and so extrapolation to domestic rabbits is cautioned. Concomitant illness may also affect circulating thyroid hormone concentrations. Euthyroid sick syndrome or nonthyroidal illness syndrome is considered an adaptive response by which the body downregulates metabolism during illness by decreasing thyroid hormone concentrations. Rabbits with known illness were recently shown to have significantly lower levels of TT_4 and FT_4 than healthy conspecifics.[32] Results suggested that bone fractures and ileus may cause greater decreases in circulating thyroxine than other types of diseases observed.[32] This may confound diagnosis of primary disorders of thyroid function, mainly hypothyroidism, in rabbits as it does in other mammals. Clinicians are advised to consider history, signalment, physical examination findings, and other clinicopathologic data when approaching potential cases of thyroid disease in rabbits rather than base a diagnosis off blood thyroxine concentrations alone.

Scintigraphy using technetium 99^{mc} pertechnetate can be used for assessment of thyroid function. This method is particularly useful for hyperthyroidism cases. In a previous study, technetium 99^{mc} pertechnetate (111 MBq [3.0 mCi]) was administered intravenously to 10 rabbits sedated with midazolam and hydromorphone.[30] Thyroid-to-salivary gland ratio at 20 minutes after technetium 99^{mc} pertechnetate was 1:1, which is similar to cats.[30] These results are also supported by a previous study investigating the protective effect of amifostine in a rabbit model.[35] Subjective evaluation of the images provided in this publication suggest a similar contrast uptake between the salivary gland and the thyroid gland.[35] There was no significant difference between time points up to 60 minutes; however, 20 minutes provided the narrowest range. Therefore, 20 minutes should be the recommended time point.[30] The findings of these studies support the presumptive diagnosis of hyperthyroidism in 2 rabbits.[28] In the suspected hyperthyroid cases, the thyroid-to-salivary ratio was approximately 4:1,[28] which is considerably higher than in euthyroid rabbits, which should be 1:1.[30]

In the 2 hyperthyroidism cases, methimazole (1.25 mg total dose by mouth every 12 hours) was initiated, and circulating thyroid hormone concentration decreased after therapy.[28] One animal died 12 months following diagnosis. Bicavitary effusion, mild myocardial fibrosis, and chronic passive congestion were identified on necropsy, which were suggestive of chronic cardiac insufficiency. There was no evidence of hyperplasia or neoplasia within the thyroid gland. The pituitary gland had cysts, but the clinical significance of these lesions was unclear. The second case was initially treated with methimazole (1.25 mg total dose by mouth every 12 hours), which led to clinical improvement. Because of the lack of client compliance, medication was discontinued, and clinical signs recurred. Route of administration was changed to transcutaneous methimazole, which led to resolution of the clinical signs, and the case was subsequently lost to follow-up.[28] The use of antithyroidal drugs in laboratory rabbits has shown effect. Methimazole (1.4 mg/kg SID) with or without atenolol (8.5 mg/kg SID) was administered to rabbits with experimentally induced hyperthyroidism. Compared with the control group, there was improved sympathetic overactivity and decreased thyroxine levels. The most significant effect was achieved when both drugs were administered.[36] Moderate hypothyroidism was induced in rabbits with 50 mg/kg by mouth SID propylthiouracil for 6 days and 20 mg/kg methimazole for 14 additional days. Circulating TT_4 and TT_3 measured by radioimmunoassay decreased by about 38% to 40% and 32% to 36%, respectively.[37] Several other experimental studies have demonstrated induced hypothyroid status using propylthiouracil and/or methimazole;[38,39] however, it is important to note that the suggested doses may not be clinically appropriate.

DISCLOSURE

The authors have nothing to disclose.

REFERENCES

1. Zarrin K. Thyroid carcinoma of a guinea pig: a case report. Lab Anim 1974;8: 145–8.
2. LaRegina C, Wightman SR. Thyroid papillary adenoma in a guinea pig with signs of cervical lymphadenitis. J Am Vet Med Assoc 1979;175:969–71.
3. Mayer J, Wagner R, Taeymans O. Advanced diagnostic approaches and current management of thyroid pathologies in guinea pigs. Vet Clin North Am Exot Anim Pract 2010;13:509–23.
4. Gibbons PM, Garner MM, Kiupel M. Morphological and immunohistochemical characterization of spontaneous thyroid gland neoplasms in guinea pigs (Cavia porcellus). Vet Pathol 2012;50:334–42.
5. Brandão J, Vergneau-Grosset C, Mayer J. Hyperthyroidism and hyperparathyroidism in guinea pigs (Cavia porcellus). Vet Clin North Am Exot Anim Pract 2013;16:407–20.
6. Thorson L. Thyroid diseases in rodent species. Vet Clin North Am Exot Anim Pract 2014;17:51–67.
7. Künzel F, Mayer J. Endocrine tumours in the guinea pig. Vet J 2015;206:268–74.
8. Künzel F, Hierlmeier B, Christian M, et al. Hyperthyroidism in four guinea pigs: clinical manifestations, diagnosis, and treatment. J Small Anim Prac 2013;54: 667–71.
9. Pignon C, Mayer J. Hyperthyroidism in a guinea pig (Cavia porcellus). Pratique médicale et chirurgicale de l'animal de compagnie 2013;48:15–20.
10. Girod-Rüffer C, Müller E, Marschang RE, et al. Retrospective study on hyperthyroidism in guinea pigs in veterinary practices in Germany. J Exot Pet Med 2019; 29:87–97.
11. Laik-Schandelmaier C, Klopfleisch R, Schöniger S, et al. Spontaneously arising tumours and tumour-like lesions of the cervix and uterus in 83 pet guinea pigs (Cavia porcellus). J Comp Pathol 2017;156:339–51.
12. Kondo H, Koizumi I, Yamamoto N, et al. Thyroid adenoma and ectopic thyroid carcinoma in a guinea pig (Cavia porcellus). Comp Med 2018;68:212–4.
13. Thompson EB. Comparison of degree of susceptibility of hyperthyroid and euthyroid animals to cardiac glycoside-induced arrhythmias. J Pharm Sci 1973;62: 1638–43.
14. Sillau AH. Capillarity and oxygen diffusion distances of the soleus muscle of guinea pigs and rats. Effects of hyperthyroidism. Comp Biochem Physiol 1985; 82A:471–8.
15. Szymanska G, Pikula S, Zborowski J. Effect of hyper- and hypothyroidism on phospholipid fatty acid composition and phospholipases activity in sarcolemma of rabbit cardiac muscle. Biochim Biophys Acta 1991;1083:265–70.

16. Goldman HM. Experimental hyperthyroidism in guinea pigs. Am J Orthod Dentofac Orthop 1943;29:B665–81.

17. Das SK, Chatterjee D, Uddin M. Induction of pro-renin converting enzyme mk9 by thyroid hormone in the guinea-pig liver. Biochem Biophys Res Commun 2002; 293:412–5.

18. Hashimoto H, Nakashima M. Influence of thyroid hormone on the positive inotropic effects mediated by α- and β-adrenoceptors in isolated guinea pig atria and rabbit papillary muscles. Euro J Pharmacol 1978;50:337–47.

19. Castro MI, Alex S, Young RA, et al. Total and free serum thyroid hormone concentrations in fetal and adult pregnant and nonpregnant guinea pigs. Endocrinology 1986;118:533–7.

20. Felzen B, Rubinstein I, Lotan R, et al. Developmental changes in ventricular action potential properties in guinea-pigs are modulated by age-related changes in the thyroid state. J Mol Cell Cardiol 1991;23:787–94.

21. Müller K, Müller E, Klein R, et al. Serum thyroxine concentrations in clinically healthy pet guinea pigs (*Cavia porcellus*). Vet Clin Pathol 2009;38:507–10.

22. Fredholm DV, Cagle LA, Johnston MS. Evaluation of precision and establishment of reference ranges for plasma thyroxine using a point-of-care analyzer in healthy guinea pigs (*Cavia porcellus*). J Exot Pet Med 2012;21:87–93.

23. Mayer J, Wagner R, Mitchell MA, et al. Use of recombinant human thyroid-stimulating hormone for evaluation of thyroid function in guinea pigs (*Cavia porcellus*). J Am Vet Med Assoc 2013;242:346–9.

24. Mayer J. Evidence-based medicine in small mammals. J Exot Pet Med 2009;18: 213–9.

25. Mayer J, Hunt K, Eshar D, et al. Thyroid scintigraphy in a guinea pig with suspected hyperthyroidism. Exot DVM 2009;11:25–9.

26. Kromka MC, Hoar RM. An improved technique for thyroidectomy in guinea pigs. Lab Anim Sci 1975;25:82–4.

27. Summa NM, Brandão J. Evidence-based advances in rabbit medicine. Vet Clin North Am Exot Anim Pract 2017;20:749–71.

28. Brandão J, Higbie C, Rick M, et al. Naturally occurring idiopathic hyperthyroidism in two pet rabbits. ExoticsCon 2015 Proceedings. San Antonio (TX), August 29-September 2, 2015. p. 341–2.

29. Rodríguez-Castelán J, Moral-Morales AD, Piña-Medina AG, et al. Hypothyroidism induces uterine hyperplasia and inflammation related to sex hormone receptors expression in virgin rabbits. Life Sci 2019;230:111–20.

30. Brandão J, Ellison M, Beaufrere H, et al. Quareportive 99M-Technetium pertechnetate thyroid scintigraphy in euthyroid New Zealand white rabbits (Oryctolagus cuniculus). Proceedings of the American College of Veterinary Radiology Conference. St Louis (MO): American College of Veterinary Radiology; 2014. p. 62.

31. Brandão J, Rick M, Tully TN. Measure of serum free and total thyroxine and triiodothyronine concentrations in rabbits. ExoticsCon 2016 Proceedings. Portland (OR), August 27 – September 1, 2016. p. 485–6.

32. Thöle M, Brezina T, Fehr M, et al. Presumptive nonthyroidal illness syndrome in pet rabbits (*Oryctolagus cuniculus*). J Exot Pet Med 2019;31:100–3.

33. Azuma H, Takeichi T, Ohara T, et al. Metabolism of plasma fibronectin in rabbits with experimental hyperthyroidism and hypothyroidism. Metabolism 1987;36: 777–80.

34. Ben Saad MM, Maurel DL. Reciprocal interaction between seasonal testis and thyroid activity in Zembra Island wild rabbits (*Oryctolagus cuniculus*): effects of

castration, thyroidectomy, temperature, and photoperiod. Biol Reprod 2004;70: 1001–9.

35. Bohuslavizki KH, Brenner W, Klutmann S, et al. Radioprotection of salivary glands by amifostine in high-dose radioiodine therapy. J Nucl Med 1998;39:1237–42.

36. Li YM, Cai-Li Z. The effects of methimazole, atenolol alone and in combination on hyperthyroidism in rabbits. Chin Pharmacol Bull 1996;5.

37. Brzezinska-Slebodzinska E. Influence of hypothyroidism on lipid peroxidation, erythrocyte resistance and antioxidant plasma properties in rabbits. Acta Vet Hung 2003;51:343–51.

38. Hussien BA, Yaser SM, Alsafy AM, et al. Histological study of hypothyroidism induced effect by methimazole on heart and blood vessels of healthy female rabbits. Indian J Pub Health Res Develop 2019;10:911–6.

39. Simsek G, Yelmen NK, Guner I, et al. The role of peripheral chemoreceptor activity on the respiratory responses to hypoxia and hypercapnia in anaesthetized rabbits with induced hypothyroidism. Chin J Physiol 2004;47:153–60.

Emerging Diseases of Avian Wildlife

Susan J. Tyson-Pello, VMD, MS[a],*, Glenn H. Olsen, DVM, MS, PhD[b]

KEYWORDS

- Emerging diseases of avian wildlife • Tick-associated diseases • West Nile virus
- Lymphoproliferative disease virus • Wellfleet Bay virus • Avian influenza
- Salmonella

KEY POINTS

- Avian wildlife diseases include *Haemaphysalis longicornis*, West Nile virus, lymphoproliferative disease virus, Wellfleet Bay virus, avian influenza, and salmonellosis.
- Previously documented avian wildlife diseases have taken a new focus with more affected species and changes in preventive medicine.
- Geographic region and climate change can influence new and existing avian wildlife diseases.

HAEMAPHYSALIS LONGICORNIS

Neotropical migratory birds have been implicated in the importation of exotic neotropical ticks to the United States.[1] The geographic range of ticks such as *Ixodes scapularis* has been expanded by migratory birds, with climate change driving the dispersion and the growth of more suitable climates because of global warming.[1] *Haemaphysalis longicornis*, the longhorned tick originally native to Asia, was introduced and quickly established in the eastern United States. The longhorned tick was originally discovered in New Jersey in 2017; however, during importation inspection and quarantine of horses, the tick was noted in 6 cases over the last 30 years by the US Department of Agriculture.[1] The longhorn tick population in the United States is parthenogenetic, with the female able to reproduce asexually. Multiple life stages coexist on a wide range of wild and domestic species (it is also referred to as the 3-host tick) so, along with the longhorned tick being parthenogenic, controlling the population is difficult. The longhorn tick has a broad zoophilic host range, including birds, rodents, ungulates, lagomorphs, carnivores, and humans. This broad range of hosts results in rapid geographic dispersion.[2–4] Ticks found in avian wildlife include the longhorn tick, *Argas* species, including *Argas giganteus*; *Ixodes scapularis*; *Ixodes brunneus*; *Argas*

[a] Mount Laurel Animal Hospital, 220 Mount Laurel Road, Mount Laurel, NJ 08054, USA; [b] USGS Patuxent Wildlife Research Center, 12302 Beech Forest Road, Laurel, MD 20708, USA
* Corresponding author.
E-mail address: TysonVMD@gmail.com

Vet Clin Exot Anim 23 (2020) 383–395
https://doi.org/10.1016/j.cvex.2020.01.002
1094-9194/20/© 2020 Elsevier Inc. All rights reserved.

americanum; and *Haemaphysalis cordeilis*. They are found cofeeding, resulting in co-infection and pathogen acquisition.[1,4]

The longhorn tick is the vector for multiple pathogens, including *Anaplasma*, *Coxiella burnetii*, *Rickettsia japonica*, *Theileria mutans*, and *Theileria orientialis*. The most common tick-associated disease is tick paralysis.[5] Ticks can be found primarily on the feet, legs, keel, and inguinal regions.[1] Edema, ecchymoses, and petechiae can be found at the attachment sites, and infested birds may show sternal recumbency, polyneuropathy, distal to proximal ascending paralysis, anemia, dehydration, respiratory distress, lethargy, ataxia, difficulty swallowing, and death.[1,3,6] The longhorned tick can be found in heavy infestations on multiple hosts and poses agronomic threat for livestock producers, horses, and humans. With the current state of the environment, global warming, and the expansion of neotropical species, expansion of this species and possibly translocation of other species into new geographic locations are expected.

WEST NILE VIRUS IN AVIAN WILDLIFE

In a recent retrospective study of raptor mortality in Ontario, Canada, West Nile virus (WNV) was found to be the most commonly diagnosed infectious disease among raptor species from 1991 to 2014.[7] WNV is an arthropod-borne, single-stranded RNA virus within the genus Flavivirus, family Flaviviridae, which contains more than 90 viruses.[8,9] The first domestic avian deaths were described in 1997 in Israel and involved hundreds of young geese (*Anser anser*).[9] In 1999, WNV emerged on the east coast of the United States, migrated to the west coast by 2003, and is now considered enzootic.[10] Up to 9 distinct lineages of WNV have been found with molecular phylogenic analysis, with lineages 1 and 2 being grossly distributed worldwide.[9] Lineage 1 viruses are especially virulent to native North American avian species, causing high mortality in corvids. The route that WNV entered the western hemisphere is still unknown.[11] Lineage 2 viruses were restricted to sub-Saharan Africa and Madagascar but have been isolated in Europe.[9,12,13] Lineage 2 spread resulted in 115 human deaths in 2018 in Europe.[9] Despite genomic variability and the discovery of 9 distinct lineages, only 1 WNV serotype has been described that would allow the development of vaccines to protect against all WNV genotypes.[9]

WNV continues to emerge as vectors move into new geographic regions and undocumented locations because of climate change.[14,15] To date, WNV has been detected in more than 300 avian species,[14] and more than 40 mosquito species are considered vectors.[16]

Domestic and wild avian species are the primary amplifying hosts of WNV, and more than 300 avian species have shown susceptibility.[8] WNV also infects more than 30 vertebrate species, including marine mammals, rodents, bats, horses, camelids, canids, felids, and reptiles.[11,12,17] The most common form of transmission is mosquito borne, *Culex* spp; however, other vectors have been implicated. Alternate routes of infection include horizontal transmission among corvids, ingestion of WNV-infected organs, and blood contamination of wounds. Bird-to-bird transmission has been confirmed by detection of viremia in magpies.[15]

Birds are the natural reservoir hosts of WNV; however, species susceptibility, morbidity, and mortality vary. Species in the order Columbiformes and Galliformes show low viremia, although other species in the orders Passeriformes, Charadriiformes, and Strigiformes show high viremia without clinical disease, making them more effective competent viral reservoirs for WNV transmission.[9,11]

Postmortem detection of WNV has been well documented in tissues such as the central nervous system (CNS), ocular, cardiac, renal, skin, and vascular feather pulp, as well as blood, oropharyngeal, and cloacal swabs.[18,19] Chronic infections are difficult to diagnose because of clearance of the virus, with the host then succumbing to chronic inflammatory sequelae of WNV with low amounts of viral antigen present.[20] Immunohistochemistry, viral isolation, and histopathology of organ tissue can be performed to diagnose WNV. In chronic infections, ocular, CNS, renal, and feather samples have yielded positive viral/antigen detection results.[8,17,21]

Clinical signs of WNV in avian species appear 10 to 12 days after infection.[22] Neurologic deficits are the most common clinical finding in WNV infection.[13] A complete blood count may reveal a moderate leukocytosis characterized by a heterophilia and lymphocytosis.[13] Other clinical findings include ataxia, head tilt, pinched-off feathers, myocarditis, myalgias, arthralgias, rashes, pancreatitis, hepatitis, and inflammation of the pecten and choroid.[21,23–26] Relapses of neurologic signs can occur for several years after infection.[23]

Viremia is often detectable 1 to 8 days after infection.[8] Cloacal and oral shedding during viremia may continue for 14 days or longer. Antibodies are produced 5 to 7 days after infection, so serology and plaque reduction neutralization test (PRNT) can be used for detection.[27,28] PRNT is the is the preferred diagnostic once the virus has been cleared by the host immune system. WNV affects multiple organ systems and can be cleared in 1 to 2 weeks; however, WNV has been documented to persist for longer periods depending on the age and immune status.[8] If the period of infection cannot be determined, running polymerase chain reaction (PCR) and paired PRNT is recommended.

Sample collection for antemortem WNV detection includes blood and oral/cloacal swabs, as well as feather, organ, and skin biopsies. Serology is useful when paired titers are run 2 to 4 weeks apart.[8] The high cross reactivity of flavivirus infections complicates the precise serologic diagnosis by immunologic techniques, such as enzyme-linked immunosorbent assay. Therefore, confirmation with PRNT is the gold standard.[9]

The mature WNV virion external protein shell is composed of 180 copies of an N-glycosylated E protein found in most WNV isolates.[9] This surface glycoprotein constitutes the major target for neutralizing antibodies, becoming the basis of many vaccine candidates. Although the lack of glycosylation influences WNV replication in experimentally infected chickens,[9] it does not compromise the induction of antibodies. The E protein carries Flavivirus cross-reactive and WNV-specific epitopes. This cross reactivity between WNV and related flaviruses results in cross-protection, which is beneficial but also results in the adverse effect of antibody-dependent enhancement of the infection.[9]

Prevention, vaccination, and vector control are important to reduce WNV in avian wildlife. WNV persists in organs for up to several months, thus playing a role in viral overwintering and enabling infections to spread through vectors and bird-to-bird transmission.[9]

Flaviviruses represent an emerging challenge because of their worldwide spread, increasing outbreaks of WNV and emergence of Zika virus in 2017.[15] Development of an effective vaccine labeled for birds is essential because of the ability of avian species to develop a competent viremia resulting in transmission of WNV to vectors.[15] Several commercial equine vaccines are used extralabel in avian species,[29] including a formalin-inactivated whole-WNV killed vaccine (formerly Fort Dodge, now Veteran), a DNA-based vaccine using the prM and E capsid proteins from Fort Dodge (West Nile Innovator DNA equine) and Merial Recombitek live canarypox vectored vaccine; the last 2 have been discontinued. Experimental vaccines have been assayed, including ChimeriVax-WN, a chimeric virus vaccine that uses yellow fever 17D vaccine strains and WNV surface proteins, and a vaccine based on WNV recombinant subviral particles. Other approaches include DNA plasmid vaccines that express modified WNV E proteins of lineage 1 and 2.[9]

Vaccination induces humoral and cellular responses, reducing WNV-related disease, viral shedding, viremia, and mortality.[9] Vaccines may not seroconvert every bird but may produce tissue-mediated immunity.[29] Vaccines have been used in avian species[28–30] and in some cases have shown antibody development. In sandhill cranes (*Grus canadensis*), vaccination resulted in reduced viremia and shedding.[21,29] Vectored WNV vaccines showed efficacy against WNV infection using a vectored vaccine for delivery of WNV genes, which provided protection in a domestic goose model.[31] Further development and research are needed to produce an avian-labeled WNV vaccine.

WNV is a zoonotic and epizootic infection of great importance in avian wildlife, which serve as critical vectors because of their high viral load. To prevent exposure, the US Centers for Disease Control and Prevention recommends reducing mosquito exposure during times of peak activity, using mosquito nets around outdoor enclosures, and removing standing water to eliminate and reduce mosquito breeding sites.[14] Supportive care and antiinflammatories are the treatment of choice for WNV-infected avian patients[13] because of the severe inflammatory sequelae WNV causes in the body. However, there is no antiviral treatment available to date. With the recent loss of marketed vaccines and the degree of infectivity of WNV, it is important to continue research to develop a labeled vaccine for avian species.

LYMPHOPROLIFERATIVE DISEASE VIRUS IN WILD TURKEYS

Lymphoproliferative disease virus (LPDV), a C-type retrovirus, is one of 3 oncogenic avian viruses and is responsible for neoplastic disease in wild and domestic turkeys (*Meleagris gallopavo*).[32–34] It was first discovered in 1978 in the United Kingdom. LPDV is characterized by rapid clinical decline with gross intracelomic lesions and generalized anorexia, lethargy, and ruffled feathers. Clinical signs are not present in all affected birds and transmission routes are unknown. Recent discovery of LPDV in wild turkeys in the United States has produced new concern for infection of wild turkeys and potential outbreaks in commercial flocks. Before 2009, the virus was considered rare, with little concern for spread to commercial poultry.[32]

LPDV targets lymphoid tissue and is the primary site of replication. Age at the time of infection determines disease manifestation. Experimental infection at 1 day of age leads to viremia with no other clinical signs, whereas infection at 4 weeks of age results in neoplastic lesions of multiple organs. Mortality begins at 10 weeks of age and steadily increases in naturally infected flocks, with mortalities as high as 25%. Chickens and turkeys are susceptible to LPDV, whereas ducks and geese are not.[32]

LPDV transmission may occur via horizontal transmission and direct contact during seasonal flocking. However, vertical transmission and vector-mediated transmission, both noted in other retroviruses, have not been shown to occur with LPDV.[33] There is potential for bidirectional pathogen spread among wild and domestic turkeys, with wildfowl, domestic fowl, and other wild avian species possibly acting as disease reservoirs for the others. Shared contaminated environmental substrates in the region of turkey farms may serve as sources of exposure to wild turkeys and other wildlife.[34] LPDV in wild turkeys is spreading from the northeast across the United States, with recent cases in Ohio and Pennsylvania, but the origin is unknown.[34]

Cutaneous tumors are noted on the head, neck, and feet of wild turkeys, and do not present in domestic turkeys. Tumor formation leads to direct mortality caused by blindness and lack of mobility resulting in starvation. It is conjectured that this tumor formation is caused by a secondary infection or novel pathogenesis.[32,33] It is rare for LPDV to cause large-scale die-offs in wild birds. Many wild turkeys test positive for LPDV without showing internal or external gross lesions, making it difficult to determine the level of effect that subclinical infection has on the wild bird population.[33] Diagnosis of LPDV is difficult because of inconsistent clinical signs. PCR of whole blood, bone marrow, or buffy coat is a viable option for testing live birds.[32]

Recent discovery of LPDV in wild turkeys leaves concern for infection to spread from these wild turkeys to commercial flocks, causing potential outbreaks. Further monitoring and research are needed to protect domestic and commercial flocks from LPDV.

WELLFLEET BAY VIRUS

Wellfleet Bay virus (WFBV) is a recently identified orthomyxovirus associated with mortality in wild avian species. The mortality events of consequence started in 1998 in and around Cape Cod, Massachusetts (41°54'15" N, 70°2'33" W),[35,36] although there were smaller, unrecognized mortality events starting as early as 1956. The virus that causes WFBV has been classified in the genus Quaranjavirus and may be an arbovirus.[35]

Mortality events have largely been confined to common eider (*Somateria mollissima dresseri*). Common eider are large (~2 kg) sea ducks that breed from Massachusetts (Boston Harbor) north to Labrador and winter from Newfoundland to the Chesapeake Bay on the eastern coast of North America. The largest concentration of wintering common eider are in the Cape Cod area, including Cape Cod Bay, Wellfleet Bay, and Nantucket Sound, where rafts of more than 100,000 birds may be found.[37] The mortality events occur in the fall, winter, and early spring, and sometimes primarily involve only 1 sex. Mortality in other subspecies of common eider found in the Hudson Bay area of Canada and along the Pacific and Arctic coasts of North America have not been reported. Other common eider subspecies occur in Europe and Asia, and no disease outbreaks have been reported from these areas.

The first documented mortality event may have occurred from September 1956 to March 1957 in the Cape Cod area.[38] Two further events occurred in the 1980s and early 1990s in midwinter and late spring associated with acanthocephaliasis.[39] The first large-scale mortality event of the current epizootic occurred in 1998, with events now occurring once or sometimes twice a year.[40]

Most common eider are found dead, with those still alive having nonspecific clinical signs of incoordination, lethargy, respiratory distress,[40]anemia, and emaciation.[35] Necropsy findings include acute hepatic necrosis with variable amounts of pancreatic necrosis, splenic necrosis, or intestinal necrosis.[40] In a study[40] to test Koch's hypothesis, 6-week-old common eider ducklings were inoculated with WFBV. Clinical signs developed in 25% of the inoculated ducklings, and weight loss alone occurred in another 18.75% compared with control ducklings. WFBV was isolated from 37.5% of the infected ducklings, and serum antibody titers were detected 5 days after inoculation in surviving ducklings.[40]

Little is known about routes of transmission, host range, and origin of WFBV. Studies in common eider subspecies, *S m dresseri* and *Somateria mollissima borealis*,[41] showed significantly higher numbers of eider with titers in Massachusetts and Rhode Island (16.3%, n = 387), compared with Maine (3%, n = 346), Nova Scotia (3%, n = 180), Quebec (1%, n = 501), Nunavut (0%, n = 530), or Iceland (0%, n = 52).

Mortality events only occur in the Cape Cod area, which may indicate exposure to a carrier, an arthropod vector, or environmental factors that favor the virus.[41] Herring gulls (*Larus argentatus*) from Massachusetts and New Jersey have tested positive for WFBV,[42] as have ring-billed gulls (*Larus delawarensis*) from Massachusetts, a single white-winged scoter (*Melanitta fusca*) from Massachusetts, and black scoters (*Melanitta americana*) also from Massachusetts.[42] Several of these positive birds were collected either from the Boston Harbor nesting islands of common eider or from Cape Cod. Herring gulls and common eider overlap in most of their range, so it is unlikely that herring gulls are the reservoir host or exposure to the disease in common eider would not just be confined to Massachusetts. However, ring-billed gulls are winter-only residents of Massachusetts, nesting at inland areas across North America.[43] White-winged and black scoters are also both winter-only residents of coastal Massachusetts, breeding in the far north.[43] Furthermore, they dive to feed on mollusks, as do eider.

The characterization and cause of WFBV have progressed since our last review,[44] but there are still some unknown factors. The virus has now been found in several other avian species but not in high incidence and not shown to cause any disease.[42] The highest incidence of disease prevalence is known to be in the Massachusetts and Rhode Island area[41,42] and centered on common eider that nest in the spring and summer on Calf Island in Boston Harbor. However, the mortality events occur during the fall, winter, and early spring in the waters surrounding Cape Cod, and can involve common eider from other nesting areas along eastern North America. The method of transmission has not been discovered. The arboviruses are normally associated with tick transmission, but, to date, no ticks have been found on the birds or in the nesting material. However, the authors have found lice on many of the common eider brought in for veterinary examination, and these lice have been submitted for analysis.

WFBV is still a mystery. The route of infection in the wild is unknown. In the duckling study,[40] inoculation was done using a standard World Organization of Animal Health procedure for determining pathogenicity of avian influenza in poultry by inoculating via 3 routes simultaneously (intravenous, intratracheal, and oral), and infection resulted. In this study,[40] there was a single contact control eider housed with the inoculated eiders. This control eider gained weight, showed no signs of illness, and did not develop detectable antibody titer, indicating lack of transmission of the virus from the inoculated eider ducklings to this control duckling.[40] There are several other Quaranjavirus species that affect avian wildlife, such as the Cygnet River virus from Kangaroo Island, South Australia,[45] that may have caused mortality in Muscovy ducks (*Cairina moschata*), and Quaranfil, Johnston Atoll, and Lake Chad viruses, which are all associated with colonial nesting avian species and ticks.[46] Quaranfil has also been isolated from 2 young children that had a mild febrile illness[47]; therefore, there are zoonotic implications with this group of viruses. Continued research is needed to learn more about WFBV and its implications for common eider, other avian wildlife, and people.

AVIAN INFLUENZA

The emergence and spread of H5N1, H5N8, and other highly pathogenic forms of avian influenza virus across Eurasia, Africa, and (for H5N8) North America has meant an increased interest in tracking and following this disease. Waterfowl (Anseriformes), along with shorebirds and gulls (Charadriiformes), are the primary reservoir hosts of the various forms of avian influenza, and these forms are normally considered of low pathogenicity.[48]

Influenza viruses are found in the *Orthomyxoviridae* family. The influenza viruses are described as enveloped, segmented, negative-stranded RNA viruses with 2 surface glycoproteins.[49] The influenza viruses are divided into types A, B, and C based on M and nucleocapsid proteins.[50] Types B and C are primarily found in humans, whereas the influenza A virus is the only form found in avian species, but it can infect humans too. Dogs and cats can be infected with influenza A virus both naturally and experimentally, but no cases of transmission to humans have occurred.[49] Influenza A is further classified by differences in the surface glycoproteins hemagglutinin (H) and neuraminidase (N). Sixteen H glycoproteins and 9 N glycoproteins are known[50] for a total of 144 subtype combinations, such as N1H1, N5H1, and N5H8. Through mutations during virus replications, new combinations with varying virulence are constantly being created. The virulence or pathogenicity is further described as being either low pathogenic avian influenza (LPAI) or highly pathogenic avian influenza (HPAI), with the pathogenicity referring to the disease as seen in chickens.

A form of avian influenza that is highly pathogenic in chickens may produce little to no clinical illness in another species, especially in the reservoir host species, such as waterfowl. Birds are capable of shedding high concentrations of influenza virus in their feces, with feces/oral transmission being the primary route of transmission in wild birds.[51] Birds carrying influenza virus may also shed virus in saliva and nasal secretions. Poultry become infected through direct contact with other birds or indirectly through contact with contaminated food, water, or inanimate objects such as equipment or even the clothing of humans. The virus can persist for 1 to 2 days on the surface of inanimate objects.[49] Some highly pathogenic H5N1 have evolved to be able to be transmitted by aerosol.[52] HPAI has a 1-day to 5-day incubation and typically manifests as lethargy; facial edema; discoloration or swelling of eyelids, comb, or wattle; swollen hocks; diarrhea; soft-shelled or misshapen eggs; decreased egg production; incoordination; and death.[49] LPAI has few clinical signs, but these include mild respiratory symptoms, such as nasal discharge, coughing, or sneezing; inappetence; and decreased egg production.[49]

The influenza viruses are always changing, using mutation, reassortment, insertion, deletion, and recombination to evolve into new viral forms.[53] Reassortment has been detected in wild waterfowl.[54] More avian influenza viral isolations have been found in mallards (*Anas platyrhynchos*) than in any other bird species.[49] Peak viral load timing and thus the spread of the influenza viruses differ among avian species.[53] In waterfowl, primarily ducks, in North America, the peak is just before fall migration during a period called staging, when there are many naive juveniles in the population. For shorebirds, the peak is during the spring migration.[53] During spring migration, shorebirds congregate along stretches of shoreline rich in seasonal food resources, such as the shores of Delaware Bay, where horseshoe crabs (*Limulus polyphemus*) come ashore to deposit eggs that literally cover the beaches. Ruddy turnstones (*Arenaria interpres*) are considered a key agent in spreading the virus.[53] It is possible that the influenza virus may overwinter in the frozen earth of the high Arctic in North America and Eurasia.[55,56]

When the authors last reported about avian influenza in *Veterinary Clinics of North America: Exotic Animal Practice*,[44] H5N1 had emerged as a pathogen in wild waterfowl, specifically bar-headed geese (*Anser indicus*) in China.[56] Avian influenza H5N1 spread across Eurasia and into Africa but was never found in the Americas. However, in the 7 years since this previous publication, new forms of avian influenza have emerged and spread around the world. In January 2014, an H5N8 HPAI emerged on a duck farm in South Korea.[57] In further studies in South Korea, H5N8 was found in 167 out of 771 dead wild birds of 8 different species.[57] Baikal teal (*Anas formosa*), bean geese (*Anser fabalis*), and whooper swans (*Cygnus cygnus*) were among the most common wild birds to die of H5N8.[57] Histopathologic findings were those associated with renal failure and gout.[57] H5N8 spread rapidly to China and Japan, then to Germany, the Netherlands, and the United Kingdom by November 2014.[58] Also, in November 2014, H5N2 influenza virus, which was a novel reassortment of the Eurasian clade of H5, appeared on a poultry farm in British Columbia, Canada, and adjacent Washington state. H5N2 was found by PCR in dead northern pintail (*Anas acuta*), several mallards, and an American widgeon (*Anas americana*) on a nearby lake 32 km from the original Washington state outbreak.[58] Four captive gyrfalcons (*Falco rusticolus*) and gyrfalcon crosses fed a dead American widgeon also died of avian influenza, H5N8. In another study, mortality caused by HPAI H5N8 was detected in 6 species of raptors from Midwestern and western US states in association with areas where HPAI outbreaks occurred in poultry.[59]

In 2017, ring-billed gulls (*L delawarensis*) in Minnesota were tested for avian influenza, with positive results in various age classes, including 57.8% of juveniles testing positive.[60] In January 2019, HPAI H5N8 was found to be the cause of mortality in several hundred African penguins (*Spheniscus demersus*) in Namibia, Africa.[61] Novel reassortment again led to outbreaks of H5N8 in Korea and Japan in 2016 to 2017, and later in China and Vietnam.[62] The recent and rapid spread of these avian influenza viruses globally through wild birds and with some mortality occurring in the wild bird populations is of some concern.[48]

The emergence with novel reassortment and movement among wild bird populations poses health risks to wild bird populations, to domestic poultry, and possibly to human health, although H5N8 has not been linked to disease in humans, unlike the H5N1 epizootic. There is need for continued determination to maintain HPAI-free domestic poultry flocks through testing, eradication programs, prevention and control methods, appropriate use of vaccinations, and postvaccination monitoring.[62] Wild bird monitoring programs that were established during the H5N1, but are not currently in place in North America, should be reestablished. The recent increase in backyard or hobby poultry in the United States poses a challenge for continued HPAI surveillance and control programs.

SALMONELLOSIS

The genus *Salmonella* is one of the most common causes of gastroenteritis and infectious diarrhea. One author estimates that less than 1% of cases are reported correctly. *Salmonella* is a genus of gram-negative, facultative, anaerobic, rod-shaped bacteria with more than 2300 serotypes or serovars associated with the genus, with *Salmonella enteritidis* and *Salmonella typhimurium* being the most common.[63] Pullorum disease (*S pullorum*) and fowl typhoid (*Salmonella galinarum*) are avian forms of salmonellosis that cause disease in poultry. Wild birds can become infected with either of these bacteria, but wild birds are more commonly infected with *S typhimurium*.[64] Outbreaks in birds are most common in colonial nesting species or concentrated around food supplies.[65] Songbirds in winter congregating at bird feeders can lead to higher transmission rates and high mortality.[66]

In birds, clinical signs can include ruffled feathers or fluffed feathers, shivering, deep or rapid respiration, weakness, diarrhea, plaques on the oral mucous membranes and crop, lethargy, and death. Enteritis is usually seen as diarrhea, although, given the nature of avian droppings in general, this is more difficult to determine than in mammals. Diarrhea can lead to soiled feathers around the vent, or the vent can be pasted with fluid feces or urates. Sometimes *S typhimurium* becomes isolated in other organs, such as joints.[67] Exposure to *Salmonella* spp may produce disease, either acute or chronic, but may also produce an asymptomatic carrier stage in the intestinal tract of the bird. Necropsy findings include emaciation, hepatic necrosis and inflammation, hemorrhagic or necrotizing enteritis or enterocolitis,[63] and arthritis.[63,67] Birds dying acutely have few gross lesions.[68] Nonspecific lesions may be seen, such as congested lungs and kidneys, and swollen, congested, mottled livers and spleen with or without small hemorrhagic or necrotic foci.[68] In more chronic disease situations, tan to white foci or nodules form in the liver, spleen, pectoral muscles, subcutaneous tissue, brain, and other locations.[68] Infection that is passed through egg transmission presents as a creamy or caseous yolk sac that is not absorbed into the celomic cavity at hatching.[68]

S typhimurium has either evolved or become more prevalent in songbirds that are frequent visitors at bird feeders.[68] Population density of the songbirds and seasonality/winter when more bird feeders are available have been factors in the spread of this form of salmonellosis. The use of bird feeders as a recreational pursuit in developed countries has led to the emergence of several diseases in songbirds, not just salmonellosis. Escherichia coli septicemia[69] and mycoplasma infections[70] are both emerging diseases also associated with songbirds and bird feeders.

Less common, Salmonella enterica subspecies enterica serovar Hessarek has been isolated from some passerines. This disease was first identified in common raven (Corvus corax) from Hessarek, Iran, and has caused epizootics killing 10 to more than 1000 passerines in Europe, and was recently identified in Piciformes, the great spotted woodpecker (Dendrocopus major), in the United Kingdom.[71] The reservoir host for this form of salmonellosis is unknown and there is no seasonal association or connection with human-supplied food sources such as bird feeders with S typhimurium.[71] Woodpeckers have a primarily insectivorous diet and, therefore, there is less possibility of a fecal-oral transmission cycle as seen with S typhimurium.

Salmonella was among the organisms that were developed and used in biowarfare from 1932 to 1945 during World War II.[66,72] S typhimurium was used by bioterrorists in Oregon in 1984 to contaminate salad bars in 10 restaurants as part of a trial for a larger attack. This bioterrorist attack sickened 750 people and hospitalized 45.[66,73] Attempts to contaminate a city water supply with Salmonella by the same bioterrorist group was not successful.[66,74] This incident highlights the danger that Salmonella spp pose to public health if used in a sophisticated bioterrorist attack. The wildlife form, S typhimurium is especially dangerous because of its capability to infect multiple domestic species and humans.[66] Salmonella spp are still listed as category B (second highest priority) critical biological agents that could be used in a bioterrorism attack.[66]

DISCLOSURE

The authors have nothing to disclose.

REFERENCES

1. Latas P, Auckland LD, Teel PD, et al. Argas (Persicargas) Giganteus Soft Tick Infection with Rickettsia Hooogstraali and Relapsin Fever Borrelia on wild avian species of the Desert Southwest, USA. J Wildl Dis 2020;56(1):113–25.

2. Burridge M. Non-native and invasive ticks: threats to human and animal health in the United States. Gainesville (FL): University Press of Florida; 2011.

3. Hutcheson HJ, Dergousoff SJ, Lindsay LR. Haemaphysalis longicornis: a tick of considerable veterinary importance now established in North America. Can Vet J 2019;60:27–8.

4. Tufts DM, VanAcker MC, Fernandez MP, et al. Distribution, host-seeking phenology, and host and habitat associations of haemaphysalis longicornis ticks, Staten Island, New York, USA. Emerg Infect Dis 2019;25(4):792–6. Available at: www.cdc.gov/eid.

5. Gonzales-Astudillo V, Hernandez SM, Yabsley MJ, et al. Mortality of selected avian orders submitted to a wildlife diagnostic laboratory (southeastern cooperative wildlife disease study, USA): a 36-year retrospective analysis. J Wildl Dis 2016;52(3):441–58.

6. Justice-Allen A, Orr K, Schuler K, et al. Bald eagle nesting mortality associated with argas radiatus and argas ricei tick infestation and successful management with nest removal in Arizona, USA. J Wildl Dis 2016;52(4):940–4.

7. Smith KA, Campbell GD, Pear DL, et al. A retrospective summary of raptor mortality in Ontario, Canada (1991-2014), including the effects of west nile virus. J Wildl Dis 2018;54(2):261–71.

8. Miller RE, Fowler ME. Fowler's zoo and wild animal medicine current therapy, vol. 7. St Louis (MO): Elsevier Saunders; 2011.

9. Jimenez de Oya N, Escribano-Romero E, Blazques AB, et al. Current progress of avian vaccines against west Nile virus. Vaccines 2019;7(126):1–23.

10. Foss L, Padgett K, Reisen WK, et al. West Nile virus-related trends in avian mortality in California, USA 2003-12. J Wildl Dis 2015;51(3):576–88.

11. Thomas NJ, Hunter DB, Atkinson CT. Infectious diseases of wild birds. Ames (IA): Blackwell Publishing; 2007. p. 1–490.

12. van der Meulen KM, Pensaert MB, Nauwynck HJ. West Nile virus in the vertebrate world. Arch Virol 2005;150:637–57.

13. Phalen DN, Dahlhausen B. West Nile virus. Semin Avian Exot Pet 2004;13(2):67–78.

14. CDC. West Nile virus: information and guidance for clinicians. CDC; 2012. p. 1–48. Available at: www.cdc.gov.

15. Jimenez de Oya N, Escribano-Romero E, Camacho EC, et al. A recombinant subviral particle-based vaccine protects Magpie (Pica pica) against West Nile virus infection. Front Microbiol 2019;10:1133.

16. Murray K, Walker C, Goulde E. The virology, epidemiology, and clinical impact of West Nile virus: a decade of advancements in research since its introduction into the Western Hemisphere. Epidemiol Infect 2011;139(6):807–17.

17. Carboni D, Nevarez J, Tully T, et al. West Nile virus infection in a sun conure (Aratinga solstitialis). J Avian Med Surg 2008;22(3):240–5.

18. Nemeth NM, Kratz GE, Bates R, et al. Clinical evaluation and outcomes of naturally acquired WNV in raptors. J Zoo Wildl Med 2009;10(1):1–13.

19. Godhardt JA, Beheler K, O'Connor MJ, et al. Evaluation of antigen-capture ELISA and immunohistochemical methods for avian surveillance of West Nile virus. J Vet Diagn Invest 2006;18:85–9.

20. Gancz AY, Smith DA, Barker IK, et al. Pathology and tissue distribution of West Nile virus in North American owls (family: strigidae). Avian Pathol 2012;35(1):17–29.

21. Nemeth NM, Young GR, Burkhalter KL, et al. West Nile virus detection in nonvascular feathers from avian carcasses. J Vet Diagn Invest 2009;21(5):616–22.

22. Hinten S, Komar N, Langevin S, et al. Experimental infection of North American birds with the New York 1999 strain of West Nile virus. Emerg Infect Dis 2003;9(3):311–22.

23. Pauli A, Cruz-Martinez L, Ponder J. Ophthalmologic and oculopathologic findings in red-tailed hawks and Cooper's hawks with naturally acquired West Nile virus infection. J Am Vet Med Assoc 2007;231(8):1241–8.

24. Wunschmann A, Shivers J, Bender J, et al. Pathologic findings in red-tailed hawks (Accipiter cooperi) naturally infected with West Nile virus. Avian Dis 2004;48(3):570–80.

25. Willis AM, Wilkie DA. Avian ophthalmology, part 2: review of ophthalmic diseases. J Avian Med Surg 1999;13(4):245–51.

26. Fitzgerald SD, Patterson JS, Kiupel M, et al. Clinical and pathologic features of West Nile virus infection in native North American owls (family Strigidae). Avian Dis 2003;47(3):602–10.

27. Busquets N, Bertran K, Costa T, et al. Experimental West Nile virus infection in gyrsaker hybrid falcons. Vector Borne Zoonotic Dis 2012;12(6):482–9.

28. Dauphin G, Zientara S. West Nile virus: recent trends in diagnosis and vaccine development. Vaccine 2007;25(30):5563–76.

29. Olsen GH, Miller KJ, Docherty DE, et al. Pathogenicity of West Nile virus and response to vaccination in sandhill cranes (Grus canadensis) using a killed vaccine. J Zoo Wildl Med 2009;40(2):263–71.

30. Okeson D, Llizo S, Miller C, et al. Antibody response of five bird species after vaccination with a killed West Nile virus vaccine. J Zoo Wildl Med 2007;38(2): 240–4.

31. Silva M, Ellis A, Karaca K, et al. Domestic goose as a model for West Nile virus vaccine efficacy. Vaccine 2013;31(7):1045–50.

32. Alger K, Bunting E, Schuler K, et al. Diagnosing lymphoproliferative disease virus in live wild Turkeys (Meleagris gallopavo) using whole blood. J Zoo Wildl Med 2015;46(4):806–14.

33. Alger K, Bunting E, Schuler K, et al. Risk factors for and spatial distribution of lymphoproliferative disease virus (LPDV) in wild Turkeys (Meleagris gallopavo) in New York State, USA. J Wildl Dis 2017;53(3):499–508.

34. MacDonald AM, Jardine CM, Bowman J, et al. Detection of lymphoproliferative disease virus in canada in a survey for viruses in Ontario Wild Turkeys (Meleagris gallopavo). J Wildl Dis 2019;55(1):113–22.

35. Ellis J, Courchesne S, Shearn-Bochsler V, et al. Cyclic mass mortality of common eiders at Cape Cod, MA: and ongoing puzzle. Pacific Seabird Group Annual Meeting, The Westin Hotel, Long Beach, California, February 17-21, 2010. p. 17–8.

36. Allison AB, Ballard JR, Tesh RB, et al. Cyclic avian mass mortality in the northeastern United States is associated with a novel orthomyxovirus. J Virol 2015; 89:1389–403.

37. Goudie RI, Robertson GJ, Reed A. Common eider (Somateria mollissima). In: Poole A, Gill F, editors. The birds of North America. No. 546. Philadelphia: Academy of Natural Sciences; 2000. p. 32.

38. Clark GM, O'Meara D, Van Weelden JW. An epizootic among eider ducks involving an acanthocephalid worm. J Wildl Manage 1958;22:204–5.

39. US Geological Survey, National Wildlife Health Center. Wildlife health information sharing partnership event reporting system (WHISPers) online data base. Available at: https://wwwnwhc.usgs.gov/whispers. Accessed November 2, 2019.

40. Shearn-Bochsler V, Ip HS, Ballmann A, et al. Experimental infection of common eider ducklings with Wellfleet Bay virus, a newly characterized orthomyxovirus. Emerg Infect Dis 2017;23(12):1974–81.

41. Ballard JR, Mickley R, Gibbs SEJ, et al. Prevalence and distribution of Wellfleet Bay virus exposure in the common eider (Somateria mollissima). J Wildl Dis 2017;53(1):81–90.

42. Ballard JR, Mickley R, Brown JD, et al. Detection of Wellfleet Bay virus antibodies in sea birds of the Northeastern USA. J Wildl Dis 2017;53(4):875–9.

43. Dickinson MB. Field guide to the birds of North America. Washington, DC: National Geographic Society; 2002.

44. Pello SJ, Olsen GH. Emerging and reemerging diseases of avian wildlife. Vet Clin North Am Exot Anim Pract 2013;16(2):357–81.

45. Kessell A, Hyatt A, Lehmann D, et al. Cygnet River virus, a novel orthomyxovirus from ducks, Australia. Emerg Infect Dis 2012;18:2044–6.

46. Presti RM, Zhao G, Beatty WL, et al. Quaranfil, Johnston Atoll, and Lake Chad viruses are novel members of the family Orthomyxoviridae. J Virol 2009;83: 11599–606.

47. Taylor RM, Hurlbut HS, Work TH, et al. Arboviruses isolated from Argas ticks in Egypt: Quaranfil, Chenuda, and Nyamanini. Am J Trop Med Hyg 1966;15:76–86.

48. Hall JS, Dusek RJ, Spackman E. Rapidly expanding range of highly pathogenic avian influenza viruses. Emerg Infect Dis 2015;21(7):1251–2.

49. Balckmore C, Rabinowitz PM. Influenza. In: Rabinowitz PM, Conte LA, editors. Human-animal medicine: clinical approaches to zoonosis, toxicants and other shared health risks. Maryland Heights (MO): Saunders; 2012. p. 177–86.

50. Knipe DM, Howley DM, editors. Fields virology. 5th edition. Philadelphia: Lippincott Williams & Wilkins; 2007.

51. Brown JD, Berghaus RD, Costa TP, et al. Intestinal secretion of a wild bird-origin H3N8 low pathogenic avian influenza virus in mallards (Anas platyrhynchos). J Wildl Dis 2012;48(4):991–8.

52. Lebarbenchon C, Feare CJ, Renaud F, et al. Persistence of highly pathogenic avian influenza viruses in natural ecosystems. Emerg Infect Dis 2010;16(7): 1057–62.

53. Webster RG, Krauss S, Hulse-Post D, et al. Evolution of influenza A viruses in wild birds. J Wildl Dis 2007;43(3):S1–6.

54. Rott R. Genetic determinants for infectivity and pathogenicity of influenza viruses. Philos Trans R Soc Lond B Biol Sci 1980;288:393–9.

55. Okazaki K, Takada A, Ito T, et al. Perpetuation of influenza A viruses in Alaskan waterfowl reservoirs. Arch Virol 1995;140:1163–72.

56. Li Y, Shi J, Qi Q, et al. H5N1 avian influenza outbreak in wild birds in Western China in 2005. J Wildl Dis 2007;43(3):S21.

57. Kim H-R, Kwon Y-K, Jang I, et al. Pathologic changes in wild birds infected with highly pathogenic avian influenza A (H5N8) viruses, South Korea, 2014. Emerg Infect Dis 2015;21(5). https://doi.org/10.3201/eid2105.141967. Accessed November 2, 2019.

58. Ip HS, Torchetti MK, Crespo R, et al. Novel Eurasian highly pathogenic avian influenza A H5 viruses in wild birds, Washington, USA, 2014. Emerg Infect Dis 2015; 21(5):886–90.

59. Shearn-Bochsler VI, Knowles S, Ip H. Lethal infection of wild raptors with highly pathogenic avian influenza H5N8 and H5N2 viruses in the USA, 2014-2015. J Wildl Dis 2019;55(1):164–8.

60. Froberg T, Cuthbert F, Jennelle CS, et al. Avian influenza prevalence and viral shedding routes in Minnesota ring-billed gulls (Larus delawarensis). Avian Dis 2019;63(1s):120–5.

61. Umberto M, Alkukutu G, Roux J-P, et al. Avian influenza H5N8 outbreak in African penguins (Spheniscus demersus), Namibia, 2019. J Wildl Dis 2020;56(1). https://doi.org/10.7589/2019-03-067. Accessed November 2, 2019.
62. Lee D-H, Bertran K, Kwon J-H, et al. Evolution, global spread and pathogenicity of highly pathogenic avian influenza H5Nx clade 2.3.4.4. J Vet Sci 2017;18(40): 269–80.
63. Rabinowitz PM, Conti LA. Salmonellosis. In: Rabinowitz PM, Conti LA, editors. Clinical approaches to zoonoses, toxicants, and other shared health risks. Maryland Heights (MO): Saunders/Elsevier; 2010. p. 248–54.
64. Friend M. Salmonellosis, Chapter 9. In: Friend M, Franson JC, editors. Field manual of wildlife diseases. Madison (WI): USGS Biological Resources Division, National Wildlife Health Center; 1999. p. 99–109.
65. Reed KD, Meece JK, Henkel JS, et al. Birds, migration and emerging zoonoses: West Nile virus, Lyme disease, influenza A and enteropathogens. Clin Med Res 2003;1(1):5–12.
66. Friend M. Disease emergence and resurgence: the wildlife-human connection. US Department of Interior, US Geological Survey; 2006. p. 388. Circular 1285.
67. Kang M-S, Jeong O-M, Kim H-R, et al. Arthritis in an egret (*Egretta intermedia*) caused by *Salmonella typhimurium* and its potential risk to poultry health. J Wildl Dis 2015;40(2):534–7.
68. Daoust P-Y, Prescott JF. Salmonellosis, Chapter 13. In: Thomas NJ, Hunter B, Atkinson CT, editors. Infectious diseases of wild birds. Ames (IA): Blackwell Publishing; 2007. p. 270–88.
69. Pennycott TW, Ross HM, McLaren IM, et al. Causes of death of wild birds of the family Fringillidae in Britain. Vet Rec 1998;143:155–8.
70. Hartup BK, Bickal JM, Dhondt AA. Dynamics of conjunctivitis and *Mycoplasma gallisepticum* infections in house finches. Auk 2001;118:327–33.
71. Wilkinson V, Fernandez JR-R, Nunez A, et al. Novel *Salmonella* variant associated with mortality in two great spotted woodpeckers (*Dendrocopos major*). J Wildl Dis 2019;55(4):874–8.
72. Harris SH. Factories of death: Japanese biological Warfare, 1932-1945, and the American cover-up. New York: Routledge; 2002. p. 385.
73. Torok TJ, Tauxe RV, Wise RP, et al. A large community outbreak of salmonellosis caused by intentional contamination of restaurant salad bars. J Am Med Assoc 1997;278:389–95.
74. McDade JE, Franz D. Bioterrorism as a public health threat. Emerg Infect Dis 1998;4:493–4.

Selected Emerging Infectious Diseases of Amphibians

La'Toya V. Latney, DVM, DECZM, DABVP (Reptile/Amphibian)[a],*,
Eric Klaphake, DVM, DACZM[b]

KEYWORDS

- Amphibian • Ranavirus • *Batrachochytrium dendrobatidis* • Chytrid • Urodele
- Caecilian • Emerging disease

KEY POINTS

- *B dendrobatidis* (Bd) and Ranavirus are the most significant infectious diseases contributing to global population declines in amphibians.
- Fluid therapy and itraconazole are the mainstays of therapy for Bd infections; however, species variations in response to itraconazole or heat therapy can cause mortality.
- Ranavirus infects several species of anurans, larval and adults, and disease susceptibility varies among species.
- Ranavirus and Bd status can influence species susceptibility to parasitic disease.

INTRODUCTION

Given their virulence, devastating impact on global amphibian populations, and genetically divergent natures, *Batrachochytrium dendrobatidis* (Bd) and Ranavirus are the primary foci of this article. The Association of Reptile and Amphibian Veterinarian's Infectious Disease Committee has a quarterly publication of newly reported infectious diseases that is an invaluable source to stay current: "Infectious Diseases of Reptiles and Amphibians: Peer-Reviewed Publications" in the *Journal of Herpetological Medicine & Surgery*.

FUNGAL DISEASE: *BATRACHOCHYTRIUM DENDROBATIDIS*

Amphibians face the gravest threat of taxa extirpation[1,2] because of numerous factors; however, the catastrophic emergence of two World Organization for Animal Health (OIE) reportable infectious diseases, the chytrid fungus Bd and virus Ranavirus, may

[a] Avian and Exotic Medicine & Surgery, The Animal Medical Center, 610 East 62nd Street, New York, NY 10065, USA; [b] Cheyenne Mountain Zoo, 4250 Cheyenne Mountain Zoo Road, Colorado Springs, CO 80906, USA
* Corresponding author.
E-mail address: latoya.latney@amcny.org

Vet Clin Exot Anim 23 (2020) 397–412
https://doi.org/10.1016/j.cvex.2020.01.003
1094-9194/20/© 2020 Elsevier Inc. All rights reserved.

be the largest collective cause. The global Bd panzootic is responsible for the greatest loss of biodiversity attributable to disease in amphibia[1] with loss of more than 40% of amphibian species in areas of Central America and widespread losses across Europe, Australia, and North America.[3] Bd is known to affect anurans, urodeles, and caecilian species.[1] It alone has caused the decline of at least 501 amphibian species over the past half century, causing 90 extinctions and at least a 90% reduction in 25% of the extant species.[1]

Batrachochytrium dendrobatidis History and Epidemiology

Several strains of Bd have been identified, with the global pandemic lineage (Bd-GPL1) recognized as a globally invasive species that has caused mass mortality, population declines, and extinctions.[4,5] A regional enzootic lineage strain isolated in Brazil (Bd-Brazil) can kill naive wild populations,[6,7] and additional lineages have been identified from east Asia (Bd-Asia), Switzerland (Bd-CH), and South Africa (Bd-CAPE),[5,8,9] with differences in virulence among these lineages.[5,6,10] Multilineage Bd coinfections occur in natural populations with competitive pressures resulting from the human movement of pathogen strains that rapidly alters the genetics, community dynamics, and spatial epidemiology of pathogens in the wild.[5] Bd can rapidly evolve novel phenotypes independent of shared ancestry through phenotypic plasticity in response to temperature and may be genetically constrained to adapt to high temperatures. Bd infects more than 700 species[11] with potentially any amphibian species able to be host, vector, or reservoir.[5] Rare Bd-free countries include Papua New Guinea, Seychelles, Fiji, and the Solomon Islands.[5,12] Reports of infection in wild-caught caecilians have originated from Cameroon,[13] South America,[14] and several African countries.[15] In a study of fossorial and aquatic South American caecilians, quantitative polymerase chain reaction (qPCR) detected Bd in preserved caecilians collected over a 109-year period from the Uruguayan savanna, Brazil's Atlantic Forest, and the Amazon basin.[14] The overall Bd prevalence of 12.4% called attention to the role caecilians may serve as a potential reservoir.[14]

In a survey of wild and captive species, 30% of Tanzanian and Cameroonian terrestrial caecilians tested Bd positive including more than six species, six genera, and four families.[15] Other infections in captivity included the terrestrial *Geotrypetes seraphini*, HYP[15,16] neotropical aquatic species *Potomotyphlus kaupii*,[16] and *Typhlonectes natans*.[17]

Species-specific susceptibility for infective spore dose has been reported in some urodeles. More than 100,000 zoospores were necessary to cause disease in the northern slimy salamander (*Plethodon glutinosus*) and the Blue Ridge Mountain dusky salamander (*Desmognathus orestes*).[18] Conversely, 1000 spores in captive Vietnamese salamanders *Tylototriton asperrimus* and *Tylototriton vietnamensis* caused severe orthokeratosis and death within 3 weeks of infection.[19]

North American cryptobranchids can harbor Bd and remain asymptomatic, as identified in asymptomatic wild hellbenders (*Cryptobranchus alleganiensis*) with Bd-GPL1.[20] Multiple studies have detected Bd in wild hellbenders.[21–26] In West Virginia, the overall prevalence of Bd in hellbenders was 52%, highest in larger individuals and from montane locations.[26]

Batrachochytrium Salamandrivorans

In 2013, reports of *Batrachochytrium salamandrivorans* (Bsal) emerged from Southeast Asia, causing severe wild and captive urodele population declines[3] especially in native European salamanders, nearly causing the extinction of fire salamanders (*Salamandra salamandra*) in the Netherlands in 2008.[27] Because North America has the greatest diversity for salamanders (10 families, 675 species), Bsal in North America would have a catastrophic impact on global salamander diversity.[28] The United States listed 201 species of salamanders as injurious wildlife under the Lacey Act in 2016 to prevent the introduction, establishment, and spread of Bsal to their native species (USFWS, accessible online at https://www.fws.gov/injuriouswildlife/pdf_files/List-of-Salamander-Species.pdf). Not long after, OIE listed Bsal as a notifiable disease in 2017. Known reservoir species include the actively traded Asian salamanders: *Cynops cyanurus*, *Cynops pyrrhogaster*, and *Paramesotriton deloustali*. Bsal originated from and still coexists within a clade of Asian salamanders that are resistant to clinical disease. Bsal seems to only infect urodeles, with European and New World species being highly susceptible to infection and clinical disease. European and New World urodeles are highly susceptible to Bsal and develop severe disease.[29] Europe has suffered mass die-offs and population declines in several species from Bsal, yet Europe is also home to at least two other species of chytrid: an endemic Swiss lineage and the invasive Bd-GPL lineage.[30] Bd has been listed as widespread throughout Europe, and as reports of Bsal continue to emerge, it has become clear that its impact in urodeles could mirror the same devastation seen by Bd.[30] Bsal has not been detected in Eastern hellbenders[31] and to date Bsal has not been detected in the US pet population of urodeles.[32]

Batrachochytrium Dendrobatidis Pathogenesis and Life Cycle

Excellent clinical reviews of chytridiomycosis are available in the veterinary literature.[29,33] Chytridiomycosis belongs to a "lower" fungal phylum: the Chytridiomycota.[34] Bd, Bsal, and the fish pathogen *Ichthyochytrium vulgare* are the only known members adapted to vertebrate hosts.[34] The Bd life cycle has two main stages: environmental and on the host. In the environmental stage, flagellated zoospores live for 24 hours and are waterborne, motile, and free living.[35] Zoospores exhibit chemotaxis with two major predilection sites: adult epidermis and tadpole mouthparts. The zoospore encysts in the epidermis and germlings develop into sporangia, which produce more zoospores that can reinfect the host or enter the environment. Reinfection contributes to high pathogen burdens, high morbidity, and high mortality. Zoospores are extremely sensitive to temperature with a 4-day life cycle at 17°C to 22°C.[36] Three hours of desiccation kills 100% of infective Bd stages. Zoospores can survive 7 weeks in sterile pond water or several weeks in a moist environment.[37,38] Zoospores are stable in dead amphibian keratin and mosquitoes can serve as mechanical vectors of Bd.[39]

Zoospore epidermal invasion in adults can induce peracute mortalities. Bd interferes with the epidermal sodium-potassium pump, inhibiting up to 50% of sodium and potassium plasma concentrations resulting in drastic declines in pH, bradycardia, and asystolic cardiac arrest.[40] Rate of skin sloughing contributes to high levels of infectivity but does not curb disease progression and may actually contribute to physiologic homoeostasis loss by further inhibiting skin water and electrolyte transport.[41] In tadpoles, keratinized mouthpart loss decreases food intake, slows metamorphosis, and contributes to sublethal morbidity and mortality. Urodeles may present with lethargy and coelomic distention.[42] Bd is transmitted within and between amphibian life stages but it has not been documented to infect egg masses.[43] The skin of the neotenic Axolotl (*Ambystoma mexicanum*) is also susceptible to Bd.[42] Other animals may serve as fomites. Bd can parasitize zebrafish (*Danio rerio*),[44] red swamp crayfish (*Procambarus clarkii*) can carry and increase Bd infections in anurans,[45] and 42% of Andean aquatic bird toe museum specimens were qPCR positive for Bd.[46]

Susceptible amphibians have ineffective constitutive and innate defenses, a late-stage response characterized by immunopathology and Bd-induced suppression of lymphocyte responses.[47] Species with better skin peptide defenses had lower infection intensity and higher survival rates, therefore Bd resistance may correlate with the presence of skin peptides.[48] Compounds produced by resident bacteria *Janthinobacterium lividum* and *Serratia* species were found on anurans and caudates from five continents. A total of 89% of tested *Serratia* isolates and 82% of *J lividum* isolates were capable of inhibiting Bd.[49] Susceptibility variation seems related to genetic variation in the major histocompatibility complex class II locus in anurans.[50] Species-specific disease susceptibility is mapped to identify and optimize conservation targets.[51–53]

Batrachochytrium Dendrobatidis Diagnostics, Clinical Signs, and Treatment

Real-time or qPCR remains the preferred method to diagnose and qualify disease burden in afflicted species for Bd and Bsal.[54,55] Bsal and Bd species-specific duplex real-time PCR allows rapid detection on noninvasively collected amphibian samples and is used in the field.[56] Histologic zoospores obtained from sloughed skin samples are identified with better sensitivity (75%)[57] than previously reported.[58] Clinical signs in adults include abnormal posture/behavior, increased soaking time, reflex loss, lethargy, excessive epidermal roughening/sloughing, epidermal hyperemia, and peracute death. Tadpoles may be asymptomatic, have abnormal swimming behavior, or show discoloration of mouthparts.[36] Urodeles infected with Bsal develop skin hemorrhage and ulcerations 5 to 15 days after exposure.[29]

Electrolyte therapy with itraconazole and/or increased temperature for tolerant species are the mainstays of therapy. The pharmacokinetic studies of topical itraconazole in Panamanian golden frogs (*Atelopus zeteki*) found that a 0.01% itraconazole concentration for 10 minutes exceeded the minimal inhibitory concentration (MIC) for itraconazole for Bd for at least 36 hours, which may suggest that daily treatment is not needed. The study also showed that 0.001% itraconazole may be too low because it remained higher than the MIC for 1 hour after application[59]

Itraconazole concentration-dependent toxicity at 0.01% has been noted in metamorphs, larvae, adult Wyoming toads (*Anaxyrus baxteri*),[60] mountain yellow-legged frogs (*Rana muscosa*), common midwife toads (*Alytes obstetricans*), and striped marsh frogs (*Limnodynastes peronii*).[61] A shallow bath treatment of 0.0025% itraconazole for 5 minutes every 24 hours for 6 days cured individuals and reduced the possible drug toxicity risk.[62] Elevated temperatures (>26°C for 5 days) cleared Bd in midwife toads.[63] Juvenile Iberian midwife toads (*Alytes cisternasii*) and some individual poison dart frogs (Dendrobatidae family) infected with low Bd zoospore burdens showed a clinical response to voriconazole (1.25 mg/mL in water) sprayed on animals every 24 hours for 7 days.[64] Infected wild green and golden bell frogs (*Litoria aurea*) preferentially chose waterbodies with higher salinity than fresh water, leading to the assumption that infected frogs benefited from improved hydration and electrolyte osmoregulation in ponds with the adjusted salinity.[65] Manipulation of water where *L aurea* are infected by Bd may be a viable management action to reduce winter mortality.[65]

Chloramphenicol as a 20 mg/mL baths every 24 hours for 14 days and temperature increases to 28°C[66] in *Litoria caerulea* clears Bd infections. Chloramphenicol increased the risk of leukemia in Egyptian toads (*Bufo regularis*).[67] In vitro therapies demonstrating Bd sensitivity being applied in vivo must be done cautiously because amphotericin B has killed tadpoles.[64]

Itraconazole safety and efficacy may vary by species, therefore repeat testing should be performed post-treatment. Persistent Bd PCR-positive results in treated green-and-black poison dart frogs (*Dendrobates auratus*, 100%), red-eyed tree frogs (*Agalychnis callidryas*, 36.4%), gray tree frogs (*Hyla versicolor*, 33.3%), and green tree frogs (*Hyla cinera*, 27.3%) were reported several months post-treatment, including at the time of death (6–8 or 12–15 months).[68] Other considerations include optimizing biosecurity during treatment to avoid relapses or failures. Bd can persist on gloves for 6 minutes and in tap and deionized water sources for 3 and 4 weeks, respectively.[37,69]

The impact of Bd is so severe that in situ field treatment options have been pursued. A large-scale field project has been performed, capturing mountain chicken frogs (*Leptodactylus fallax*) in Montserrat that were treated for 5 minutes in a 0.01% aqueous itraconazole bath for 24 weeks. There was evidence of prophylactic effect during the treatment period, infection probability was lower for treated versus untreated animals, although the study was cut short by volcanic eruption. In situ individual animal treatment using said bath was effective in reducing Bd-induced mortality rate short term; however, it is labor intensive and requires high recapture rates. In situ individual treatment could be a useful short-term measure to augment other conservation actions for Bd-threatened amphibian species or to facilitate population survival during high disease risk periods.[70]

Bd treatment protocols and outcomes for urodeles vary, with some treatment protocols resulting in high mortality (**Table 1**).

In caecilians, successful treatment of Bd infection was reported in the terrestrial African *G seraphini* and the aquatic neotropical *P kaupii*, using 30-minute immersions in 0.01% solution of itraconazole every 24 hours for 11 days.[16] Captive aquatic *T nata* were successfully cleared of infection by elevating to and then holding water temperatures at 32.2°C (90°F) for 72 hours; however, another died despite treatment with a 0.01% itraconazole bath.[17] Treatment was successful for Bsal-infected fire salamanders, with a 10-minute daily submersion bath of polymyxin E (2000 IU/mL) and voriconazole (12.5°μF06Dg/mL spray every 12°h) at an ambient temperature of 20°C for 10 days.[55]

Batrachochytrium Dendrobatidis Biosecurity

Disinfection protocols for Bd and Bsal (**Table 2**) are also outlined in the OIE manual (https://www.oie.int/index.php?id=2439&L=0&htmfile=chapitre_batrachochytrium_dendrobatidis.htm) and in the previous review.[37] The Northeast Partnership for the Amphibians and Reptile Conservation, provides a user-friendly and detailed overview of biosecurity recommendations freely accessible at http://www.northeastparc.org/products/pdfs/NEPARC_Pub_2014-02_Disinfection_Protocol.pdf.

VIRAL DISEASE: RANAVIRUS

The OIE lists ranaviruses as reportable, because they can cause population decline and extinction, affecting entire communities[76,77] Ranaviruses are notifiable because of their potential severe host impact and the likely role of international trade facilitating emergence.[78] Ranaviruses are large, double-stranded DNA viruses of the family Iridoviridae with broad geographic and host ranges. They infect and cause disease in fish and reptiles but are most concerning for their ability to cause lethal disease in amphibians in the Americas, Europe, Asia, and Australia.[77]

Responsible for amphibian die-offs worldwide, ranaviruses have infected greater than 100 species in 18 taxonomic families.[79] Systemic hemorrhage and mortality

Table 1
Bd treatment outcomes in urodeles

Species	Medication	Submersion Time	Duration	Outcome
Axolotls[42]	0.002%–0.0025% itraconazole bath	5 min	q 24 h × 10 d	Disease clearance, PCR negative for 6 mo
Rough-skinned newts (Taricha granulosa)[42]	0.002%–0.0025% itraconazole bath	5 min	q 24 h × 10 d	Disease clearance, PCR negative for 6 mo
Japanese giant salamanders (Andrias japonicus)[71]	0.01% itraconazole bath	5 min	q 24 h × 10 d	Eradication of disease
Ambystoma andersoni[72]	0.01% itraconazole buffered with 1 teaspoon of sodium chloride in 5 L of tap water to maintain pH 7	5 min	q 24 h × 6 d at 16°C–20°C	50% mortality
Ambystoma dumerilii[72]	0.01% itraconazole baths	15 min	q 24 h × 11 d at 16°C	No adverse effects
Ambystoma mexicanum[72]	0.01% itraconazole baths	7 min	q 24 h × 7 d at 18°C	100% mortality
A mexicanum[72]	0.005% baths	7 min	q 24 h × 7 d at 18°C	100% mortality

Data from Refs. [42,71,72]

Table 2 Disinfection protocols for Bd and Bsal spores		
Surface	**Disinfectants**	**Contact Time**
Bd spores, soil[36]	Heat	37°C for 4 h inactivating zoospores or 60°C for 5 min
Bd spores, hard surfaces[36,73]	Path-X, 1:500 dilution Benzalkonium chloride 1:1500 dilution 1% sodium hypochlorite 70% ethanol Virkon 1 mg/mL	30 s 1 min 20 s 20 s 20 s
Bsal spores[74,75]	1% Virkon S, 4% sodium hypochlorite and 70% ethanol	5 min
Bsal, Bd, and Ranavirus[74,75]	Biocidal, 0.5% and 1% chloramine-T, 1:20 dilution of Dettol medical, Disolol, 70% ethanol, F10 75%, 76%, 4% chlorhexidine, 1% or 2% potassium permanganate, and 3% or 5% benzalkonium chloride	1 min

Data from Refs.[36,73–75]

can occur 3 days following pathogen water exposure.[80,81] Ranaviruses contribute to population decimation because (1) they can infect multiple host species with different susceptibilities[81,82]; (2) viral particles can persist outside the host[83,84]; and (3) several amphibian host life stages naturally cluster, which leads to density-independent transmission.[85,86] Details of ranavirus ecology and the unique threat it poses to several vertebrate orders are found in a freely accessible manuscript: *Ranaviruses: lethal pathogens of ectothermic vertebrates* (available at https://www.ranavirus.org/).

In North America, disease-associated amphibian community die-offs are most frequently caused by ranaviruses (43%–58% of die-offs),[87,88] and can involve large numbers of individuals.[89] In populations with reoccurring die-offs, recruitment may be nonexistent.[90] Negative effects of ranavirus outbreaks could be reduced in populations with a metapopulation structure through the rescue of affected populations by immigration.[86,90] It is unusual for a pathogen to exploit a broad range of host species and extremely rare for multiple host species to suffer synchronous mass mortality and declines when infection emerges.[91,92] In the last 30 years, exceptions include West Nile virus in North America, *Pseudogymnoascus destructans* (white-nose syndrome in North American bats), and Bd.[77] Ranaviruses meet the conditions required to cause similar host extinction.[85]

Ranavirus challenge laboratory trials and stage-structured population matrix models applied survival estimates to simulate potential population consequences of ranavirus exposure in dusky gopher frogs (*Lithobates sevosus*) and boreal toads (*Anaxyrus boreas boreas*). They found that both species were highly susceptible to ranaviruses in environmentally relevant ranavirus concentrated water. Dusky gopher frogs experienced 100% mortality in four of six life stages, whereas boreal toads experienced 100% mortality when exposed as tadpoles or metamorphs, the only life stages tested.[86] Extinction risk from ranavirus exposure was not mitigated by low levels of immigration, suggesting that open and closed population fates may be similar. Preventing ranavirus introduction by restricting public access to breeding ponds should be a priority and a component of species conservation plans.

According to the International Committee of Viral Taxonomy, the genus Ranavirus includes three fully sequenced viruses: Frog virus 3 (FV3), Ambystoma tigrinum virus, and Common midwife toad virus and several partially sequenced viruses. The official OIE listing is available at https://www.oie.int/index.php?id=2439&L=0&htmfile=chapitre_ranavirus.htm.

Ranavirus Pathogenesis and Diagnosis

A freely accessible, detailed overview of the viruses' ecopathology and impact on amphibians is available.[85] North American amphibians reflect the highest numbers of reported morbidities and mortalities in comparison with other locales.[85] Given the viruses' virulence, diagnosis is restricted to mortality being the only clinical finding. Other clinical signs include erratic swimming, buoyancy problems, lethargy, anorexia, leg and body swelling, leg and ventrum erythema, pericloacal/urostyle ecchymoses, skin and internal organ petechiation/ecchymoses, and irregular patches of skin discoloration.[85] In metamorphs and adults, the gastrointestinal tract may be empty or contain minimal ingesta and the gallbladder may be enlarged, both consistent with anorexia. Although hemorrhage and swellings are the most common gross lesions noted in larvae/tadpoles, cutaneous erosions and ulcerations are more frequently seen in adult European anurans and adult North American caudates.[85]

Transmission is indirect or direct, including contaminated water or soil; casual or direct contact with infected individuals; and ingestion of infected tissue during predation, cannibalism, or necrophagy.[36] As with Bd, mosquitoes have also been identified as vectors.[93] Recent widespread amphibian population die-offs from ranaviruses may be an interaction of suppressed and naive host immunity, anthropogenic stressors, and novel strain introduction. Susceptibility to ranaviruses differs among amphibian developmental stages, even in the same species. Adults tend to be least susceptible, likely because of more competent immune function. Several studies have shown that the most susceptible stage varies among species, with some most vulnerable during metamorphosis and others, such as the eastern spadefoot toad (Scaphiopus holbrookii), which are most susceptible as hatchlings because of delayed immune system development associated with rapid growth.[85] North American amphibian species that develop faster as larvae, have restricted distributions, or inhabit semipermanent breeding sites tend to be more susceptible than slow developing, widespread species that live in temporary wetlands.

FV3 causes tadpole edema syndrome, with adults as subclinical carriers. Free-ranging American bullfrog metamorphs may present with the one eye approximately 50% larger than the other and granulomas within the orbit caused by FV3 viral particles.[80] Bohle-like iridovirus was identified in captive magnificent tree frogs (Litoria splendida) and green tree frogs (Litoria caerulea) in Australia that had died or were euthanized after becoming lethargic or developing skin lesions.[80] In caudates, Ambystoma tigrinum virus infection manifests as gular edema, and plantar and tail hemorrhages. Raised skin plaques or polyps have been described in tiger salamanders and Chinese giant salamanders.[94,95] Clinical disease has not been reported in cryptobranchids; however, in eastern Tennessee, one study found the overall DNA prevalence of Bd, Ranavirus, and coinfections were 26%, 19%, and 5%, respectively.[25]

Necrosis of the hematopoietic tissues, vascular endothelium, and epithelial cells; hemorrhage; and intracytoplasmic basophilic inclusion bodies are common histopathologic lesions in all hosts.[80] Antemortem versus postmortem tissue PCR results may not match. A common lethal sampling technique is to test liver samples to estimate ranavirus prevalence because of pathogen targeting predilection and the ease of collection. To avoid euthanizing population-limited species, tail clips or skin swabs are more practicable for ranavirus surveillance programs, although infection prevalence by these methods may be underestimated compared with liver sampling.[96] The most appropriate test is dependent on the question that needs to be answered. Individual animal verification to be ranavirus-free is not possible, especially using nonlethal sampling.[80]

Ranavirus Control and Biosecurity

There are no OIE-recommended treatments, but control measures are outlined. Amphibians may harbor quiescent ranavirus, with macrophages serving as a hiding spot for FV3 in immunocompetent adult African clawed frogs (Xenopus laevis).[97] FV3 is detected within macrophages for up to 3 weeks postinfection, well after the kidneys clear the virus (14 days). Infected macrophages remain unaffected by the virus, suggesting a possible antiantigen (permissive) response to FV3. Immunocompetent adult African clawed frogs were found to shed FV3 into water, resulting in immunosuppressed cohabitant infection, highlighting the existence and potential role of carrier animals.[97] Ranavirus has a large genome and evidence of recombination events are being reported.[98] A chimeric strain of ranavirus has been identified in the state of Georgia, and models estimate it has the highest reported basic reproduction number of any amphibian pathogen and is one of the most virulent pathogens reported in wildlife populations.[99]

In reviewing the host response, ectotherms have less effective adaptive immune responses, displaying poorer T-lymphocyte expansion, fewer antibody isoforms, and a less developed immunologic memory response than mammals.[100] Ranaviruses have highly efficient strategies for evading and using host immune components to achieve persistence, facilitate dissemination, and expand host range. In 2007, adaptive responses were demonstrated in the Xenopus model.[101] Earlier proliferation and infiltration associated with faster viral clearance were observed during a secondary infection. These results provide in vivo evidence of protective antigen-dependent CD8$^+$ T-cell proliferation, recognition, and memory in fighting a natural pathogen. Prior infection with a ranavirus led to enhanced immunity against subsequent exposure.[102]

Although use of a vaccine might have limited field utility, it could be valuable in captive populations. Two different DNA vaccines were developed that targeted the viral envelope proteins, ADRV 2L and 58L genes, to protect Chinese giant salamanders against ADRV infection.[103] Chinese giant salamanders vaccinated with pcDNA-2L showed a relative survival of 66.7%, and pcDNA-58L of only 3.3%. Antibodies against pcDNA-2L were detected 14 and 21 days after infection. Vaccination with pcDNA-2L significantly suppressed virus replication, seen by a low splenic viral load in survivors after ADRV challenge. These results suggest that pcDNA-2L could induce a significant innate immune response and an adaptive immune response involving humoral and cell-mediated immunity that confer effective protection against ADRV infection.[103] An insect vector and a recombinant baculovirus of AcNPV-MCP elicited robust and specific humoral immune responses detected by enzyme-linked immunosorbent assay and neutralization assays and potent cellular immune responses in Chinese giant salamanders.[104] Immunization conferred highly protective immunity for Chinese giant salamanders against CGSIV challenge with a survival rate of 84%.[104]

Ranaviruses infect at least 175 species across 53 families of ectothermic vertebrates on every continent except Antarctica.[99] Viral persistence is highest in sterilized pond water, then unsterilized pond water, and lowest in soil. Infective doses of ranaviruses can survive at low temperatures (4°C) for 102 to 182 days in sterile pond water, 58 to 72 days in unsterile pond water, and 30 to 48 days in soil. At 20°C, virus survival was 22 to 31 days in sterile pond water and 22 to 34 days in unsterile pond water.[83] In captive ranavirus mortalities, aggressive sterilization/removal of substrate and cleaning is advised. Effective cleansers to inactive ranaviruses after 1 minute of exposure include chlorhexidine (0.75%), sodium hypochlorite (3.0%), and Virkon S (1.0%). Potassium permanganate was ineffective at inactivating virus at 5 ppm.[105]

A clinical reference is freely available online, accessible at http://www.northeastparc.org/products/pdfs/NEPARC_Pub_2014-02_Disinfection_Protocol.pdf, with an overview for ranavirus and Bd control because of coinfection prevalence.[52]

DISCLOSURE

The authors have nothing to disclose.

REFERENCES

1. Scheele BC, Pasmans F, Skerratt LF, et al. Amphibian fungal panzootic causes catastrophic and ongoing loss of biodiversity. Science 2019;363(6434): 1459–63.
2. Stegen G, Pasmans F, Schmidt BR, et al. Drivers of salamander extirpation mediated by *Batrachochytrium salamandrivorans*. Emerg Infect Dis 2016; 22(7):1286–8.
3. Martel A, Spitzen-van der Sluijs A, Blooi M, et al. *Batrachochytrium salamandrivorans* sp. nov. causes lethal chytridiomycosis in amphibians. Proc Natl Acad Sci USA 2013;110(38):15325–9.
4. Farrer RA, Weinert LA, Bielby J, et al. Multiple emergences of genetically diverse amphibian-infecting chytrids include a globalized hypervirulent recombinant lineage. Proc Natl Acad Sci USA 2011;108(46):18732–6.
5. Jenkinson TS, Rodriguez D, Clemons RA, et al. Globally invasive genotypes of the amphibian chytrid outcompete an enzootic lineage in coinfections. Proc R Soc Lond 2018;285(1893):20181894.
6. Becker CG, Greenspan SE, Tracy KE, et al. Variation in phenotype and virulence among enzootic and panzootic amphibian chytrid lineages. Fungal Ecol 2017; 26:45–50.
7. Carvalho T, Becker CG, Toledo LF. Historical amphibian declines and extinctions in Brazil linked to chytridiomycosis. Proc Biol Sci 2017;284(1848):20162254.
8. O'Hanlon SJ, Rieux A, Farrer RA, et al. Recent Asian origin of chytrid fungi causing global amphibian declines. Science 2018;360(6389):621–7.
9. Kolby JE. Amphibia: global amphibian declines caused by an emerging infectious disease and inadequate immune responses. In: Cooper EL, editor. Advances in comparative immunology. Cham (Switzerland): Springer; 2018. p. 981–90.
10. Greenspan SE, Lambertini C, Carvalho T, et al. 2018 hybrids of amphibian chytrid show high virulence in native hosts. Sci Rep 2018;(8):9600.
11. Olson DH, Aanensen DM, Ronnenberg KL, et al. Mapping the global emergence of *Batrachochytrium dendrobatidis*, the amphibian chytrid fungus. PLoS One 2013;8:e56802.
12. Labisko J, Maddock ST, Taylor ML, et al. Chytrid fungus (*Batrachochytrium dendrobatidis*) undetected in the two orders of Seychelles amphibians. Herpetol Rev 2015;46(1):41–5.
13. Doherty-Bone TM, Gonwouo NL, Hirschfeld M, et al. *Batrachochytrium dendrobatidis* in amphibians of Cameroon, including first records for caecilians. Dis Aquat Org 2013;102:187–94.

14. Lambertini C, Becker CG, Bardier C, et al. Spatial distribution of *Batrachochytrium dendrobatidis* in South American caecilians. Dis Aquat Org 2017;124(2): 109–16.

15. Gower DJ, Doherty-Bone T, Loader SP, et al. *Batrachochytrium dendrobatidis* infection and lethal chytridiomycosis in caecilian amphibians (Gymnophiona). Ecohealth 2013;10(2):173–83.

16. Rendle ME, Tapley B, Perkins M, et al. Itraconazole treatment of *Batrachochytrium dendrobatidis* (Bd) infection in captive caecilians (Amphibia: Gymnophiona) and the first case of Bd in a wild neotropical caecilian. J Zoo Aquar Res 2015;3(4):137–40.

17. Churgin SM, Raphael BL, Pramuk JB, et al. *Batrachochytrium dendrobatidis* in aquatic caecilians (*Typhlonectes natans*): a series of cases from two institutions. J Zoo Wildl Med 2013;44(4):1002–9.

18. Chinnadurai SK, Cooper D, Dombrowski DS, et al. Experimental infection of native North Carolina salamanders with *Batrachochytrium dendrobatidis*. J Wild Dis 2009;45(3):631–6.

19. Thien TN, Martel A, Brutyn M, et al. A survey for *Batrachochytrium dendrobatidis* in endangered and highly susceptible Vietnamese salamanders (*Tylototriton* spp.). J Zoo Wildl Med 2013;44(3):627–33.

20. Tominaga A, Irwin KJ, Freake MJ, et al. *Batrachochytrium dendrobatidis* haplotypes on the hellbender *Cryptobranchus alleganiensis* are identical to global strains. Dis Aquat Org 2013;102(3):181–6.

21. Simpson H, Petokas P. Occurrence of the fungal pathogen *Batrachochytrium dendrobatidis* among eastern hellbender populations (*Cryptobranchus a. alleganiensis*) within the Allegheny-Ohio and Susquehanna river drainages, Pennsylvania, USA. Herpetol Rev 2012;43(1):90–3.

22. Briggler JT, Larson KA, Irwin KJ. Presence of the amphibian chytrid fungus (*Batrachochytrium dendrobatidis*) on hellbenders (*Cryptobranchus alleganiensis*) in the Ozark Highlands. Herpetol Rev 2008;39:443–4.

23. Gonynor JL, Yabsley MJ, Jensen JB. A preliminary survey of *Batrachochytrium dendrobatidis* exposure in hellbenders from a stream in Georgia, USA. Herpetol Rev 2011;42:58–9.

24. Williams LA, Groves JD. Prevalence of the amphibian pathogen *Batrachochytrium dendrobatidis* in eastern hellbenders (*Cryptobranchus a. alleganiensis*) in western North Carolina, USA. Herpetol Conserv Bio 2014;9(3):454–67.

25. Souza MJ, Gray MJ, Colclough P, et al. Prevalence of infection by *Batrachochytrium dendrobatidis* and Ranavirus in eastern hellbenders (*Cryptobranchus alleganiensis alleganiensis*) in eastern Tennessee. J Wild Dis 2012;48(3):560–6.

26. Seeley KE, D'Angelo M, Gowins C, et al. Prevalence of *Batrachochytrium dendrobatidis* in Eastern Hellbender (*Cryptobranchus alleganiensis*) populations in West Virginia, USA. J Wild Dis 2016;52(2):391–4.

27. Spitzen-van der Sluijs A, Spikmans F, Bosman W, et al. Rapid enigmatic decline drives the fire salamander (*Salamandra salamandra*) to the edge of extinction in the Netherlands. Amphib Reptil 2013;34(2):233–9.

28. Yap TA, Koo MS, Ambrose RF, et al. Averting a North American biodiversity crisis. Science 2015;349(6247):481–2.

29. Mutschmann F. Chytridiomycosis in amphibians. J Exot Pet Med 2015;24(3): 276–82.

30. Lips KR. Overview of chytrid emergence and impacts on amphibians. Philos Trans R Soc Lond B Biol Sci 2016;371(1709):20150465.

31. Bales EK, Hyman OJ, Loudon AH, et al. Pathogenic chytrid fungus *Batrachochytrium dendrobatidis*, but not *B. salamandrivorans*, detected on eastern hellbenders. PLoS One 2015;10(2):e0116405.
32. Klocke B, Becker M, Lewis J, et al. *Batrachochytrium salamandrivorans* not detected in US survey of pet salamanders. Sci Rep 2017;7(1):13132.
33. Baitchman EJ, Pessier AP. Pathogenesis, diagnosis, and treatment of amphibian chytridiomycosis. Vet Clin North Anim Exot Anim Prac 2013;16(3): 669–85.
34. Martel A, Pasmans F, Fisher MC, et al. Chytridiomycosis. In: Seyedmousavi S, de Hoog GS, Guillot J, et al, editors. Emerging and epizootic fungal infections in animals. Cham (Switzerland): Springer; 2018. p. 309–35.
35. Rosenblum EB, Stajich JE, Maddox N, et al. Global gene expression profiles for life stages of the deadly amphibian pathogen *Batrachochytrium dendrobatidis*. Proc Natl Acad Sci USA 2008;105(44):17034–9.
36. Latney LV, Klaphake E. Selected emerging diseases of amphibia. Vet Clin North Anim Exot Anim Prac 2013;16(2):283–301.
37. Johnson ML, Speare R. Survival of *Batrachochytrium dendrobatidis* in water quarantine and disease control implications. Emerg Infect Dis 2003;9:922–5.
38. Johnson ML, Speare R. Possible modes of dissemination of the amphibian chytrid *Batrachochytrium dendrobatidis* in the environment. Dis Aquat Organ 2005; 65:181–6.
39. Gould J, Valdez J, Stockwell M, et al. Mosquitoes as a potential vector for the transmission of the amphibian chytrid fungus. Zool Ecol 2019;29:38–44.
40. Voyles J, Berger L, Young S, et al. Electrolyte depletion and osmotic imbalance in amphibians with chytridiomycosis. Dis Aquat Org 2007;77(2):113–8.
41. Ohmer ME, Cramp RL, White CR, et al. Skin sloughing rate increases with chytrid fungus infection load in a susceptible amphibian. Funct Ecol 2015;29(5): 674–82.
42. Del Valle JM, Eisthen HL. Treatment of chytridiomycosis in laboratory axolotls (*Ambystoma mexicanum*) and rough-skinned newts (*Taricha granulosa*). Comp Med 2019;69(3):204–11.
43. Rachowicz LJ, Vredenburg VT. Transmission of *Batrachochytrium dendrobatidis* within and between amphibian life stages. Dis Aquat Org 2004;61:75–83.
44. Liew N, Moya MJ, Wierzbicki CJ, et al. Chytrid fungus infection in zebrafish demonstrates that the pathogen can parasitize non-amphibian vertebrate hosts. Nat Commun 2017;8:15048.
45. Oficialdegui FJ, Sánchez MI, Monsalve-Carcaño C, et al. The invasive red swamp crayfish (*Procambarus clarkii*) increases infection of the amphibian chytrid fungus (*Batrachochytrium dendrobatidis*). Biol Invasions 2019;21(11): 3221–31.
46. Burrowes PA, De la Riva I. Detection of the amphibian chytrid fungus *Batrachochytrium dendrobatidis* in museum specimens of Andean aquatic birds: implications for pathogen dispersal. J Wild Dis 2017;53(2):349–55.
47. Grogan LF, Robert J, Berger L, et al. Review of the amphibian immune response to chytridiomycosis, and future directions. Front Immunol 2018;9:2536.
48. Woodhams DC, Ardipradja K, Alford RA, et al. Resistance to chytridiomycosis varies among amphibian species and is correlated with skin peptide defenses. Anim Conserv 2007;10(4):409–17.
49. Woodhams DC, LaBumbard BC, Barnhart KL, et al. Prodigiosin, violacein, and volatile organic compounds produced by widespread cutaneous bacteria of

amphibians can inhibit two *Batrachochytrium* fungal pathogens. Microb Ecol 2018;75(4):1049–62.

50. Fu M, Waldman B. Major histocompatibility complex variation and the evolution of resistance to amphibian chytridiomycosis. Immunogenetics 2017;69(8–9): 529–36.

51. Borteiro C, Cruz JC, Kolenc F, et al. Dermocystid-chytrid coinfection in the Neotropical frog *Hypsiboas pulchellus* (Anura: Hylidae). J Wild Dis 2014; 50(1):150–3.

52. Watters JL, Davis DR, Yuri T, et al. Concurrent infection of *Batrachochytrium dendrobatidis* and ranavirus among native amphibians from northeastern Oklahoma, USA. J Aquat Anim Health 2018;30(4):291–301.

53. Longo AV, Fleischer RC, Lips KR. Double trouble: co-infections of chytrid fungi will severely impact widely distributed newts. Biol Invasions 2019;21(6): 2233–45.

54. Boyle DG, Boyle DB, Olsen V, et al. Rapid quantitative detection of chytridiomycosis (*Batrachochytrium dendrobatidis*) in amphibian samples using real-time Taqman PCR assay. Dis Aquat Org 2004;60(2):141–8.

55. Blooi M, Pasmans F, Longcore JE, et al. Duplex real-time PCR for rapid simultaneous detection of *Batrachochytrium dendrobatidis* and *Batrachochytrium salamandrivorans* in amphibian samples. J Clin Microbiol 2013;51(12):4173–7.

56. Thomas V, Blooi M, Van Rooij P, et al. Recommendations on diagnostic tools for *Batrachochytrium salamandrivorans*. Transbound Emerg Dis 2018;65(2): e478–88.

57. Borteiro C, Kolenc F, Verdes JM, et al. Sensitivity of histology for the detection of the amphibian chytrid fungus *Batrachochytrium dendrobatidis*. J Vet Diagn Invest 2019;31(2):246–9.

58. Kriger KM, Hines HB, Hyatt AD, et al. Techniques for detecting chytridiomycosis in wild frogs: comparing histology with real-time Taqman PCR. Dis Aquat Org 2006;71(2):141–8.

59. Rifkin A, Visser M, Barrett K, et al. The pharmacokinetics of topical itraconazole in Panamanian golden frogs (*Atelopus zeteki*). J Zoo Wildl Med 2017;48(2): 344–51.

60. Pessier A. Management of disease as a threat to amphibian conservation. Int Zoo Yearbk 2008;42(1):30–9.

61. Woodward A, Berger L, Skerratt LF. In vitro sensitivity of the amphibian pathogen *Batrachochytrium dendrobatidis* to antifungal therapeutics. Res Vet Sci 2014;97:364–5.

62. Brannelly LA, Richards-Zawacki CL, Pessier AP. Clinical trials with itraconazole as a treatment for chytrid fungal infections in amphibians. Dis Aquat Org 2012; 101(2):95–104.

63. Schmidt B, Küpfer E, Geiger C, et al. Elevated temperature clears chytrid fungus infections from tadpoles of the midwife toad, alytes obstetricans. Amphib Reptil 2011;32(2):276–80.

64. Martel A, Van Rooij P, Vercauteren G, et al. Developing a safe antifungal treatment protocol to eliminate *Batrachochytrium dendrobatidis* from amphibians. Med Mycol 2011;49(2):143–9.

65. Klop-Toker KL, Valdez JW, Stockwell MP, et al. Assessing host response to disease treatment: how chytrid-susceptible frogs react to increased water salinity. Wildl Res 2018;44(8):648–59.

66. Young S, Speare R, Berger L, et al. Chloramphenicol with fluid and electrolyte therapy cures terminally ill green tree frogs (*Litoria caerulea*) with chytridiomycosis. J Zoo Wildl Med 2012;43(2):330–7.

67. El-Mofty MM, Abdelmeguid NE, Sadek IA, et al. Induction of leukaemia in chloramphenicol-treated toads. East Mediterr Health J 2000;6:1026–34.

68. Georoff TA, Moore RP, Rodriguez C, et al. Efficacy of treatment and long-term follow-up of *Batrachochytrium dendrobatidis* PCR-positive anurans following itraconazole bath treatment. J Zoo Wildl Med 2013;44(2):395–403.

69. Mendez DR, Webb LB, Speare R. Survival of the amphibian chytrid fungus *Batrachochytrium dendrobatidis* on bare hands and gloves: hygiene implications for amphibian handling. Dis Aquat Org 2008;82:97–104.

70. Hudson MA, Young RP, Lopez J, et al. In-situ itraconazole treatment improves survival rate during an amphibian chytridiomycosis epidemic. Biol Conserv 2016;195:37–45.

71. Une Y, Matsui K, Tamukai K, et al. Eradication of the chytrid fungus *Batrachochytrium dendrobatidis* in the Japanese giant salamander *Andrias japonicus*. Dis Aquat Org 2012;98(3):243–7.

72. Michaels CJ, Rendle M, Gibault C, et al. *Batrachochytrium dendrobatidis* infection and treatment in the salamanders *Ambystoma andersoni*, *A. dumerilii* and *A. mexicanum*. Herpetol J 2018;28(2):87–92.

73. Gold KK, Reed PD, Bemis DA, et al. Efficacy of common disinfectants and terbinafine in inactivating the growth of *Batrachochytrium dendrobatidis* in culture. Dis Aquat Org 2013;107(1):77–81.

74. Van Rooij P, Pasmans F, Coen Y, et al. Efficacy of chemical disinfectants for the containment of the salamander chytrid fungus *Batrachochytrium salamandrivorans*. PLoS One 2017;12(10):e0186269.

75. De Jong MS, Van Dyk R, Weldon C. Antifungal efficacy of F10SC veterinary disinfectant against *Batrachochytrium dendrobatidis*. Med Mycol 2017;56(1):60–8.

76. Earl JE, Gray MJ. Introduction of ranavirus to isolated wood frog populations could cause local extinction. Ecohealth 2014;11:581–92.

77. Price SJ, Garner TW, Nichols RA. Collapse of amphibian communities due to an introduced Ranavirus. Curr Biol 2014;24(21):2586–91.

78. Schloegel LM, Daszak P, Cunningham AA, et al. Two amphibian diseases, chytridiomycosis and ranaviral disease, are now globally notifiable to the World Organization for Animal Health (OIE): an assessment. Dis Aquat Org 2010;92(2–3):101–8.

79. Duffus AL, Waltzek TB, Stöhr AC, et al. Distribution and host range of ranaviruses. In: Gray MJ, Chinchar VG, editors. Ranaviruses: lethal pathogens of ectothermic vertebrates. Secaucus (NJ): Springer; 2015. p. 9–57.

80. Miller DL, Pessier AP, Hick P, et al. Comparative pathology of ranaviruses and diagnostic techniques. In: Gray MJ, Chinchar VG, editors. Ranaviruses: lethal pathogens of ectothermic vertebrates. Secaucus (NJ): Springer; 2015. p. 171–208.

81. Hoverman JT, Gray MJ, Haislip NA, et al. Phylogeny, life history, and ecology contribute to differences in amphibian susceptibility to ranaviruses. Ecohealth 2011;8:301–19.

82. Brenes R, Miller DL, Waltzek TB, et al. Susceptibility of fish and turtles to three ranaviruses isolated from different ectothermic vertebrate classes. J Aquat Anim Health 2014;26:118–26.

83. Nazir J, Spengler M, Marschang RE. Environmental persistence of amphibian and reptilian ranaviruses. Dis Aquat Org 2012;98(3):177–84.

84. Johnson AF, Brunner JL. Persistence of an amphibian ranavirus in aquatic communities. Dis Aquat Org 2014;111:129–38.

85. Miller DL, Gray MJ, Storfer A. Ecopathology of ranaviruses infecting amphibians. Viruses 2011;3:2351–73.

86. Earl JE, Chaney JC, Sutton W, et al. Ranavirus could facilitate local extinction of rare amphibian species. Oecologia 2016;182(2):611–23.

87. Green DE, Converse KA, Schrader AK. Epizootiology of sixty-four amphibian morbidity and mortality events in the USA, 1996-2001. Ann N Y Acad Sci 2002;969(1):323–39.

88. Muths E, Gallant AL, Grant EHC, et al. The amphibian research and monitoring initiative (ARMI): 5-year report. U.S. Department of the Interior, US Geological Survey Scientific Investigations Report 2006-5224; 2008. p. 68–77.

89. Wheelwright NT, Gray MJ, Hill RD, et al. Sudden mass die-off of a large population of wood frog (*Lithobates sylvaticus*) tadpoles in Maine, USA, likely due to ranavirus. Herpetol Rev 2014;45:240–2.

90. Petranka JW, Harp EM, Holbrook CT, et al. Long-term persistence of amphibian populations in a restored wetland complex. Biol Conserv 2007;138:371–80.

91. Woolhouse MEJ, Taylor LH, Haydon DT. Population biology of multihost pathogens. Science 2001;292:1109–12.

92. Smith KF, Acevedo-Whitehouse K, Pedersen AB. The role of infectious diseases in biological conservation anim. Conserv Biol 2009;12:1–12.

93. Kimble SJ, Karna AK, Johnson AJ, et al. Mosquitoes as a potential vector of ranavirus transmission in terrestrial turtles. Ecohealth 2015;12(2):334–8.

94. Jancovich JK, Davidson EW, Morado JF, et al. Isolation of a lethal virus from the endangered tiger salamander *Ambystoma tigrinum stebbinsi*. Dis Aquat Org 1997;31:161–7.

95. Geng Y, Wang KY, Zhou ZY, et al. First report of a ranavirus associated with morbidity and mortality in farmed Chinese giant salamanders (*Andrias davidianus*). J Comp Pathol 2011;145(1):95–102.

96. Gray MJ, Miller DL, Hoverman JT. Reliability of non-lethal surveillance methods for detecting ranavirus infection. Dis Aquat Org 2012;99(1):1–6.

97. Robert J, George E, De Jesús Andino F, et al. Waterborne infectivity of the Ranavirus frog virus 3 in *Xenopus laevis*. Virology 2011;2:410–7.

98. Claytor SC, Subramaniam K, Landrau-Giovannetti N, et al. Ranavirus phylogenomics: signatures of recombination and inversions among bullfrog ranaculture isolates. Virology 2017;511:330–43.

99. Peace A, O'Regan SM, Spatz JA, et al. A highly invasive chimeric ranavirus can decimate tadpole populations rapidly through multiple transmission pathways. Ecol Model 2019;410:108777.

100. Robert J, Ohta Y. Comparative and developmental study of the immune system in *Xenopus*. Dev Dyn 2009;238:1249–70.

101. Morales HD, Robert J. Characterization of primary and memory CD8 T-cell responses against ranavirus (FV3) in *Xenopus laevis*. J Virol 2007;81(5):2240–8.

102. Majj S, LaPatra S, Long SM, et al. Rana catesbeiana Virus Z (RCV-Z): a novel pathogenic Ranavirus. Dis Aquat Organ 2006;73:1–11.

103. Chen ZY, Li T, Gao XC, et al. Protective immunity induced by DNA vaccination against ranavirus infection in chinese giant salamander *Andrias davidianus*. Viruses 2018;10(2):52, p1-12.

104. Zhou X, Zhang X, Han Y, et al. Vaccination with recombinant baculovirus expressing ranavirus major capsid protein induces protective immunity in Chinese giant salamander, *Andrias davidianus*. Viruses 2017;9(8):195, p1-15.
105. Bryan LK, Baldwin CA, Gray MJ, et al. Efficacy of select disinfectants at inactivating Ranavirus. Dis Aquat Org 2009;84:89–94.

Updates on Selected Emerging Infectious Diseases of Ornamental Fish

Colin McDermott, VMD, CertAqV[a],*,
Brian Palmeiro, VMD, DACVD, CertAqV[b]

KEYWORDS

- Goldfish herpesvirus • Koi herpesvirus • Carp edema virus • *Erysipelothrix*
- *Edwardsiella* • *Francisella*

KEY POINTS

- New emerging infectious diseases of ornamental fish include carp edema virus, *Erysipelothrix, E ictaluri,* and *E piscicida.*
- Our understanding of previously discussed emerging infectious diseases have improved. Clinical updates on goldfish herpesvirus, koi herpesvirus, and *Francisella* are provided.
- Currently, the best practices for preventing outbreaks of emerging diseases in ornamental fish populations involves exceptional husbandry, biosecurity, and disease surveillance protocols.
- With improved molecular diagnostics, our understanding of ornamental fish diseases continues to evolve both in detecting new diseases and advancing our understanding of known pathogens.

INTRODUCTION

By their nature, emerging diseases are always changing. Since the publication of "Selected Emerging Infectious Diseases of Ornamental Fish" in 2013,[1] much has changed in the world of ornamental fish diseases. As our ability to detect and classify pathogens improves, we are discovering both novel pathogens and previously well-described pathogens that have the potential to infect other species. This article focuses on important emerging infectious diseases that affect ornamental fish in the aquarium, research, and aquaculture industries. New emerging diseases are described, and clinical updates to some diseases in the 2013 edition are provided where applicable. Some of these diseases are listed by the World Organization for Animal Health (**Box 1**).

---
[a] Zodiac Pet and Exotic Hospital, Victoria Centre, Shop 101A, 1/F, 15 Watson Road, Fortress Hill, Hong Kong; [b] Lehigh Valley Veterinary Dermatology & Fish Hospital, Pet Fish Doctor, 4580 Crackersport Road, Allentown, PA 18104, USA
* Corresponding author.
E-mail address: Cmcd.vmd@gmail.com

Vet Clin Exot Anim 23 (2020) 413–428
https://doi.org/10.1016/j.cvex.2020.01.004
1094-9194/20/© 2020 Elsevier Inc. All rights reserved.

vetexotic.theclinics.com

> **Box 1**
> **World Organization for Animal Health listed diseases of fish 2019**
>
> Epizootic hematopoietic necrosis[a]
>
> Epizootic ulcerative syndrome (*A invadans*)
>
> Infection with *Gyrodactylus salaris*
>
> Infectious hematopoietic necrosis
>
> HPR-deleted or HPRO infectious salmon anemia
>
> KHV[a]
>
> Red sea bream iridoviral disease[a]
>
> Spring viremia of carp
>
> Viral hemorrhagic septicemia
>
> Salmonid alphavirus
>
> [a] Discussed in this article or 2013 VCNA article.
> *Modified from* McDermott C, Palmeiro B. Selected emerging infectious diseases in ornamental fish. Vet Clin North Am Exot Anim Pract. 2013; 16(2):261-282; with permission.

VIRAL DISEASES

Owing to the changing nature of viral taxonomy and classification, all viruses are named and discussed using the current nomenclature from the International Committee on Taxonomy of Viruses (International Committee on Taxonomy of Viruses 2018 Master Species List Version 2).[2] Novel and unassigned viruses are discussed as applicable.

Alloherpesviruses

Herpesviruses show strong host specificity, but some can infect multiple species with varying clinical signs. The order Herpesvirales contains 3 distinct families: Herpesviridae that infect mammals, birds, and reptiles; *Alloherpesviridae* that infect fish and amphibians; and *Malacoherpesviridae* that infect bivalve mollusks (oysters and abalone).[2,3] Cyprinid herpesvirus-2 (CyHV-2) and cyprinid herpsevirus-3 continue to be important emerging diseases in the ornamental fish trade.

Cyprinid Herpes Virus-2: Clinical Updates[a]

CyHV-2 (Goldfish herpesvirus or herpesviral hematopoietic necrosis virus) affects goldfish worldwide. Prevalence studies in the United States have shown viral detection by polymerase chain reaction (PCR) from goldfish production facilities nationwide, with 1 publication finding 78% of goldfish commercial farms in 3 eastern states having detectable levels of CyHV-2.[4] Recent studies have focused on the effect of water temperature on clinical disease.

In experimental infections, cumulative mortality rates at 15°C, 20°C, and 25°C (59°F, 68°F, and 77°F) were 10%, 90%, and 60% respectively; the authors concluded that a

---

[a] Clinical updates are provided for some diseases discussed in the previous 2013 VCNA article "Selected Emerging Diseases of Ornamental Fish."[1] Readers are encouraged to refer to that article for information about these diseases. Diseases in the 2013 article are all still important emerging diseases that continue to affect ornamental fish.

temperature range of 20°C to 25°C (68°F–77°F) is highly permissible for CyHV-2 infection.[5] Fish that recover from infection are considered carriers that can infect naïve fish.[6] Another study found that most fish infected with CyHV-2 at 13°C to 15°C (55.4°F –59°F) were able to develop resistance to clinical disease.[5,6]

Cyprinid Herpesvirus 3 (Koi Herpesvirus)

Koi herpesvirus (KHV, CyHV-3, CyHV-3, carp interstitial nephritis, and gill necrosis virus) infects and causes massive mortality in koi and common carp (*Cyprinus carpio*).[7] KHV was first reported as a cause of massive fish mortality in Israel in 1998 and is now global in distribution.[8,9] It is listed as a reportable disease by the World Organization for Animal Health.[10]

Clinical signs

Clinical signs of KHV can be found in **Box 2**. On post mortem examination, all fish have mild to severe gill necrosis (**Fig. 1**). In more mild cases, loss of gill epithelium with exposed lamellar cartilage is seen. Other gross necropsy changes are nonspecific, including darkening or mottling of internal organs, coelomic effusion, and adhesion formation.[8,10] Wet mount examination of the gills shows necrosis with a complete loss of normal lamellar architecture. Secondary skin and gill parasitic and bacterial infections are extremely common.

Virulent virus is shed via the feces, urine, and skin/gill mucus.[10] The main portal of entry for KHV in koi is through the skin,[11] with systemic spread of the virus from the skin and gills through the bloodstream (via white blood cells) to the kidney, spleen, liver, and intestines.[12,13] Branchitis and interstitial nephritis are seen histologically as early as 2 days after infection, but mortality typically occurs 6 to 8 days after infection.[12,13] The virus causes lysis of infected cells (**Fig. 2**).[12] Different strains that vary in virulence have been reported.[14]

Box 2
Clinical Signs of KHV Infection

- Piping (gasping at water surface)
- Elevated opercular rate
- Gathering near the surface and in well aerated areas such as near waterfalls/filter input
- Excessive mucus from the gills
- Mottled areas of gill necrosis/discoloration (see **Fig. 1**)
- Skin changes including ulcers, hemorrhages, sloughing of scales, and increased or decreased mucus production
- Lethargy
- Anorexia
- Sunken eyes (enophthalmos) (see **Fig. 1**)
- Notched appearance dorsal to the nares (notched nose) (see **Fig. 1**)
- Erratic swimming
- "Hanging" with a head down position in the water column
- High mortality rate (typically 70%–100%)

Modified from McDermott C, Palmeiro B. Selected emerging infectious diseases in ornamental fish. Vet Clin North Am Exot Anim Pract. 2013; 16(2):261-282; with permission.

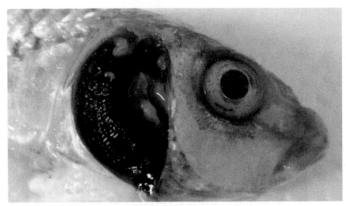

Fig. 1. Koi infected with KHV. Note patchy white areas of gill necrosis, notched nose, and hyphema. (*Courtesy* Brian Palmeiro, VMD, DACVD, Allentown, PA.)

Water temperature contributes significantly to the course of the disease, both directly by affecting viral replication and indirectly by modulating the fish's immune response.[10] The permissive range for clinical infection with KHV is 16°C to 28°C (61°F–82°F),[15] and clinical disease is only seen within this temperature range.[12] Fish seem most susceptible to clinical disease and mortality between 21°C and 27°C (72°F–81°F).[8] Typically, mortality approaches 70% to 100% over a course of 7 to 21 days.[15] The virus can replicate in common carp at 13°C (55°F) and in cell culture at 4°C (39°F), supporting the hypothesis that the virus can overwinter with the fish.[15,16] No growth occurs in cell culture at or above 30°C (86°F).[15]

Fish surviving infection, including those subjected to elevated water temperatures after infection, develop partial or complete resistance to reinfection.[15] Fish that survive KHV infection are considered life-long carriers of the virus, although it is currently unknown what percentage become carriers. In an effort to determine site of latency, normal fish from facilities with a history of KHV infection or exposure have been studied.[17] KHV DNA, but not infectious virus or messenger RNAs from lytic infection, was

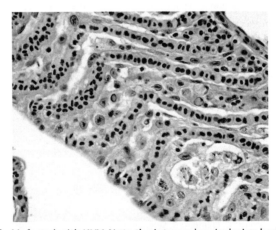

Fig. 2. Gill from koi infected with KHV. Note the intranuclear inclusion bodies and hyperplasia. (*Courtesy* Thomas B. Waltzek, MS, DVM, PhD, Gainesville, FL.)

detected in white blood cells from koi, suggesting that leukocytes are a possible site of latency for KHV.[17] Further research has documented the B-lymphocyte as the main site for KHV latency.[18]

Common carp that recover from KHV infection can become persistently infected and may shed the virus to infect naïve fish at water temperatures greater than 20°C (68°F).[19] In 1 study, the virus became reactivated and infected naïve fish up to 30 weeks after initial infection.[19] Given that persistently infected fish are created, exposing fish to KHV at nonpermissive temperatures is not considered a safe method of disease prevention.[19]

Diagnosis

The diagnosis of KHV is based on clinical signs and detection of the virus via virus isolation (on KF-1 cell line) or DNA identification via PCR. PCR is considered the most sensitive diagnostic modality available[20] and, in cases of an acute infection, PCR is the most practical and rapid method of diagnosis. Because KHV is most abundant in gill, kidney, and spleen, these organs should be submitted for virologic testing.[20] Detection of KHV DNA via PCR is extremely difficult more than 64 days after exposure.[16]

Currently, the most challenging aspect in the diagnosis of KHV is the ability to detect carrier fish. Detection of KHV antibodies is currently the only method of determining previous exposure to the virus if viral DNA is not detectable via PCR assays.[10] An enzyme-linked immunosorbent assay (ELISA) was shown to detect antibodies in the serum of koi for up to 1 year after previous exposure.[21] In a study of KHV-exposed fish, antibodies were detected by ELISA for up to 65 weeks.[19] Serum antibodies have been shown to peak 3 to 4 weeks after infection with high levels maintained for several months, followed by a gradual and continuous decrease with time.[22] A quantitative KHV ELISA is currently commercially available at the University of California Davis Veterinary Teaching Hospital.

False-negative serology results may occur early in the course of exposure as development of positive titers may take several weeks to develop. False-positive results may occur owing to cross-reactions on ELISA testing between KHV and CyHV-1, but occur more commonly at lower serum dilutions.[19]

A KHV real-time PCR has been shown to detect DNA from white blood cells in 9 of 10 fish previously exposed to KHV, potentially providing for an alternate mechanism for detecting KHV carrier fish.[17] Other research on KHV latency has found that the ORF6 messenger RNA and protein are expressed by the virus in latently infected koi, which could be a potential target for latency testing in the future.[23]

Treatment

There is no effective treatment for KHV. Depopulation and disinfection are recommended because fish that survive infection are considered carriers. In private collections, some owners may elect to treat their pet fish. The authors recommend that the water temperature be increased to greater than 29°C (84°F) to help decrease morbidity and mortality. Secondary bacterial and parasitic infections are extremely common and must be treated accordingly. Prolonged bath immersion with salt (0.1%–0.3%) can be used to decrease osmotic stresses associated with gill necrosis and cutaneous ulceration. The owners must be thoroughly educated by the veterinarian that surviving fish are considered carriers and should not be mixed with naïve fish.

Prevention

Methods to control and prevent KHV include avoiding exposure to the virus, good hygiene and biosecurity practices, and vaccination. Fish should be purchased from reputable sources and quarantined for a minimum of 4 to 6 weeks at permissive temperatures. Quarantine should be combined with blood testing to aid in detection of carrier fish.

Goldfish housed with infected koi have been shown to harbor KHV without developing clinical disease, implicating their role as a possible vector in spreading of KHV.[24] Another study found that goldfish carry the genome of KHV, and that the genome can persist in goldfish for long periods after an outbreak.[25] An ante mortem test to screen for the presence of the KHV carrier state in goldfish is not currently available and duration of carriage in goldfish is unknown; therefore, caution should be taken when introducing goldfish into any existing koi population.

The first report of successful vaccination of carp for KHV involved an attenuated virus; koi exposed to this attenuated virus were resistant to the disease.[26] The attenuated virus was then irradiated to decrease its pathogenicity and formulated into a modified live vaccine delivered by immersion.[26] Short-term immersion was found to be sufficient for infection and immunization, and the attenuated virus was found to be active in the water for at least 2 hours.[26] A modified live KHV vaccine has been approved by the US Department of Agriculture for use in koi (Cavoy, Novartis Animal Health, Greensboro, NC); however, this vaccine is no longer commercially available in the United States. The vaccine is manufactured by Kovax Ltd (Jerusalem, Israel) and has been approved and used successfully by large koi producers in Israel since 2005.

Several studies have found success with various other methods of KHV vaccination including injection with a DNA vaccine containing the recombinant plasmid IRES–ORF25,[27] an oral vaccine containing liposome-entrapped formalin-killed KHV antigens,[28] and genetically engineered *Lactobacillus plantarum* coexpressing glycoprotein (G) of Spring Viremia of Carp Virus and ORF81 protein of KHV as an oral vaccine.[29]

KHV can survive in pond water for at least 4 hours at temperatures around 22°C (72°F)[22] and probably survives for much longer periods in feces and pond mud.[30,31] Its ability to survive in water likely plays an important role in its rapid spread between fish.[12] Common disinfectants that can be used on the system and equipment include chlorine (such as household bleach) at 200 mg/L and quaternary ammonium compounds.[8] Other disinfectants that are reported to inactivate the virus include iodophores at 200 mg/L for 20 minutes, benzalkonium chloride at 60 mg/L for 20 minutes, and 30% ethyl alcohol for 20 minutes.[12] Ponds and equipment can also be drained and dried, but the virus may survive in mud and pond sediment; therefore, complete drying for a minimum of 2 weeks is recommended.

Poxvirus

Carp edema virus disease (CEVD), also referred to as koi sleepy disease, is an emerging disease worldwide that may cause high morbidity and mortality in ornamental koi and common carp (*C carpio*).[32,33] CEVD is caused by a double-stranded DNA virus that is believed to belong to the *Poxviridae* family.[32]

Clinical Signs

The most common clinical signs are behavioral abnormalities, including lethargy and a lack of responsiveness, with fish often lying on their sides or ventrum on the bottom of the tank or pond.[32] When disturbed, affected fish swim for short bursts, but quickly become inactive. Other clinical signs include decreased appetite or anorexia, erosions or ulcers of the skin with edema, cutaneous hemorrhages, enophthalmos, pale swollen gills with areas of gill necrosis, and mortality (**Fig. 3**).[32,33] Gill damage can result in respiratory symptoms, including increased opercular or respiratory rate, gathering near well-aerated areas, and gasping for air at the surface. Mortality rates may be

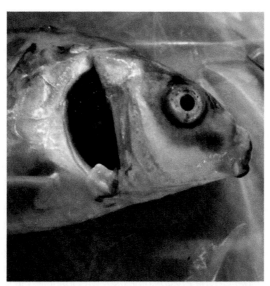

Fig. 3. Koi infected with Carp Edema Virus. Note pale and swollen gills with areas of necrosis and cutaneous hemorrhages. (*Courtesy* Brian Palmeiro, VMD, DACVD, Allentown, PA.)

higher in younger or juvenile fish and younger fish may hang below the water surface.[32,33] Given the clinical findings of gill necrosis and enophthalmos, this disease must be differentiated from KHV.

The disease is most commonly seen at water temperatures of 15°C to 25°C (59°F–77°F), but outbreaks are reported outside this temperature.[32–35] Strains that cause outbreaks in colder temperatures 6°C to 9°C (43°F–48°F) have been reported in the UK, and in Austria at temperatures of 7°C to 15°C (44°F–59°F).[34,35] In Japan, CEVD is most commonly seen in juvenile koi after they are moved from mud or earthen ponds into concrete-lined tanks.[32] Mortality in naive koi begins as soon day 6 and continues up to 16 days after infection via bath challenge.[36] It is unknown if CEV-exposed fish can carry and shed the virus.

Diagnosis

Supportive histopathologic findings include hypertrophy and hyperplasia of gill epithelium, necrotizing branchitis with interstitial edema, inflammation or ulceration and edema of the skin and underlying tissues.[33,36] Definitive diagnosis requires PCR testing.[32,33] The virus has not been propagated in cell culture.[32] Transmission electron microscopy of the gill may show hypertrophied epithelial cells and poxvirus-like particles.[36]

Treatment and prevention

Methods to control and prevent CEVD include avoiding exposure to the virus, good hygiene, and biosecurity practices. Fish should be purchased from reputable sources and quarantined for a minimum of 4 to 6 weeks at permissive temperatures. Koi producers in Japan often use 0.5% (5 g/L) salt to prevent disease in young harvest koi; salinity of 0.3% to 0.5% has been reported to improve clinical symptoms and decrease mortality in koi infected with CEVD.[32,33,37] Treatment of concurrent parasite and bacterial infections is important to reduce morbidity and mortality.

BACTERIAL DISEASES
Erysipelothrix

Bacteria in the genus *Erysipelothrix* are gram positive, non–spore-forming, facultative intracellular, and facultatively anaerobic rods.[38] There are currently 4 recognized species of *Erysipelothrix*, namely, *E rhusiopathiae*, *E tonsillarum*, *E inopinata*, and *E larvae sp. nov.*, although recent genetic studies have proposed new species with several serotypes.[38] The most well-known of these recognized species, *E rhusiopathiae*, has been described in a variety of animal hosts, most importantly in mammals and birds. *E rhusiopathiae* can readily be recovered from soil, freshwater, and marine environments with a long environmental persistence.[38] *E rhusiopathiae* infection in humans is well-described, with 3 distinct forms—localized cutaneous (erysipeloid), diffuse cutaneous, and septicemia with possible endocarditis. Case reports of all 3 forms have been linked to exposure to pet fish or food fish handling.[39,40]

Until recently, fish were only viewed as carriers for *Erysipelothrix* without signs of pathology.[41] *Erysipelothix spp.* can routinely be cultured from the mucus of fish, fish tanks, and in seafood products.[42,43] The first report of pathology in fish attributed to *E rhusiopathiae* was from a 2004 outbreak in farmed cultured Australian eels, *Anguilla reinhardtii* and *A australis.*[43] In the past several years, an infectious outbreak of surface protective antigen (*spa*) C-type *Erysipelothrix sp.* was identified in several species of ornamental fish from the southeastern United States and in mosquito fish (*Gambusia affinis*) from catfish ponds in Mississippi.[44,45] A new species, *E piscicarius sp. nov.*, was recently described for these *spaC* fish isolates based on molecular analysis.[46] A summary of fish with documented clinical infections of *Erysipelothrix* can be found in **Box 3**.

Clinical signs

In *spaC Erysipelothrix* infections, most affected fish presented with orofacial ulceration and necrosis with dermal ulcerations.[44] Ulcers were commonly found along

---

Box 3
List of fish reported to be clinically affected by *Erysipelothrix sp*

Anguillidae
  Anguilla australis
  Anguilla reinhardtii

Characidae
  Aphyocharax anistisi
  Hyphessobrycon eques
  Hyphessobrycon pulchripinnis
  Hyphessobrycon colombianus
  Hasemania nana
  Hemigrammus ocellifer
  Nematobrycon palmeri
  Moenkhausia pitteri

Cyprinidae
  Puntius titteya
  Puntigrus tetrazona
  Danio rerio[a]

Poeceliidae
  Gambusia affinis

[a] Experimental infection.

the trunk. In experimental infections in zebrafish, 10% challenged by bath died in 10 days, and 90% by intraperitoneal injection died within 10 days. No lesions were noted in zebrafish challenged by immersion.[44] Experimental infections in Nile tilapia resulted in only 10% mortality with injection challenge and no lesions observed on histopathology.[44]

E rhusiopathiae infection in *A reinhardtii* caused hemorrhage in the liver, gill arches, and operculum, localized ecchymoses with superficial erosion over the flanks and hemorrhagic intestinal mucosa. Infections in *A australis* presented with severe, multifocal skin and tail ulcerations with discoloration, petechiation, and sloughing of the perianal and ventral coelomic epidermis. Gills were congested and hemorrhagic. Gross lesions included petechial hemorrhage and yellow discoloration to the liver, hemorrhage of the caudal kidney, and loss of myocardial tone in the heart.[43] The mortality rate was 10% to 20% for *A reinhardtii* and 5% for *A australis*.[43]

Diagnosis

Disease in ornamental fish resulted in necrotizing dermatitis, myositis and cellulitis of the face with abundant intralesional gram-positive bacterial colonies. Bacteria were localized to areas of necrosis and inflammation involving intramuscular capillaries of epaxial skeletal muscles. Bacteria were present in the olfactory organ, gill arch, and bulbus arteriosus, frequently without inflammatory infiltrates. The kidney was the most commonly affected coelomic organ.[44]

In experimental infections in *Danio rario*, widespread epithelial loss, moderate to large numbers of free bacteria distributed throughout scale pockets and dermal collagen were noted in the first 4 days. Myofiber necrosis was widespread after day 8. Bacterial laden macrophages reached and expanded the subperitoneal adventitia, and in some fish the epicardium, submesothelium of the pericardial cavity, peripharyngeal mucosa, extrameningeal lining of the spinal canal and swim bladder serosa. Severe granulomatous coelomitis was present by days 8 to 10. The mesenteric adipose tissue was infiltrated with large numbers of bacterial laden macrophages. In some fish, the esophageal and intestinal subepithelial basement membranes, lamina, propria and submucosa were infiltrated with bacteria and macrophages, with necrosis and sloughing of the mucosal epithelium.[44]

In *A reinhardtii*, multifocal hemorrhage of the liver along the periphery of the lobes, congestion of hepatic vessels, and occasional lipid vacuolation of hepatocytes were observed. Gills were affected by distal filament epithelial hyperplasia, lamellar fusion, epithelial necrosis, focal bronchitis, or thrombus formation in the central vessel. Intestinal submucosa was hemorrhagic. Abundant gram-positive bacilli were present along the collagen fibers of the bulbus arteriosis and within endothelial macrophages of the ventricle and atrium. Renal glomeruli were disrupted, enlarged, and infiltrated with macrophages.[43] In *A australis*, Gram-positive bacilli were abundant in the heart, liver, kidney, and spleen, but not present in the gills. Marked interstitial hemorrhage was present in the kidneys with bacteria in macrophages of the glomeruli. Severe, necrotizing, and ulcerative hemorrhage with acute myositis occurred in superficial layers of underlying muscle.[43]

Aerobic culture of affected lesions can be used to isolate *Erysipelothrix*.[43] PCR testing targeting the 16S rRNA gene can be used to identify *Erysipelothrix*, but is poor at differentiating between species.[45] Further genetic testing aimed at the surface protective antigen and gyrB genes are more specific at positively identifying species of *Erysipelothrix*.[44,45] *Spa* isoform testing can be used to differentiate serotypes, because spaC seems to be more virulent in fish, and *spaA* and *spaB* are more likely to cause clinical disease in mammals and birds.[44]

Treatment and prevention

In *A australis*, initial bath treatment with oxytetracycline was unsuccessful (dose not listed). *A australis* adults were depopulated and the farms disinfected.[43] Clinical signs and mortalities in *A reinhardtii* stopped after treatment with erythromycin (dose and route not specified).[43] In humans, the treatments of choice are penicillins or macrolides.[47]

The spread of *Erysipelothrix* can be controlled by regular disinfection of contaminated sources. *E rhusiopathiae* can persist in the environment for extended periods under harsh conditions. Disinfection of surfaces with a benzalkonium chloride has been shown to be extremely effective.[47] Occupational health risk can be mitigated by wearing gloves and practicing good hygiene with proper hand washing.[39,43]

Edwardsiella

Bacteria in the genus *Edwardsiella* are Gram-negative facultatively anaerobic, flagellated rods. Before 2012, there were 3 primary species recognized under the genus *Edwardsiella*: *E hoshinae*, *E ictauluri*, and *E tarda*. *E hoshinae* is primarily associated with birds and reptiles. *E ictaluri* is economically important as the causative agent of enteric septicemia of catfish. *E tarda* had been described as a worldwide pathogen infecting a wide range of species, including fish and humans.[48]

Over the past 2 decades, advances in genomic testing have redefined our understanding of the genus *Edwardsiella*. Through gene sequencing (specifically evaluating 16S rRNA and the *gyrB* gene, among others), new species and strains of *Edwardsiella* have been described.[49] *E tarda* has been split into 2 species, namely, *E tarda* and *E piscicida*. Many previously described infections attributed to *E tarda* in fish may have been *E piscicida*.[48] As a result, *E piscicida* infections may have been underreported. Despite the reclassification into 2 species, *E tarda* is still responsible for disease outbreaks in fish. *E tarda* has been described as a zoonotic pathogen, although recent molecular data call into question the zoonotic potential of the current classification of the bacteria. More studies are needed to determine the true zoonotic potential between species. A fifth species of *Edwardsiella* has since been described as *Edwardsiella anguillarum sp nov*.[50] Both *E ictaluri* and *E piscicida* are emerging diseases of ornamental fish.

Edwardsiella ictaluri in zebrafish

Although *E ictaluri* was originally thought to be host specific to Channel catfish (*Ictalurus punctatus*), white catfish (*Ameiurus catus*) and Brown Bullhead (*Ameiurus nebulosus*), but it has been documented in an increasing number of catfish worldwide. Natural infection has been described in a number of nonictalurid species.[51–53] Previous experiments have shown susceptibility to infection in zebrafish (*Danio rerio*) by bath immersion and intraperitoneal injection.[54] Recently, natural infection in several research populations of *D rerio* were reported in Louisiana, Pennsylvania, and Massachusetts.[55]

Clinical signs

Early signs of infection with *E ictaluri* in *D rerio* included lethargy and hemorrhage in the skin along the eyes, opercula, base of fins, and ventral coelom. Mortalities began 3 days after clinical signs started. Lesions progressed to skin ulceration in several fish. Coelomic distension and ascites were present in advanced disease. Within 10 days of the first clinical signs, the mortality rate was 60%, at which point the remaining fish were culled.[55] Clinical signs were all observed after a stress event, either shortly after shipping or after an accidental large volume water change.[55]

Diagnosis
Histopathology showed severe encephalitis, nephritis, and splenitis associated with acute bacterial disease. Affected fish showed severe, multifocally extensive to diffuse systemic disease characterized by tissue necrosis and large numbers of bacteria often within macrophages.[55] The kidney and spleen were most commonly and severely affected. Diffuse and severe inflammation and necrosis of the nasal pits was observed in all cases. Inflammation extended form the nasal pits to the telencephalon via the olfactory nerve. Less common lesions included skeletal muscle necrosis with liquefaction and dermatitis with epidermal ulceration.[55]

Culture of liver, kidney, spleen, and brain of moribund specimens on TSAB [Tryptic soy agar with 5% sheep blood] at 28°C (82.4°F) exhibited growth at 48 hours. Contaminants are often cultured owing to the slow growth of *E ictaluri*. Edwardsiella is characterized as a gram-negative rod approximately 0.75 × 1.0 μm. Samples from zebrafish were slightly different than channel catfish as the bacteria was weakly motile at 28°C (82.4°F).[55] PCR testing for the *gyrB* gene can be used to identify to the species level and is more specific than 16S rRNA testing.[49]

Treatment and prevention
Administration of florfenicol in medicated feed was successful in controlling morbidity and mortality in 1 outbreak. However, fish were humanely killed 3 days after treatment ended.[55] In 1 research colony, enrofloxacin treatments stopped mortalities in affected fish (dose and route not specified). An outbreak of *E ictaluri* occurred several months later at the same facility.[55]

All isolates from *D rerio* were susceptible to Romet (Aquatactics, Kirkland, WA), oxytetracycline, florfenicol, and enrofloxacin, although clinical breakpoints for these drugs have not been determined for zebrafish.[55] This is similar to antimicrobial profiles tested in limited *E ictaluri* samples; however, samples tested from Nile tilapia infections showed no susceptibility to ormetoprim/suladimethoxine and trimethoprim/sulphamethoxazole concentrations tested.[49] Culture and sensitivity of all suspected bacterial infections is recommended.

Proper quarantine for research specimens is essential and is the best practice for aquaculture and keeping ornamental fish. Morbidity and mortality in cases of natural infection in ornamental fish has been precipitated by a stress event (including transport or sudden water quality changes).[55]

Edwardsiella piscicida
Since its formal description in 2012, *E piscicida* has been identified in numerous freshwater and marine fish with a global distribution.[56] A review of previous literature and sampling of archived isolates using current genetic techniques have identified several cases of atypical *E tarda* that were reclassified as *E piscicida*.[48] However, it should be noted that *E tarda* is still being diagnosed and is a potential zoonotic concern.[57] In ornamental fish, *E piscicida* has been reported in koi (*C carpio*) and a blotched fantail stingray (*Taeniura meyeni*).[48,58]

Clinical signs
Clinical signs seem to be consistent for *E piscicida*, even with infection in multiple species. Externally, fish show discolored areas of skin with depigmentation, external hemorrhage, and signs of septicemia. Exophthalmia, ascites, and petechiae throughout internal organs has been described in turbot (*Scophthalmus maximus*).[59] Abscesses and nodules throughout the visceral organs in sharp snout seabream have been recorded.[60] External lesions of barramundi affected with *E tarda* and *E piscicida* were nearly identical.[57]

Diagnosis

Histopathology in largemouth bass showed multifocal necrosis throughout the heart, liver, spleen, and the anterior and posterior kidney.[61] In affected barramundi, histopathology showed granulomatous splenitis, hepatitis, and nephritis with intrahistiocytic intracytoplasmic bacteria.[57] Culture of bacteria from lesions can be used to isolate *Edwardsiella* and identify to the genus level. Further molecular testing targeted at the *gyrB* gene is needed to identify the bacteria to a species level and differentiate between *E tarda* and *E piscicida*.[48,49,56]

Treatment and prevention

In all examined strains, culture and sensitivity results have been comparable with other *Edwardsiella* species.[48,56] However, genetic variation and resistance patterns may be possible.[56] Aerobic culture and sensitivity of all suspected bacterial infections is recommended. Prevention of disease outbreaks may best be accomplished by good husbandry and biosecurity protocols.

FRANCISELLA: CLINICAL UPDATES[a]

Although the majority of infections with *Francisella* ssp. have been documented in Nile tilapia and other farmed fish, *Francisella noatunensis subsp. orientalis* (Fno) has been associated with low-level mortalities in multiple species of Malawi cichlids in an Austrian breeding facility.[62] A previous survey of formalin-fixed samples has identified the presence of a *Francisella*-like bacterium in ornamental cichlid fish in Taiwan from 1998 to 2002.[63]

In 2013, Camus and colleagues[64] documented infection of Fno in Indo-Pacific reef fish imported into the United States from 2 aquarium facilities on the east coast. Species affected included fairy wrasses (*Cirrhilabrus spp.*) and blue green damselfish (*Chromis viridis*). Clinical signs included lethargy, anorexia, and spiral or circular swimming with significant mortalities. Lesions on gross necropsy and histopathology were consistent with francisellosis. Multifocal to coalescing granulomas were present throughout the coelom, most consistently in the spleen and anterior kidney.[64] French grunts (*Haemulon flavolineatum*) and Caesar grunts (*Haemulon carbonarium*) wild caught off the coast of Florida have been found to be host species for Fno.[65]

Experimental infection of striped catfish (*Pangasianodon hypothalamus*) and common carp (*C carpio*) with Fno by intraperitoneal injection failed to induce morbidity and mortality, but Fno was recovered from the fish 21 days after infection. This may indicate a subclinical infective carrier state in these fish that warrants further study.[66] Experimental infection in sunfish (*Lepomis gibbosus*) and common carp (*C carpio*) with Fno via intraperitoneal injection induced mortality and *Francisella*-like lesions in sunfish, with no clinical signs of disease in carp.[67]

A novel strain of *Francisella* sp. was isolated from infection in cultured spotted rose snapper (*Lujanus guttatus*) in Central America. *Francisella marina sp. nov.* was found to cause similar granulomatous inflammation to other species of *Francisella*, but with a lower pathogenicity in experimentally infected tilapia compared with Fno.[68]

---

[a] Clinical updates are provided for some diseases discussed in the previous 2013 VCNA article "Selected Emerging Diseases of Ornamental Fish."[1] Readers are encouraged to refer to that article for information about these diseases. Diseases in the 2013 article are all still important emerging diseases that continue to affect ornamental fish.

As molecular diagnostics improve, *Francisella* may be found in more species and geographic locations. As with other infectious diseases, good husbandry and biosecurity practices are key in prevention. Treatment with florenfenicol and oxytetracycline has proven effective in outbreaks, but culture and sensitivity are indicated for ideal treatment recommendations.[68]

DISCLOSURE

The authors have nothing to disclose.

REFERENCES

1. McDermott C, Palmeiro B. Selected emerging infectious diseases of ornamental fish. Vet Clin North Am Exot Anim Pract 2013;16(2):261–82.
2. ICTV master species list 2018 version 2. International Committee on the Taxonomy of Viruses. 2019. Available at: https://talk.ictvonline.org/files/master-species-lists/m/msl/8266. Accessed November 17, 2019.
3. van Beurden SJ, Bossers A, Voorbergen-Laarman MH, et al. Complete genome sequence and taxonomic position of anguillid herpesvirus 1. J Gen Virol 2010; 91(4):880–7.
4. Goodwin A, Merry G, Sadler J. Detection of the herpesviral hematopoietic necrosis disease agent (Cyprinid herpesvirus 2) in moribund and healthy goldfish: validation of a quantitative PCR. Dis Aquatic Organ 2006;69:137–43.
5. Ito T, Maeno Y. Effects of experimentally induced infections of goldfish *Carassius auratus* with cyprinid herpesvirus 2 (CyHV-2) at various water temperatures. Dis Aquat Org 2014;110:193–200.
6. Ito T, Kurita J, Ozaki A, et al. Growth of cyprinid herpesvirus 2 (CyHV-2) in cell culture and experimental infection of goldfish *Carassius auratus*. Dis Aquat Org 2013;105:193–202.
7. Waltzek TB, Kelley GO, Stone DM, et al. Koi herpesvirus represents a third cyprinid herpesvirus (CyHV-3) in the family Herpesviridae. J Gen Virol 2005; 86(6):1659–67.
8. Hartman K, Yanong R, Pouder D, et al. Koi Herpesvirus (KHV) disease 2004. p. 1–9. Available at: http://edis.ifas.ufl.edu/pdffiles/VM/VM11300.pdf. Accessed November 18, 2019.
9. Gilad O, Yun S, Andree K, et al. Initial characteristics of koi herpesvirus and development of a polymerase chain reaction assay to detect the virus in koi, Cyprinus carpio koi. Dis Aquat Org 2002;48:101–8.
10. Way K. Koi herpesvirus and goldfish herpesvirus: an update of current knowledge and research at Cefas. Fish Vet J 2008;10:62–73.
11. Costes B, Raj S, Michel B, et al. The major portal of entry of koi herpesvirus in *Cyprinus carpio* is the skin. J Virol 2009;83(7):2819–30.
12. Walster C. Koi Herpesvirus: The International Perspective. In: WAVMA Conference/29th World Veterinary Congress. Vancouver, Canada, July 27-31, 2008.
13. Pikarsky E, Ronen A, Abramowitz J, et al. Pathogenesis of acute viral disease induced in fish by carp interstitial nephritis and gill necrosis virus. J Virol 2004; 78(17):9544–51.
14. Aoki T, Hirono I, Kurokawa K, et al. Genome sequences of three koi herpesvirus isolates representing the expanding distribution of an emerging disease threatening koi and common carp worldwide. J Virol 2007;81(10):5058–65.

15. Gilad O, Yun S, Adkison M, et al. Molecular comparison of isolates of an emerging fish pathogen, koi herpesvirus, and the effect of water temperature on mortality of experimentally infected koi. J Gen Virol 2003;84(10):2661–7.

16. Gilad O, Yun S, Zagmutt-Vergara F, et al. Concentrations of a Koi herpesvirus (KHV) in tissues of experimentally-infected *Cyprinus carpio* koi as assessed by real-time TaqMan PCR. Dis Aquat Organ 2004;60:179–87.

17. Eide K, Miller-Morgan T, Heidel J, et al. Investigation of Koi Herpesvirus latency in Koi. J Virol 2011;85(10):4954–62.

18. Reed AN, Izume S, Dolan BP, et al. Identification of B cells as a major site for cyprinid herpesvirus 3 latency. J Virol 2014;88:9297–309.

19. St-Hilaire S, Beevers N, Way K, et al. Reactivation of koi herpesvirus infections in common carp *Cyprinus carpio*. Dis Aquat Organ 2005;67:15–23.

20. Haenen O, Way K, Bergmann S, et al. The emergence of koi herpesvirus and its significance to European aquaculture. Bull Eur Assoc Fish Pathol 2004;24(6): 293–307.

21. Adkison M, Gilad O, Hedrick R. An enzyme linked immunosorbent assay (ELISA) for detection of antibodies to the koi herpesvirus (KHV) in the serum of koi *Cyprinus carpio*. Fish Pathol 2005;40(2):53–62.

22. Perelberg A, Ilouze M, Kotler M, et al. Antibody response and resistance of *Cyprinus carpio* immunized with cyprinid herpes virus 3 (CyHV-3). Vaccine 2008; 26(29):3750–6.

23. Reed A, Lin L, Ostertag-Hill C, et al. Detection of ORF6 protein associated with latent KHV infection. Virology 2017;500:82–90.

24. El-Matbouli M, Saleh M, Soliman H. Detection of cyprinid herpesvirus type 3 in goldfish cohabiting with CyHV-3-infected koi carp (*Cyprinus carpio koi*). Vet Rec 2007;161(23):792–3.

25. Sadler J, Bluff A, Marecaux E, et al. Detection of koi herpes virus (CyHV-3) in goldfish, *Carassius auratus* (L.), exposed to infected koi. J Fish Dis 2008; 31(1):71–2.

26. Ronen A, Perelberg A, Abramowitz J, et al. Efficient vaccine against the virus causing a lethal disease in cultured *Cyprinus carpio*. Vaccine 2003;21(32): 4677–84.

27. Zhou J, Wang H, Li X, et al. Construction of KHV-CJ ORF25 DNA vaccine and immune challenge test. J Fish Dis 2014;37(4):319–25.

28. Miyazaki T, Yasumoto S, Kuzuya Y, et al. A primary study on oral vaccination with liposomes entrapping koi herpesvirus (KHV) antigens against KHV infection in carp. Dis Asian Aquac 2008;6:99–104.

29. Cui L, Guan X, Liu Z, et al. Recombinant lactobacillus expressing G protein of spring viremia of carp virus (SVCV) combined with ORF81 protein of koi herpesvirus (KHV): a promising way to induce protective immunity against SVCV and KHV infection in cyprinid fish via oral vaccination. Vaccine 2016;33(27):3092–9.

30. Hutoran M, Ronen A, Perelberg A, et al. Description of an as yet unclassified DNA virus from diseased Cyprinus carpio species. J Virol 2005;79(4):1983–91.

31. Dishon A, Davidovich M, Ilouze M, et al. Persistence of cyprinid herpesvirus 3 in infected cultured carp cells. J Virol 2007;81(9):4828–36.

32. Hesami S, Viadanna P, Steckler N, et al. Carp edema virus disease (CEVD)/Koi sleepy disease (KSD). University of Florida IFAS Extension Publication FA189; 2018. Available at: https://edis.ifas.ufl.edu/pdffiles/FA/FA18900.pdf. Accessed November 18, 2019.

33. Stevens B, Michel A, Liepnieks M, et al. Outbreak and treatment of carp edema virus in Koi (cyprinus carpio) from Northern California. J Zoo Wildl Med 2018;49: 755–64.
34. Way K, Stone D. Emergence of carp edema virus-like (CEV-like) disease in the UK. Finfish News 2013;15:32–5.
35. Lewisch E, Gorgoglione B, Way K, et al. Carp edema virus/koi sleepy disease: an emerging disease in central-east Europe. Transbound Emerg Dis 2015;62:6–12.
36. Oyamatsu T, Hata N, Yamada K, et al. An etiological study on mass mortality of cultured colorcarp juveniles showing edema. Fish Pathol 1997;32:81–8.
37. Seno R, Hata N, Oyamatsu T, et al. Curative effect of 0.5% salt water treatment on Carp, *Cyprinus carpio*, infected with Carp Edema Virus (CEV) results mainly from reviving the physiological condition of the host. Suisan Zoshoku 2003;51:123–4.
38. Forde T, Biek R, Zadoks R, et al. Genomic analysis of the multi-host pathogen *Erysipelothrix rhusiopathiae* reveals extensive recombination as well as the existence of three generalist clades with wide geographic distribution. BMC Genomics 2016;17(1):461.
39. Vasagar B, Jain V, Germinario A, et al. Approach to aquatic skin infections. Prim Care 2018;45(3):555–66.
40. Asimaki E, Nolte O, Overesch G, et al. A dangerous hobby? *Erysipelothrix rhusiopathiae* bacteremia most probably acquired from freshwater aquarium fish handling. Infection 2017;45(4):557–62.
41. Boylan S. Zoonoses associated with fish. Vet Clin North Am Exot Anim Pract 2011;14(3):427–38.
42. Wang Q, Chang BJ, Riley TV. Erysipelothrix rhusiopathiae. Vet Microbiol 2010; 140(3–4):405–17.
43. Chong RM, Shinwari MW, Amigh MJ, et al. First report of *Erysipelothrix rhusiopathiae*-associated septicaemia and histologic changes in cultured Australian eels, *Anguilla reinhardtii* (Steindachner, 1867) and *A. australis* (Richardson, 1841). J Fish Dis 2015;38(9):839–47.
44. Pomaranski EK, Reichley SR, Yanong R, et al. Characterization of spaC-type *Erysipelothrix sp.* isolates causing systemic disease in ornamental fish. J Fish Dis 2018;41(1):49–60.
45. Stilwell JM, Griffin MJ, Rosser TG, et al. First detection of *Erysipelothrix sp.* infection in western mosquitofish *Gambusia affinis* inhabiting catfish aquaculture ponds in Mississippi, USA. Dis Aquat Organ 2019;133(1):39–46.
46. Pomaranski EK, Griffin MJ, Camus AC, et al. Description of *Erysipelothrix piscisicarius sp. nov.*, an emergent fish pathogen, and assessment of virulence using a tiger barb (*Puntigrus tetrazona*) infection model. Int J Syst Evol Microbiol 2019. https://doi.org/10.1099/ijsem.0.003838.
47. Fidalgo SG, Longbottom CJ, Riley TV. Susceptibility of *Erysipelothrix rhusiopathiae* to antimicrobial agents and home disinfectants. Pathology 2002;34(5): 462–5.
48. Reichley SR, Ware C, Steadman J, et al. Comparative phenotypic and genotypic analysis of *Edwardsiella* isolates from different hosts and geographic origins, with emphasis on isolates formerly classified as *E. tarda*, and evaluation of diagnostic methods. J Clin Microbiol 2017;55(12):3466–91.
49. Griffin MJ, Reichley SR, Greenway TE, et al. Comparison of *Edwardsiella ictaluri* isolates from different hosts and geographic origins. J Fish Dis 2016;39(8): 947–69.
50. Shao S, Lai Q, Liu Q, et al. Phylogenomics characterization of a highly virulent *Edwardsiella* strain ET080813T encoding two distinct T3SS and three T6SS

gene clusters: propose a novel species as *Edwardsiella anguillarum sp. nov.* Syst Appl Microbiol 2015;38(1):36–47.

51. Waltman WD, Shotts EB, Blazer VS. Recovery of *Edwardsiella ictaluri* from danio (*Danio devario*). Aquaculture 1985;46(1):63–6.

52. Soto E, Griffin M, Arauz M, et al. *Edwardsiella ictaluri* as the causative agent of mortality in cultured Nile tilapia. J Aquat Anim Health 2012;24(2):81–90.

53. Baxa DV, Groff JM, Wishkovsky A, et al. Susceptibility of nonictalurid fishes to experimental infection with Edwardsiella ictaluri. Dis Aquat Organ 1990;8(2):113–7.

54. Petrie-Hanson L, Romano CL, Mackey RB, et al. Evaluation of zebrafish *Danio rerio* as a model for enteric septicemia of catfish (ESC). J Aquat Anim Health 2007;19(3):151–8.

55. Hawke JP, Kent M, Rogge M, et al. Edwardsiellosis caused by *Edwardsiella ictaluri* in laboratory populations of zebrafish *Danio rerio*. J Aquat Anim Health 2013;25(3):171–83.

56. Buján N, Toranzo AE, Magariños B. *Edwardsiella piscicida*: a significant bacterial pathogen of cultured fish. Dis Aquat Organ 2018;131(1):59–71.

57. Loch TP, Hawke JP, Reichley SR, et al. Outbreaks of edwardsiellosis caused by *Edwardsiella piscicida* and *Edwardsiella tarda* in farmed barramundi (*Lates calcarifer*). Aquaculture 2017;481:202–10.

58. Camus A, Dill J, McDermott A, et al. Edwardsiella piscicida-associated septicaemia in a blotched fantail stingray *Taeniura meyeni* (Müeller & Henle). J Fish Dis 2016;39(9):1125–31.

59. Castro N, Toranzo AE, Barja JL, et al. Characterization of *Edwardsiella tarda* strains isolated from turbot, *Psetta maxima* (L.). J Fish Dis 2006;29(9):541–7.

60. Katharios P, Kokkari C, Dourala N, et al. First report of Edwardsiellosis in cage-cultured sharpsnout sea bream, *Diplodus puntazzo* from the Mediterranean. BMC Vet Res 2015;11(1):155.

61. Fogelson SB, Petty BD, Reichley SR, et al. Histologic and molecular characterization of *Edwardsiella piscicida* infection in largemouth bass (*Micropterus salmoides*). J Vet Diagn Invest 2016;28(3):338–44.

62. Lewisch E, Dressler A, Menanteau-Ledouble S, et al. Francisellosis in ornamental African cichlids in Austria. Bull Eur Assoc Fish Pathol 2014;34:63–70.

63. Hsieh CY, Wu ZB, Tung MC, et al. PCR and in situ hybridization for the detection and localization of a new pathogen *Francisella*-like bacterium (FLB) in ornamental cichlids. Dis Aquat Organ 2007;75(1):29–36.

64. Camus AC, Dill JA, McDermott AJ, et al. *Francisella noatunensis subsp. orientalis* infection in Indo-Pacific reef fish entering the United States through the ornamental fish trade. J Fish Dis 2013;36(7):681–4.

65. Soto E, Primus AE, Pouder DB, et al. Identification of *Francisella noatunensis* in novel host species French grunt (*Haemulon flavolineatum*) and Caesar grunt (*Haemulon carbonarium*). J Zoo Wildl Med 2014;45(3):727–31.

66. Dong HT, Nguyen VV, Kayansamruaj P, et al. *Francisella noatunensis subsp. orientalis* infects striped catfish (*Pangasianodon hypophthalmus*) and common carp (*Cyprinus carpio*) but does not kill the hosts. Aquaculture 2016;464:190–5.

67. Lewisch E, Menanteau-Ledouble S, Tichy A, et al. Susceptibility of common carp and sunfish to a strain of *Francisella noatunensis subsp. orientalis* in a challenge experiment. Dis Aquat Organ 2016;121(2):161–6.

68. Soto E, Griffin MJ, Morales JA, et al. *Francisella marina sp. nov.*, etiologic agent of systemic disease in cultured spotted rose snapper (Lutjanus *guttatus*) in Central America. Appl Environ Microbiol 2018;84(16):e00144-18.

Emerging and Re-emerging Diseases of Selected Avian Species

Anthony A. Pilny, DVM, DABVP (Avian Practice)[a],*,
Drury Reavill, DVM, DABVP (Avian and Reptile/Amphibian Practice), DACVP[b]

KEYWORDS

- Emerging disease • Re-emerging disease • Avian • Infection • Welfare

KEY POINTS

- The identification of emerging and re-emerging diseases of birds relates not only to scientific discovery, research, and species survival—but holds significant human health implications also.
- Emerging infections can be caused by numerous factors, including previously unknown infectious agents, previously known agents whose role in specific diseases has been unrecognized, and re-emergence of agents whose incidence of disease had declined or disappeared in the past and whose incidence has reappeared.
- Emerging and re-emerging diseases can have impacts on avian welfare, livestock production, and entire ecosystem health, and their recognition is of critical importance.

INTRODUCTION

The identification and significance of emerging and re-emerging diseases of birds relates not only to scientific discovery and research, but holds significant human health implications also. Two examples are bromethalin rodenticide toxicosis in wild birds living in urban areas and the worldwide disease of cercarial dermatitis (swimmer's itch). Diseases may be zoonotic or have farm production implications, present as large die-offs, and can affect zoo collections. Often, identification comes after large losses are seen and some require elimination of hosts, such as infection with exotic Newcastle disease in the poultry industry. Others can affect wild populations and affect smaller ecosystems when large die-offs are seen. Also, bird migration provides a mechanism for the establishment of new endemic disease at distances from where an infection was initially acquired.

Emerging diseases can be caused by numerous factors, including previously undetected or unknown infectious agents, known agents that have spread to new

[a] Arizona Exotic Animal Hospital, 20040 N 19th Avenue Suite C, Phoenix, AZ 85027, USA;
[b] ZNLabs, 525 E 4500 South Suite F200, Salt Lake City, UT 84107, USA
* Corresponding author.
E-mail address: apilny@azeah.com

Vet Clin Exot Anim 23 (2020) 429–441
https://doi.org/10.1016/j.cvex.2020.01.013
1094-9194/20/© 2020 Elsevier Inc. All rights reserved.

vetexotic.theclinics.com

geographic locations or populations, and previously known agents whose role in specific diseases had previously been unrecognized. Agents whose incidence of disease had declined or disappeared in the past, but whose incidence has reappeared are known as re-emerging infectious diseases. The identification and our understanding of these diseases remains critical.

This article summarizes selected emerging and re-emerging diseases of selected avian species and complements other avian articles in this issue. Many more diseases exist than the scope of this article allows, and many more currently remain undiscovered.

Bromethalin Toxicity

Bromethalin is an odorless lipid soluble chemical, used as a rodenticide since the 1980s and designed to kill with a single ingestion. It is rapidly absorbed from the digestive tract and once demethylated to its more potent metabolite, desmethyl-bromethalin it readily crosses the blood-brain barrier. It acts by uncoupling oxidative phosphorylation resulting in decreased adenosine triphosphate (ATP).[1,2] A decline in ATP leads to intracellular accumulation of sodium and an influx of water (cytotoxic edema) and splitting of myelin sheaths (intramyelinic edema).[2–5] The salient histologic feature is of vacuolar degeneration primarily of cerebellar white matter (**Fig. 1**). There is no specific antidote for the toxin.

Susceptibility to bromethalin varies by species, with domestic cats (*Felis catus domestica*) being particularly susceptible, whereas guinea pigs (*Cavia porcellus*) are considered resistant. In 1 tested avian species, adult Quail (*Coturnix coturnix*), the medium oral lethal dose is similar to domestic mice and domestic dogs. Acute toxicosis in domestic dogs and cats present with hyperexcitability, seizures, diffuse fine tremors, pelvic limb ataxia and weakness, anisocoria, blindness, abnormal nystagmus, coma, and death from respiratory arrest.[2–5] Seizures tend to occur in the later stages of intoxication and are more commonly seen in cats than dogs. Chronic toxicosis appears similar to acute with a delay in the development of the clinical signs. It is possible that these domestic species could survive with subacute or chronic exposure.[3,5]

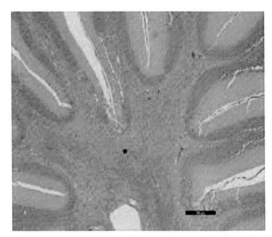

Fig. 1. Conure (Aratinga species). The prominent and consistent lesion of bromethalin toxicosis is of cerebellar white matter vacuolization (*asterisk*) with increased cellularity due to gliosis (hematoxylin-eosin stain). (*Courtesy of* D. R. Reavill, DVM, DABVP (Avian and Reptile & Amphibian Practice), DACVP, Salt Lake City, UT.)

The public noticed birds with neurologic clinical signs in a feral conure population in San Francisco monitored since the 1990s. In 2003, these birds were brought to Mickaboo Companion Bird Rescue, which arranged for veterinary care at area hospitals. A concerted effort was made in 2013 to determine a cause for the symptoms in these birds with chronic neurologic signs that seldom resolved even with aggressive supportive care. Based on clinical signs, histologic lesions in the brain, and positive tests for desmethyl-bromethalin in the feces, and brain and liver tissues, it has been determined that these birds were suffering chronic bromethalin toxicity. A definitive source has not been identified.[6]

The birds develop paresis, circling, ataxia, and seizures that are progressive until they are unable to feed themselves. The differential diagnosis based on the clinical signs includes aberrant migration of *Baylisascaris*, protozoal infections, such as sarcocystis, and less likely toxoplasma, paramyxoviruses, West Nile virus, avian bornavirus, lead toxicity, and trauma.[6] Positive testing for bromethalin was found in all examined birds.

There has been at least 1 incidence where bromethalin toxicity was suspected in bald eagles (*Haliaeetus leucocephalus*) and American coots (*Fulica americana*). The eagles were observed overflying perches or colliding with rock walls. Limb paresis and incoordination were observed in American coots. Increased mortality occurred over 2 winters in Arkansas. The consistent histologic finding was of the spongy degeneration of the white matter of the central nervous system.[7]

Antemortem testing is possible by bromethalin quantification in fecal samples in acute cases. Postmortem testing requires frozen tissue samples of brain and liver and seems to be diagnostic in chronic cases. Treatment of bromethalin toxicity is based on decontamination (emesis and activated charcoal) if possible, control of central nervous system signs, and supportive care.

Virulent Newcastle Disease

Virulent Newcastle disease is one of the most serious reportable poultry diseases worldwide.[8] Until this re-emergence, the US poultry industry was considered disease-free since the last outbreak in 2002 to 2003, the only exception being some species of wild birds implicated as reservoirs. Formerly known as exotic Newcastle disease, this is a contagious and fatal viral disease affecting the respiratory, nervous, and digestive systems of birds. The disease is so virulent that many birds die without showing any clinical signs. A death rate of almost 100% can occur in unvaccinated poultry flocks; moreover, it can infect and cause death even in vaccinated poultry. Virulent Newcastle disease spreads when healthy birds come in direct contact with bodily fluids from sick birds. In addition, the virus can travel on manure, egg flats, crates, other farming materials or equipment, and people who have picked up the virus on their hands or clothing. It has been shown to replicate in the reproductive tract of adult hens.[9]

Clinical signs in chickens include:

- Sudden death and increased death loss in flocks
- Respiratory symptoms, including sneezing, gasping for air, nasal discharge, and coughing
- Greenish, watery diarrhea, lethargy, tremors, and drooped wings
- Torticollis, circling, complete stiffness, and swelling around the eyes and neck

Understanding the potential risks of transmission of chicken- and wild bird-origin virulent Newcastle disease in poultry is critical in outbreak response and control. Inadequate biosecurity measures poses a risk to the poultry industry of a Newcastle disease-free country, with the possibility of transmission due to contacts at the wildlife-poultry interface.[10] Suspected cases should be tested or verified with necropsy and reported to the respective state veterinarian or the United States Department of Agriculture (USDA).

As of October 2019 the USDA has confirmed 451 premises as infected in California and 1 premises each in Utah and Arizona. This disease is not a food safety concern but more so of biosecurity for the poultry industry.

Sarcocystis calchasi

The apicomplexan parasite *Sarcocystis calchasi* has been identified as the causative agent of pigeon protozoal encephalitis (PPE), an emerging, severe neurologic disease in domestic pigeons (*Columba livia* f. *domestica*).[11,12] Pigeons serve as intermediate hosts in the lifecycle of *S calchasi*, and the European subspecies of the Northern goshawk (*Accipiter g. gentilis*) and the European sparrowhawk (*Accipiter nisus*) have so far been identified as definitive hosts.[13]

Also, several psittacine species, including princess parrots and cockatoos, have been reported as susceptible intermediate host species to natural infections.[14] Clinical signs and pathologic lesions in these psittacines closely resemble PPE and include central nervous system signs of torticollis, nystagmus, ataxia, inability to stand, and star-gazing. Experimental infection in cockatiels showed development of disease similar to PPE also, and suggests possible ongoing dissemination of the parasite.[15]

Pigeons infected with *S calchasi* show a biphasic disease initially with polyuria, diarrhea, and lethargy. In the later periods of infection, central nervous signs, such as torticollis and opisthotonos associated with severe brain lesions, have been observed. Mature tissue cysts can be observed in skeletal muscles in the postinfection stage and the encephalitis is associated with the schizont stage of the parasite's development (**Fig. 2**). A recent report described acute death in 4 Roller pigeons naturally infected at a zoo that had schizonts and free merozoites in the liver and spleen without lesions or protozoa in the brain and muscles.[16] Histologic and molecular characterization of this disease are described in white winged and Eurasian collared doves.[17] All these reports suggest the disease has been found in wide-ranging areas and it is likely the parasite has been present for some time and only recently described and recognized.

Baylisascaris procyonis

The nematodes of *Baylisascaris* species are well recognized as causes of cerebrospinal nematodiasis of North American animals. *Baylisascaris procyonis* is the most common cause of visceral, ocular larva migrans (OLM), and neural larva migrans (NLM),

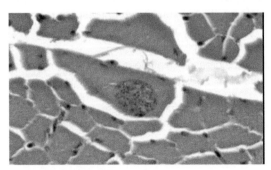

Fig. 2. An intramyocytic thin-walled sarcocyst filled with numerous bradyzoites in skeletal muscle of a dove.

using the raccoon (*Procyon lotor*) as the primary host. There are 2 other *Baylisascaris* species that have been infrequently incriminated; *Baylisascaris columnaris* that cycles through skunks, and *B melis* of badgers. These nematode parasites have less tendency to result in OLM and NLM.[18] Over 130 species of mammals and birds, as well as man, can serve as paratenic hosts.[18,19] This indicates that the parasite is highly nonspecific for paratenic hosts. Larva migrans from *B procyonis* has also been reported in Europe and Japan where raccoons have been imported as part of zoo collections and/or have become part of the wildlife fauna.[20]

These large ascarid nematodes mature in the intestines of the host. Infected raccoons can shed millions of parasitic eggs per day. These will typically accumulate within communal defecation sites, which are described as latrines. The shed eggs from the primary host can survive for extended periods within the environment as well as within contaminated cages and enclosures. Birds and small mammals serve as paratenic (transport) hosts. They are infected when they ingest the eggs from contaminated environments. These eggs hatch and larval nematodes will aggressively migrate through the tissues of the paratenic hosts, commonly resulting in neurologic damage. It takes very few migrating larvae to result in a fatal central nervous system disease.[20] The life cycle is completed when raccoons eat infected animals with the larvae either within the central nervous system or encapsulated in visceral tissues.[18]

In avian species, there have been many outbreaks within ranching situations, such as with pheasants, emus, ostriches, bobwhites, and chucker partridges.[21–24] A variety of zoo birds have also succumbed to NLM when coming in contact with raccoon latrines.[25] Some pet bird species have been exposed by contact to contaminated environment and/or transport containers. These have included cockatoos, macaws, Patagonian conures, and cockatiels.[26,27]

The clinical signs are typical for central nervous system infections: loss of equilibrium, increasing ataxia, circling, torticollis, head tilts, visual defects, and being unable to stand or walk. There may be grossly noticeable malacia and hemorrhage in the brains, although absent to minimal lesions are more common. Histologically there will be a nonsuppurative inflammatory reaction with gliosis and perivascular proliferations of lymphocytes and plasma cells. In some cases, the migration tracks can be identified. Although this is a large nematode larva, these can be very difficult to identify within sections of the brain (**Fig. 3**). In histologic sections, the third-stage larvae of *Baylisascaris* species are all similar, so species determination in cases is near impossible without epidemiologic study[27–29] or molecular diagnostics. In general, it is very uncommon to see visceral lesions of the larval migrations in birds. It has been suspected in some cases where there have been granulomas identified in the heart, liver, and kidney.[19,26] Experimentally in chickens extraneural lesions were limited to focal choroiditis and a larval granuloma in an extrinsic ocular muscle.[30]

If there are identified cases of *Baylisascaris* encephalitis, it is important to clean the environment. This includes identifying where there are raccoon latrines. Removal of contaminated soil or contaminated bedding material is necessary. It is also important that any cages that have housed raccoons as well as skunks and badgers should be thoroughly and fastidiously cleaned to remove any fecal material that may be supporting the nematode eggs.

Schistosomes

Schistosomes belong to a large family of trematodes that use snails as the intermediate host and are found worldwide. The definitive hosts include many avian species as well as mammalian species. Some schistosomes will infect both avian and mammalian species and others are more restricted. For example, the genus *Allobilharzia* has been

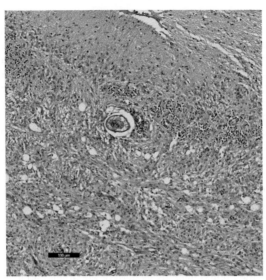

Fig. 3. Scarlet macaw (*Ara macao*) cerebellum with a cross-section through a *Baylisascaris* species. This parasite is within the white matter and is supporting bilateral alae, a thin eosinophilic cuticle, and a pseudocoelomic body cavity lined by a low musculature (hematoxylin-eosin stain). (*Courtesy of* D. R. Reavill, DVM, DABVP (Avian and Reptile & Amphibian Practice), DACVP, Salt Lake City, UT.)

isolated only from swans[31] and *Anserobilharzia* isolated only from geese. Avian schistosomes have been described in at least 10 orders of birds, most commonly Charadriiformes (gulls, terns, plovers) and Anseriformes (swans, geese, and ducks). *Gigantobilharzia huronensis* is most commonly found in passerine birds, such as red-winged blackbirds (*Agelaius phoeniceus*), grackles (*Quiscalus* spp.), and mourning doves (*Zenaida macroura*) that frequent freshwater habitats.[32] Currently there are 20 avian schistosome species representing at least 8 genera; *Allobilharzia*, *Ornithobilharzia*, *Austrobilharzia*, *Macrobilharzia*, *Trichobilharzia*, *Dendritobilharzia*, *Anserobilharzia*, and *Gigantobilharzia*.[33] Morphologic classification of schistosomes has proven difficult in both the primary and secondary hosts and further classification may rely on molecular biology and phylogenetic analyses to fully understand their life cycle.[34] In humans, cercarial dermatitis is considered an important emerging disease that is driving more research in the biology of these trematodes, particularly *Trichobilharzia*. *Trichobilharzia* represents the largest genus within the family Schistosomatidae.

Schistosomes are digenetic trematodes with a 2-host life cycle. They colonize many families of snails as first intermediate hosts. Most schistosome species are transmitted by the freshwater pulmonate snail families Physidae, Lymnaeidae, and Planorbidae. The cercarial stage penetrates the epithelial surface of the definitive host (mammalian and avian). They then spend their adult lives primarily within the vasculature of their host. All the members of these blood flukes live as separate males and females within the vascular system of their vertebrate definitive hosts. Most known schistosomes have a fresh water-based life cycle. This is true of all known mammalian schistosomes and most of the avian schistosomes. However, there are genera that have life cycles based in marine environments with marine snail hosts and definitive hosts primarily being Charadriiformes (gulls and terns).[35]

Most of the schistosomes penetrate mucosal and/or epithelial surfaces directly. The parasite may continue to migrate to other tissues, although the precise path is not fully described in many species. Based on their predilection site, *Trichobilharzia* spp. can be divided in visceral and nasal species.[35] Visceral species migrate through the viscera and can be found in mesenteric, renal, cloacal, and portal blood vessels, whereas nasal species also may display a neurotropic mode of migration.[35] With nasal schistosomes, the migration can involve blood vessels or peripheral nerves leading to the spinal cord and brain of the host. Once they reach the preadult stage in the meninges, they will start to feed on blood and then migrate via an intravascular route back to the nasal cavity. In some duck species, *Trichobilharzia* live in veins of the nasal mucosa where they mature and produce eggs. The miracidia hatch from the eggs directly in the tissue and leave the host during drinking/feeding by the infected birds.[36]

For visceral routes, many of the *Trichobilharzia* species will migrate to the intestinal portal veins where there may be a development of hyperplastic endophlebitis, which is characterized by severe myointimal hyperplasia that often obliterates the vascular lumen. From here, the schistosome eggs will migrate across the intestinal mucosa.[31,37–39] Associated lesions in some ducks can include portal fibroplasia in the liver, nonviable schistosomes in the bile ducts, and viable adult schistosomes in the portal veins.[40] The main lesions of *Trichobilharzia brantae* infection in Atlantic Brant geese (*Branta bernicla hrota*) included thrombosis of the caudal mesenteric veins with adult schistosomes in serosal and mesenteric blood vessels. The eggs in the intestinal wall elicited a fibrinohemorrhagic colitis.[41] For parasite life cycles involving the digestive tract, fecal examination can identify the trematode eggs.[34]

The clinical signs for trematode species migrating to the central nervous system include behavioral changes, disorientation, paralysis, and death in some hosts.[42]

For species with intestinal vasculature migration, the vascular lesions may contribute to emaciation and death by obstruction of venous return in the intestinal and portal veins.[38] The pathogenicity of the infection depends on many factors, such as parasite load, duration of infection, and preferred site of the adult trematode. The host inflammatory reactions are more significant with the immature schistosomes (dermatitis) and the eggs (usually a granulomatous inflammatory reaction).[35]

An unexpected natural schistosome infection was described in a pet 8-month-old female Nanday conure (*Aratinga nenday*). She presented for weight loss and blood-flecked diarrhea before death. A fecal examination found eggs (large 83–134 × 65–78 μm) containing a miracidium. The smooth shell supported the characteristic small terminal spine or knob. On histologic evaluation, the colon and cloaca had variable epithelial hyperplasia, masses of parasitic eggs, and severe chronic inflammation. Trematode eggs were present in the lungs, liver, and kidney associated with granulomas.[43]

Treatment of the infection in the final avian host has been studied in an attempt to reduce the parasite load and attempt to control swimmer's itch (cercarial dermatitis). High doses (200 mg/kg IM) of praziquantel reduced the parasite load in common mergansers[44] and 1 oral dose of 34 mg/bird was effective in reducing the parasites in mallards.[45]

Orthoreovirus

Avian orthoreoviruses belong to the family Reoviridae, genus *Orthoreovirus*. They infect wild and farm-raised birds and are important fowl pathogens associated with various syndromes, such as gastrointestinal malabsorption syndrome, tenosynovitis/arthritis, delayed growth, and sudden death. They have also been isolated from asymptomatic birds.

Scientists at the National Wildlife Health Center (NWHC), USGS, Madison, WI, have identified reovirus as the cause of death in American Crows at several locations from east to west across the United States, beginning in 2000. In January and February 2004, American Crows were found dead at the Pittock Conservation Area in Woodstock in southwestern Ontario.[46] Hemorrhage and inflammation of the intestines was the most common abnormality noted, and often was accompanied by inflammation and necrosis in the spleen. In 2008, an aggressive avian virus killed thousands of crows across New York state over several weeks, according to an investigation by the state Department of Environmental Conservation alerting its significance and linking it to reovirosis. A case report of a wild hooded crow also diagnosed with the virus was seen in Finland.[47]

Epizootic mortalities in American Crows (*Corvus brachyrhynchos*) during the winter months have been recorded in North America for almost 20 years with common postmortem findings, including necrotizing enteritis, fibrinous splenic necrosis, and colitis. These findings are consistent with infection with a *Reovirus* sp. Reovirosis shows a clear seasonal presentation with cases occurring almost exclusively in winter months. Data from 2016 to 2017 showed that reovirosis caused up to 70% of all recorded crow deaths during winter months.[48] Crows with positive orthoreovirus isolation from the spleen or intestine were 32 times more likely to die with characteristic histologic lesions of enteritis or enterocolitis and splenic necrosis than crows with negative isolation results. A new study suggested that a novel orthoreovirus was the cause of winter mortality (or reovirosis) of American Crows and placed the New York isolates in the genus of *Corvid orthoreovirus*.

RENAL TREMATODES

Several trematode genera of the families Eucotylidae (genera *Paratanaisia* and *Tanaisia*) and Renicolidae (genera *Renicola*) have been identified within the upper urinary tract of a variety of avian species.[49]

The digenetic trematode genus *Paratanasia* are known parasites of the urinary tract of neotropical birds and have been identified in other regions of the world. The genus consists of 3 species: *Paratanaisia bragai*, *P robusta*, and *P confusa*. These have a heteroxenous cycle with gastropod mollusks acting as the intermediate hosts. These trematodes do not seem to be host-specific and have been identified in many species of birds. Most intermediate hosts are land snails. The birds acquire the infection when feeding on the mollusks affected with the metacercariae, the infective form. The adult trematodes are found developing in the ureters, collecting ducts, and renal tubules of the kidney. The birds reported as having this genus of trematodes parasitizing the kidneys include: several species of Columbiformes, Galliformes, many Passeriformes, Psittaciformes,[50,51] Strigiformes, Cuculiformes, Tinamiformes, and Ciconiiformes.[52,53]

Renicolids are trematodes that inhabit the renal tubules and ureters of molluscivorous and piscivorous birds. The Manx shearwater (*Puffinus puffinus*), a migratory seabird, and the king penguin (*Aptenodytes patagonicus*) have been identified as the definitive hosts of *Renicola sloanei*. Only mild renal lesions were noted in a case report of 2 dead Manx shearwaters. Macroscopically, small black multifocal areas in the kidney were noted containing pairs of trematodes inside cyst-like structures and microscopic findings were dilation of the collecting ducts associated with accumulation of paired renicolids in the dilated ducts.[54] Many other penguin groups and several terns have been identified as supporting renal Renicola, although the species was not determined. Clinically the infections were not interpreted as causing any significant disease.[55]

The basic life cycle consists of the excreted embryonated eggs from the host that passively infect a mollusk. After the miracidium hatches, 2 generations of sporocysts, cercariae, and metacercariae develop within the snail. The definitive host acquires the infection by eating the parasitized mollusk.

In general, infected birds may have few if any clinical signs. Clinical signs noted have included poor body condition, hypothermia, inactivity, and in some cases other concurrent infections. In species considered the usual definitive hosts, the infections are considered incidental. In accidental hosts, infections with *P bragai* and *P robusta* may result in death in a variety of psittacines (South American to Australian), white-eared pheasants (*Crossoptilon crossoptilon*), and red bird-of-paradise (*Paradisaea rubra*).[50–52,56]

On gross evaluation, there may be no significant lesions noted to enlarged kidneys with a nodular appearance and urate stasis. With histology, these trematodes may be identified with dilated cystic spaces of the distended ureters, collecting ducts, and tubules. The adjacent renal parenchyma is generally compressed, and there may be a variable amount of inflammation, primarily lymphocytic and in some cases heterophilic with macrophages and other degenerative changes. The tubular lining cells are typically flattened and there may be interstitial fibrosis. Occasionally, eggs of this trematode can be noted within the interstitial tissue, and these typically elicit more significant inflammation.[53] It seems that the primary inflammation is usually directed against the eggs as opposed to the adult trematodes. The adult trematodes may also be associated with some variable hyperplasia of the renal tubular epithelium (**Fig. 4**). This is suspected due to the irritation of the lining epithelium by the integument of the trematodes.

Diagnosis of this infection has primarily been on necropsy. From a search of the literature, there are no reports of antemortem diagnosis, such as identifying the trematode eggs within the urine or urates. Once this trematode infection has been identified with histology, controlling access to the intermediate host is the best form of control.

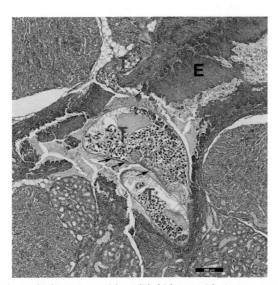

Fig. 4. Brown pelican (*Pelecanus occidentalis*) kidney with intraureter trematodes (T), possibly *Paratanasia confusa*-based morphologically on the spines (*arrows*). There is extensive epithelial hyperplasia (E) of the ureter (hematoxylin-eosin stain). (*Courtesy of* D. R. Reavill, DVM, DABVP (Avian and Reptile & Amphibian Practice), DACVP, Salt Lake City, UT.)

Prophylactic treatment of praziquantel has been used in collections/aviaries.[56] With birds in conservation programs, eliminating or preventing infections is important when considering release of infected/exposed birds and exposing naive populations to the trematodes, especially in areas supporting appropriate intermediate hosts.

DISCLOSURE

The authors have nothing to disclose.

REFERENCES

1. Dorman DC. Toxicology of selected pesticides, drugs, and chemicals. Anticoagulant, cholecalciferol, and bromethalin-based rodenticides. Vet Clin North Am Small Anim Pract 1990;20(2):339–52.
2. van Lier RBL, Cherry LD. The toxicity and mechanism of action of bromethalin: a new single-feeding rodenticide. Fundam Appl Toxicol 1988;11:664–72.
3. Dorman DC, Parker AJ, Buck WB. Bromethalin toxicosis in the dog. Part I: clinical effects. J Am Anim Hosp Assoc 1990;26(6):589–94.
4. Dorman DC, Parker AJ, Buck WB. Bromethalin toxicosis in the dog. Part II: selected treatments for the toxic syndrome. J Am Anim Hosp Assoc 1990;26(6):595–8.
5. Dorman DC, Zachary JF, Buck WB. Neuropathologic findings of bromethalin toxicosis in the cat. Vet Pathol 1992;29(2):139–44.
6. VanSant F, Hassan SM, Reavill D, et al. Evidence of bromethalin toxicosis in feral San Francisco "Telegraph Hill" conures. PLoS One 2019;14(3):e0213248.
7. Thomas NJ, Meteyer CU, Sileo L. Epizootic vacuolar myelinopathy of the central nervous system of bald eagles (*Haliaeetus leucocephalus*) and American coots (*Fulica americana*). Vet Pathol 1998;35(6):479–87.
8. Miller PJ, Koch G. Newcastle disease. In: Swayne D, editor. Diseases of poultry. Ames (IA): John Wiley & Sons, Inc; 2013. p. 120–30.
9. Dimitrov K, Ferreira H, Pantin-Jackwood M, et al. Pathogenicity and transmission of virulent Newcastle disease virus from the 2018–2019 California outbreak and related viruses in young and adult chickens. Virology 2019;531:203–18.
10. Wajid A, Dimitrov M, Wasim SF, et al. Repeated isolation of virulent Newcastle disease viruses in poultry and captive non-poultry avian species in Pakistan from 2011 to 2016. Prev Vet Med 2017;142:1–6.
11. Olias P, Gruber AD, Hafez HM. *Sarcocystis calchasi* sp. nov. of the domestic pigeon (*Columba livia* f. *domestica*) and the Northern goshawk (*Accipiter gentilis*): light and electron microscopical characteristics. Parasitol Res 2010;106:577–85.
12. Wünschmann A, Armien AG, Reed L. *Sarcocystis calchasi*-associated neurologic disease in a domestic pigeon in North America. Transbound Emerg Dis 2011;58:526–30.
13. Olias P, Olias L, Krücken J, et al. High prevalence of *Sarcocystis calchasi* sporocysts in European *Accipiter* hawks. Vet Parasitol 2011;175:230–6.
14. Rimoldi G, Speer B, Wellehan JFX Jr, et al. An outbreak of *Sarcocystis calchasi* encephalitis in multiple psittacine species within an enclosed zoological aviary. J Vet Diagn Invest 2013;25(6):775–81.
15. Olias P, Maier K, Wuenschmann A, et al. *Sarcocystis calchasi* has an expanded host range and induces neurologic disease in cockatiels (*Nymphicus hollandicus*) and North American rock pigeons (*Columbia livia* f. *dom.*). Vet Parasitol 2014;200(1–2):59–65.

16. Trupkiewicz JG, Calero-Bernal R, Verma SK, et al. Acute, fatal *Sarcocystis cal-chasi*-associated hepatitis in Roller pigeons (*Columba livia* f. *dom.*) at Philadelphia zoo. Vet Parasitol 2016;216(30):52–8.

17. Hodo C, Whitley D, Hamer S, et al. Histopathologic and molecular characterization of *Sarcocystis calchasi* encephalitis in white-winged doves (*Zenaida asiatica*) and Eurasian collared doves (*Streptopelia decaocto*), East-central Texas, USA, 2010–13. J Wildl Dis 2016;52(2):395–9.

18. Kazacos KR. *Baylisascaris procyonis* and related species. In: Samuel WM, Pybus MJ, Kocan AA, editors. Parasitic diseases of wild mammals. 2nd edition. Ames (IA): Iowa State University; 2001. p. 301–41.

19. Evans RH. *Baylisascaris procyonis* (Nematoda: Ascarididae) larva migrans in free-ranging wildlife in Orange County, California. J Parasitol 2002;88(2):299–301.

20. Page LK. Parasites and the conservation of small populations: the case of *Baylisascaris procyonis*. Int J Parasitol Parasites Wildl 2013;2:203–10.

21. Kazacos KR, Fitzgerald SD, Reed WM. *Baylisascaris procyonis* as a cause of cerebrospinal nematodiasis in ratites. J Zoo Wildl Med 1991;22(4):460–5.

22. Kazacos KR, Reed WM, Thacker HL. Cerebrospinal nematodiasis in pheasants. J Am Vet Med Assoc 1986;189(10):1353–4.

23. Reed WM, Kazacos KR, Dhillon AS, et al. Cerebrospinal nematodiasis in bobwhite quail. Avian Dis 1981;25:1039–104.

24. Sass B, Gorgacz EJ. Cerebral nematodiasis in a chukar partridge. J Am Vet Med Assoc 1978;173:1248–9.

25. Kazacos KR, Kazacos EA, Render JA, et al. Cerebrospinal nematodiasis and visceral larva migrans in an Australian (Latham's) brush turkey. J Am Vet Med Assoc 1982;181(11):1295–8.

26. Wolf KN, Lock B, Carpenter JW, et al. *Baylisascaris procyonis* infection in a Moluccan Cockatoo (*Cacatua moluccensis*). J Avian Med Surg 2007;21(3):220–5.

27. Thompson AB, Glover GJ, Postey RC, et al. *Baylisascaris procyonis* encephalitis in Patagonian conures (*Cyanoliseus patagonus*), crested screamers (*Chauna torquata*), and a western Canadian porcupine (*Erethizon dorsatum epixanthus*) in a Manitoba zoo. Can Vet J 2008;49:885–8.

28. Stringfield CE. Baylisascaris neural larva migrans in zoo animals. In: Fowler ME, Miller RE, editors. Zoo and wild animal medicine current therapy. 6th edition. St. Louis (MO): Elsevier Saunders; 2008. p. 284–8.

29. Campbell GA, Hoover JP, Russell WC, et al. Naturally occurring cerebral nematodiasis due to baylisascaris larval migration in two black-and-white ruffed lemurs (*Varecia variegata variegata*) and suspected cases in three emus (*Dromaius novaehollandiae*). J Zoo Wildl Med 1997;28(2):204–7.

30. Kazacos KR, Wirtz WL. Experimental cerebrospinal nematodiasis due to *Baylisascaris procyonis* in chickens. Avian Dis 1983;27(1):55–65.

31. Brant SV. The occurrence of the avian schistosome *Allobilharzia visceralis* Kolakrova, Rudolfova, Hampl et Skirnisson, 2006 (Schistosomatidae) in the tundra swan, *Cygnus columbianus* (Anatidae), from North America. Folia Parasitol (Praha) 2007;54(2):99–104.

32. Sweazea KL, Simperova A, Juan T, et al. Pathophysiological responses to a schistosome infection in a wild population of mourning doves (*Zenaida macroura*). Zoology (Jena) 2015;118(6):386–93.

33. Flores V, Brant SV, Loker ES. Avian schistosomes from the South American endemic gastropod genus Chilina (Pulmonata: Chilinidae), with a brief review of South American schistosome species. J Parasitol 2015;101(5):565–76.

34. Aldhoun JA, Horne EC. Schistosomes in South African penguins. Parasitol Res 2015;114(1):237–46.
35. Horak P, Kolarova L, Adema CM. Biology of the schistosome genus *Trichobilharzia*. Adv Parasitol 2002;52:155–233.
36. Horak P, Kolarova L, Dvorak J. *Trichobilharzia regenti* n. sp. (Schistosomatidae, Bilharziellinae), a new nasal schistosome from Europe. Parasite 1998;5(4):349–57.
37. Brant SV, Loker ES. Discovery-based studies of schistosome diversity stimulate new hypotheses about parasite biology. Trends Parasitol 2013;29(9):449–59.
38. van Bolhuis GH, Rijks JM, Dorrestein GM, et al. Obliterative endophlebitis in mute swans (*Cygnus olor*) caused by *Trichobilharzia* sp. (Digenea: Schistosomatidae) infection. Vet Pathol 2004;41(6):658–65.
39. Akagami M, Nakamura K, Nishino H, et al. Pathogenesis of venous hypertrophy associated with schistosomiasis in whooper swans (*Cygnus cygnus*) in Japan. Avian Dis 2010;54(1):146–50.
40. Pence DB, Rhodes MJ. *Trichobilharzia physellae* (Di-genea: Schistosomatidae) from endemic waterfowl on the high plains of Texas. J Wildl Dis 1982;18:69–74.
41. Wojcinski ZW, Barker IK, Hunter DB, et al. An outbreak of schistosomiasis in Atlantic Brant geese, *Branta bernicla* hrota. J Wildl Dis 1987;23:248–55.
42. Kolarova L, Horak P, Cada F. Histopathology of CNS and nasal infections caused by *Trichobilharzia regenti* in vertebrates. Parasitol Res 2001;87:644–50.
43. Greve JH, Sakla AA, McGehee EH. Bilharziasis in a Nanday conure. J Am Vet Med Assoc 1978;172(10):1212–4.
44. Blankespoor CL, Reimink RL, Blankespoort HD. Efficacy of praziquantel in treating natural schistosome infections in common mergansers. J Parasitol 2001;87(2):424–6.
45. Reimink RL, DeGoede JA, Blankespoor HD. Efficacy of praziquantel in natural populations of mallards infected with avian schistosomes. J Parasitol 1995;81(6):1027–9.
46. Campbell D, Barker DIK, Wobeser G. Reovirus in crows—an emerging disease? Wildlife Health Centre Newsletter. Can Cooperative Wildlife Centre 2004;10(1):8.
47. Huhtamo E, Uzcategui NY, Manni T, et al. Novel orthoreovirus from diseased crow, Finland. Emerg Infect Dis 2007;13(12):1967–9.
48. Forzan M, Renshaw R, Bunting E, et al. A novel orthoreovirus associated with epizootic necrotizing enteritis and splenic necrosis in American crows (*Corvus brachyrhynchos*). J Wildl Dis 2019;55:812–22.
49. Olson PD, Cribb TH, Tkach VV, et al. Phylogeny and classification of the Digenea (Platyhelminthes: Trematoda). Int J Parasitol 2003;33(7):733–55.
50. Alfaro-Alarcón A, Morales JA, Veneziano V, et al. Fatal *Paratanaisia bragai* (Digenea: Eucotylidae) infection in scarlet macaws (*Ara macao*) in Costa Rica. Acta Parasitol 2015;60(3):548–52.
51. Luppi MM, de Melo AL, Motta ROC, et al. Granulomatous nephritis in psittacines associated with parasitism by the trematode *Paratanaisia* spp. Vet Parasitol 2007;146(3–4):363–6.
52. De Santi M, André MR, Hoppe EGL, et al. Renal trematode infection in wild birds: histopathological, morphological, and molecular aspects. Parasitol Res 2018;117(3):883–91.
53. Xavier VB, Oliveira-Menezes A, Dos Santos MAJ, et al. Histopathological changes in the kidneys of vertebrate hosts infected naturally and experimentally with *Paratanaisia bragai* (Trematoda, Digenea). Rev Bras Parasitol Vet 2015;24(2):241–6.

54. de Matos AMRN, Lavorente FLP, Lorenzetti E, et al. Molecular identification and histological aspects of *Renicola sloanei* (Digenea: Renicolidae) in *Puffinus puffinus* (Procellariiformes): a first record. Rev Bras Parasitol Vet 2019;28(3):367–75.
55. Jerdy H, Baldassin P, Werneck MR, et al. First report of kidney lesions due to *Renicola* sp. (Digenea: Trematoda) in free-living Magellanic penguins (*Spheniscus magellanicus* Forster, 1781) found on the coast of Brazil. J Parasitol 2016; 102(6):650–2.
56. Unwin S, Chantrey J, Chatterton J, et al. Renal trematode infection due to *Paratanaisia bragai* in zoo housed Columbiformes and a red bird-of-paradise (*Paradisaea rubra*). Int J Parasitol Parasites Wildl 2013;2:32–41.

Selected Emerging Diseases of Pet Hedgehogs

Emma Keeble, BVSc (Hons), DECZM (Mammalian), MRCVS[a],*,
Bronwyn Koterwas, BA, BVM&S, MRCVS[b]

KEYWORDS

- African pygmy hedgehog • Acariasis • *Caparinia tripilis* • Central brain neoplasm
- Emerging disease

KEY POINTS

- Acariasis has been previously reported in hedgehogs as a major health problem worldwide but has more recently been identified as a significant issue in pet African pygmy hedgehogs.
- Heavy mite infestation is often associated with severe and widespread fungal infection within a hedgehog population.
- Subclinical infections are reported to occur and may explain why this condition is so common in pet hedgehogs.
- Among hedgehogs investigated for wobbly hedgehog syndrome, 6.7% had primary brain tumors.
- Recently, a growing number of reports have been published on central nervous system neoplasms in pet African hedgehogs, with astrocytomas representing the most reported brain neoplasm.

 Video content accompanies this article at http://www.vetexotic.theclinics.com.

GENERAL INTRODUCTION

Worldwide, 14 species of spiny hedgehog have been recorded, and although primarily wild animals, 1 species in particular, the African pygmy hedgehog (also known as the white-bellied or 4-toed hedgehog [*Atelerix albiventris*]) is now commonly kept as a pet, as well as in zoologic collections[1] (**Fig. 1**A). This article primarily focuses on the African pygmy hedgehog, with some references, where appropriate, to European free-living hedgehogs (*Erinaceus europaeus*) (**Fig. 1**B).

[a] The Dick Vet Rabbit and Exotic Practice, The University of Edinburgh, The Royal (Dick) School of Veterinary Studies, The Roslin Institute, Easter Bush Campus, Midlothian EH25 9RG, UK;
[b] The Dick Vet Rabbit and Exotic Practice, The University of Edinburgh, The Royal (Dick) School of Veterinary Studies, The Roslin Institute, Easter Bush Campus, Midlothian EH25 9RG, UK
* Corresponding author.
E-mail address: emma.keeble@ed.ac.uk

Vet Clin Exot Anim 23 (2020) 443–458
https://doi.org/10.1016/j.cvex.2020.01.010
1094-9194/20/© 2020 Elsevier Inc. All rights reserved.

vetexotic.theclinics.com

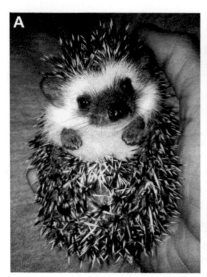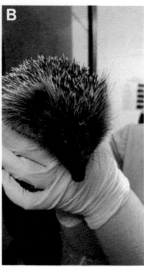

Fig. 1. (*A*) African pygmy hedgehog (*A albiventris*). (*B*) European hedgehog (*E europaeus*). ([*A*] *Courtesy of* Louise Ross, Edinburgh, Scotland.)

Veterinarians should make full use of the resources available to familiarize themselves with hedgehog-specific husbandry and diet.[2–7]

A REVIEW OF COMMON DISEASES IN HEDGEHOGS

Several retrospective studies of disease incidence in pet hedgehogs have recently been published with a wide geographic distribution, including North America, Asia, and Europe.[1,8–10] Many retrospective studies and case report series have focused primarily on neoplastic disease or clinical diagnoses and have been based on zoopathologic research,[10,11] most of which are from the United States.[1]

A review of 106 African pygmy hedgehog cases (both pet animals and those from zoologic collections) presented over a 19-year period to a veterinary hospital in the United States (Kansas) was performed to determine the most commonly occurring disease in this species. Skin diseases were most commonly seen (66.04%), specifically ectoparasites (65.71% of skin cases), with gastrointestinal disease second (33.02%).[1] Skeletal diseases were third most common, accounting for 15.09% of animals seen. Common causes of gastrointestinal disease were dental disease and oral squamous cell carcinoma, and causes of skeletal disease were degenerative joint disease, annular pedal constriction, and spondylosis.

A review of histologic samples submitted over a 5-year period from 100 pet African pygmy hedgehogs to 2 Japanese laboratories identified endometrial stromal nodules (benign uterine neoplasia) as the most common histologic diagnosis (13.33%).[8] The most common tissues included in this study were female reproductive tracts (31.43%), skin (19.05%), and oral mucosa (18.1%). The most common histologic diagnoses for the skin samples were fibrosarcomas (7.62%) and mammary tumors (7.62%), and for the oral mucosal samples were gingival hyperplasia and chronic suppurative inflammation (10.48%). Overall neoplasia accounted for 60% of all histologic cases, 74.6% of which were malignant.

A review of 63 African hedgehog clinical cases from 1 institution in Taiwan presented over an 8-year period concluded that neoplastic conditions were the most common cause of death in the group studied (35.9% of cases). Oral squamous cell carcinoma was the most commonly reported neoplasm (35.7%). Average life span in this group of hedgehogs was 3.4 ± 1.1 years.[12] The second most common cause of death was respiratory disease (25.6%), consisting of pneumonia, emphysema, pulmonary edema, and pulmonary hemorrhage, followed by digestive disorders (10.3%), consisting of intestinal obstruction, gastritis, duodenitis, and gastric ulceration. More than 50% of the respiratory cases had concurrent diseases, such as neoplasia, hepatitis, and cardiac disease.

It is speculated that the increase in life span in captivity leads to an increase in neoplastic conditions seen in this pet species.[12,13]

A recent review of hedgehog diseases in Spain (species not specified) presented to a veterinary clinic over a 7-year period found that gastrointestinal and skin diseases were most commonly seen.[9]

These findings indicate how disease presentation differs geographically; however, it can be concluded that skin disease, gastrointestinal disease, and neoplasia are commonly found in African pygmy hedgehogs worldwide. This review article discusses the new and emerging diseases occurring in 2 of the most commonly reported systems: skin disease and neoplasia. Gastrointestinal disease caused by salmonellosis is another commonly reported disease in hedgehogs and is discussed in Emma Keeble and Bronwyn Koterwas's article "Salmonellosis in Hedgehogs," in this issue.

CAPARINIA TRIPILIS INFECTIONS IN PET HEDGEHOGS
Introduction

Acariasis has previously been reported in hedgehogs as a major health problem worldwide[14–16] but has more recently been identified as a significant issue in pet African pygmy hedgehogs.[17] Skin diseases are among the most commonly presented health problems in pet African pygmy hedgehogs,[1,9] with mite infestation the most common cause.[1]

Caparinia infections were first reported in hedgehogs in Europe, Africa, and New Zealand[14,18] and have since been introduced to South and North America via the pet trade.[17,19] In Asia, an outbreak of *Caparinia tripilis* infestation in a colony of African pygmy hedgehogs from Korea was reported in 2012,[20] indicating that this is a common problem in hedgehogs regardless of geographic location. More recently, cases have been reported in eastern Europe (Poland, Romania)[17,21] and Costa Rica.[19]

Cause

Mite infestations in hedgehogs have been reported belonging to the genera *Sarcoptes*, *Notoedres*, *Otodectes*, *Chorioptes*, and *Caparinia*.[22] Mite infestation is common in both wild and rehabilitated European hedgehogs (*E europaeus*) and pet African pygmy hedgehogs (*A albiventris*), often with concurrent disease such as dermatophyte infection[6,7,17] (**Fig. 2**). In healthy animals, small numbers of mites may be considered normal; however, in immunocompromised or ill animals, infestations often occur.[1] The most common species encountered are *Caparinia* spp (nonburrowing psoroptid mites), but *Chorioptes* spp and sarcoptid species (burrowing mites) are also reported.[2,6,7,18] It has been suggested that, in past publications, there has been possible misidentification and reporting of the exact mite species involved.[14]

Hedgehogs with heavy mite infestations often have concurrent significant fungal infections (*Trichophyton erinacei*, *Microsporum canis, and Microsporum gypseum*), and fungal spores have been isolated from mite droppings, with mites suggested to be

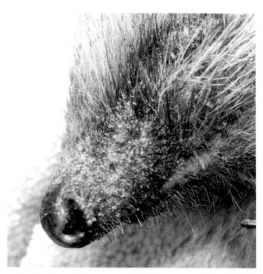

Fig. 2. Wild European hedgehog (*E europaeus*) with severe *C tripilis* infestation of the face. Visible mites are present on the rostrum, as well as scaling. (*Courtesy of* David Couper, BVM&S, Taunton, England.)

facilitating fungal growth because of their effects on the skin surface resulting in scale and crust formation.[14,23] Clinical relapse is common in nonhibernating hedgehogs that are overwintered in captivity.[14]

Many other species of mites have been reported in wild European and African hedgehogs and their nests[6,7] (for details of species and geographic location see Ref.[18]).

Epidemiology

Subclinical infections are reported to occur and may explain why this condition is so common in pet hedgehogs.[2] In stressful situations the host-parasite relationship becomes imbalanced and parasite levels may increase.[24] It is thought that factors such as stress, hormonal changes, and immune system dysfunction may all contribute to the development of clinical disease in pet hedgehogs.[21] Ectoparasite load depends on many different behavioral, physiologic, and ecological factors.[25] Stress may occur in wild hedgehogs (eg, at times of prolonged bad weather, high population densities, shortage of food sources, habitat changes,[26] or concurrent disease/ill-health) or in pet hedgehogs because of poor nutrition/husbandry, addition of a new animal, reproduction, or concurrent disease processes.[25,27] Underlying causes should always be investigated in clinical cases.

The *C tripilis* mite has a direct 3-week life cycle from egg to larva to protonymph to deutonymph (none of these are sexually dimorphic), developing into either an adult male or an adult female.[28] It feeds off epidermal debris and sloughed skin cells. The direct life cycle of *C tripilis* may facilitate its establishment in a novel environment.[21] *C tripilis* is not zoonotic.[28] The prevalence of this parasite in hedgehog populations varies between 40% and 100%,[17,22] with 1 study reporting 87% of normal pygmy hedgehogs as carriers of mites.[21] *C tripilis* could be considered a normal commensal skin inhabitant of hedgehogs without causing any clinical signs; however, it seems more likely that it is a low-pathogenicity parasite that manifests with concurrent disease or stress.[19]

Caparinia mites have been implicated in the spread of dermatophyte infection in hedgehogs, because *Trichophyton erinacei* has been cultured from mite feces.[23]

Heavy mite infestation is often associated with severe and widespread fungal infection within a hedgehog population. Hedgehogs with no mites or only small numbers of mites are rarely found to have concurrent dermatophytosis.[14,23]

C tripilis mites are classified in the Astigmata order, Psoroptidae family. Identification keys based on morphologic features for both sexes of the different life stages for identification of this mite species have been described.[17,20,29]

Clinical Signs

Clinical signs vary greatly from subclinical, to mild, to severe. Infections may be subclinical, but in severe infestations dry flaky skin, crusting, seborrhea, erythema, lichenification, and loss of quills may occur (alopecia), which may be extensive[19,30] (**Fig. 3**). White or brown hyperkeratosis may be seen at the quill base over the body, around the eyes, and behind the ears (**Fig. 4**). Crusts contain detritus produced by the burrowing mites. Animals may also be pruritic and attempt to scratch themselves or rub up against objects in their environment.[2] In some cases, self-trauma can be significant and results in secondary bacterial or fungal infection.[31] Mites within the external ear canal may lead to otitis externa with secondary bacterial infection.[32] Lethargy, weight loss, reduced appetite, and dehydration have also been reported,[2,6,19] with death occurring in severe untreated animals.[14,28] Affected animals are often in poor body condition[19] (**Fig. 5**). Wild hedgehogs with end-stage mite infestation may be seen out during the daytime and are unable to curl up in a ball.[14] Chronic cases can present in acute crisis because hedgehogs may hide signs until clinically severely debilitated.[27] Severe cases in wild animals may eventually resolve with obvious areas of alopecic quill loss evident.[14] Animals as young as 4 months old may be infected. Even without obvious clinical signs, careful examination of all hedgehogs for evidence of ectoparasites is recommended at first presentation because this condition is so common.[3] Hedgehogs usually present when the owner notices an unusual increase in the number of quills being shed or has noticed the skin appears dryer than normal and flaky. Observation of the animal in the consultation room often reveals many quills and dry skin shed into the accompanying bedding and on the consultation table. The authors always wear disposable gloves when handling pet hedgehogs because of the risk of dermatophyte infection and its zoonotic potential. Clinical signs are similar with both mite and fungal skin infections[33] and can be concurrent.[34,35] *Caparinia* mites are just visible without magnification and appear as white powdery material.[36]

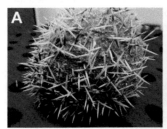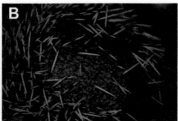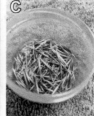

Fig. 3. (*A*) Extensive quill loss with a small amount of associated scaling in an African pygmy hedgehog (*A albiventris*) associated with *Caparinia* infestation. (*B*) This African pygmy hedgehog (*A albiventris*) presented with chronic quill loss that had occurred over a long period of time before the owner presented the animal for veterinary examination. The skin was not excessively scaly, but mites were confirmed microscopically. (*C*) Quills collected by an owner from an individual African pygmy hedgehog over a 3-week period. *Caparinia* infestation was diagnosed.

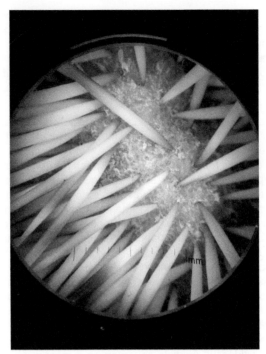

Fig. 4. Dermatoscopic view of skin at the quill base of an affected African pygmy hedgehog (*A albiventris*). Note the extensive scaling and crusting present. Mites are also easily visible feeding at the base of the quills (millimeter scale shown). (*Courtesy of* Tim Nuttall, BSc, BVSc, PhD, Edinburgh, Scotland.)

Differential diagnoses for *Caparinia* infestations include infection with other mite species (*Demodex*, *Notoedres* spp) and dermatophytosis (*Trichophyton erinacei*, *Trichophyton mentagrophytes*, *Microsporum* spp, *Arthroderma benhamiae*, *Paecilomyces variotii*, disseminated histoplasmosis, and dermal aspergillosis).[30,37–40]

Diagnosis

Diagnosis is based on suspicious clinical signs and demonstration of mites. Examination of the skin with magnification (eg, using a dermatoscope or hand lens) may reveal obvious mites (**Fig. 6**, Video 1), but skin scrapes and hair/spine samples may also be

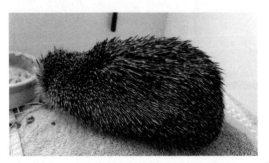

Fig. 5. This emaciated wild European hedgehog (*E europaeus*) presented with scaling and crusting lesions around the face associated with *Caparinia* infection.

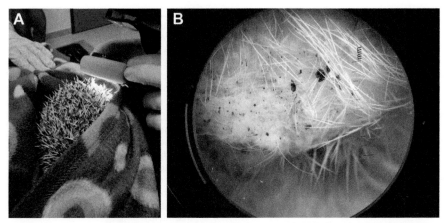

Fig. 6. (*A*) Dermatoscopic examination of the skin of an affected African pygmy hedgehog (*A albiventris*). (*B*) View through dermatoscope (millimeter scale shown). Generalized erythema of the skin indicates inflammation related to mite infestation. Light-colored material is likely plant debris and dark material is seborrheic debris. Adult and larval mite forms can be seen. ([*B*] *Courtesy of* Tim Nuttall, BSc, BVSc, PhD, Edinburgh, Scotland.)

taken and examined with direct microscopy for adult and larval stages or eggs (nits). Multiple samples should ideally be taken from various sites. The highest density of mites has been reported in the external ear canals, with less occurring on the dorsum, and lowest densities occurring on the ventrum.[28] Samples can be preserved in 70% ethanol.[19] Identification of mite species is of interest but is often not complete, and mixed infestations have been reported[31,41] (see also Ref.[42] for *Chorioptes* spp identification, for which *Caparinia* spp are often confused).

Concurrent dermatophyte infection and secondary bacterial skin infections are common, therefore dermatophyte culture and skin cytology are also recommended.[17] In cases with suspicious clinical signs but no evidence of mites on skin samples, the authors recommend trial treatment of acariasis. Anecdotally it has been suggested that some hedgehogs may develop a hypersensitivity reaction to the mites, presenting with obvious clinical signs but very low mite numbers that are often not identified.[43]

Treatment in Pet Hedgehogs

Published articles outlining treatments, their efficacy, and effective dose rates are few and usually involve limited hedgehog numbers. Drug side effects, safety data, and toxicology studies have not been properly investigated in this species, although side effects are reportedly uncommon. **Table 1** lists antiparasitic agents and dose rates for the treatment of mite infections in pet hedgehogs.

Treatment of mite infections is similar for all mite species, with response to treatment a useful guide for veterinary practitioners.[5] Various treatment options have been described, with variable efficacy,[2,5,6,32] and more recently a single oral dose of fluralaner.[30] Moxidectin (1%) combined with imidacloprid (10%) topical preparation has also been used as a once-off topical dose with excellent results and no observed side effects[28] as well as weekly topical application of a combination of ivermectin and 0.3% amitraz.[44] Systemic ivermectin is usually highly effective,[21,29] although there are reports of treatment failure with this drug.[28,30,32]

Affected hedgehogs undergoing treatment should be housed on newspaper that can be changed daily during the treatment period. It is important to treat in-contact

Table 1
Antiparasitic agents for the treatment of mite infections in pet hedgehogs

Drug	Dose Rate	Comments	Reference
Amitraz 0.03% topically	Apply topically every 7–14 d	2–3 treatments required Ophthalmic ointment applied before spray. Animals left to air dry Wear gloves No toxicity studies performed in this species; use with caution	5,28,32
Fipronil topical spray (0.25%)	Apply topically every 14 d	3 treatments required	6
	Apply topically every 10 d	2 treatments required for (*Ornithonyssus bacoti*)	67
	1 spray per hedgehog	Topical spray along dorsum (note: care with hypothermia and ensure adequate ventilation after treatment)	5,68
Fluralaner	15 mg/kg PO	Once off dose. Effective by 21 d after treatment. New quill growth 30 d after treatment Safety and toxicity in hedgehogs still to be evaluated Dose allometrically calculated from dog dose	30
Ivermectin	0.2–0.4 mg/kg SC every 14 d	3 treatments usually required	6
	0.30.4 mg/kg PO, SC every 10–14 d	3–5 treatments required. May need to be combined with topical amitraz	2,5
	1% topically at 200 μL	Administered at 21-d intervals, until clinical signs resolved May not fully clear mite infection	21,28
	0.2–0.5 mg/kg spot-on preparation	Repeat after 10 d	7
10% Imidacloprid + 1.0% moxidectin spot-on	Dosage level of 0.1 mL/kg (10 mg imidacloprid and 1 mg moxidectin)	Single topical dose Effective after 3 d No side effects observed, n = 25 Lowest effective dose trialed in study	28
Moxidectin 1% injectable	0.3 mg/kg SC injection	Repeat after 10 d *Notoedres cati* infection	34
1% Permethrin	Topical once off dose	Apply as a fine mist; change bedding at same time	69
Selamectin	6–18 mg/kg topically every 30 d	2 treatments required	5,6
	4.5 mg/kg topically, repeat after 3 wk	—	44
	12 mg per hedgehog	Once off treatment, clinical signs resolved after 21 d	17

Dose rates are often extrapolated from other species, and drug efficacy, effective dose rate, drug side effects, safety data, and toxicology studies may not have been properly investigated in this species. In the United Kingdom, prescribing of unlicensed drugs should follow the veterinary cascade system.

Abbreviations: PO, by mouth; SC, subcutaneous.
Data from Refs.[2,5–7,17,21,28,30,32,34,44,67–69]

animals concurrently, and the environment should be thoroughly cleaned and disinfected at the time of treatment.[2,5] Treatment options should be discussed with the owner, and ease of administration is an important consideration in hedgehogs because they tend to ball up when handled. In 1 case report, a single dose of fluralaner 15 mg/kg by mouth was effective at clearing mites 21 days after treatment, with cessation of pruritus and erythema at day 14 after treatment and new quill growth observed 30 days after treatment.[30] No adverse drug effects were noted in this case.

Failure to respond fully to treatment could be as a result of untreated concurrent dermatophyte infection.[35] Response to treatment and treatment efficacy should always be monitored, with repeat microscopic examination of skin samples for the presence of mites or eggs. The authors advocate at least 2 negative samples before treatment can be deemed effective and stopped.

Control

Gloves should be routinely worn by veterinarians when handling pet hedgehogs because of the risk of zoonotic transfer of disease and the inability to distinguish clinical signs from mite infestation and dermatophytosis.[45] It is important to disinfect the hedgehog's living area and bedding at the start and end of any treatment course to eliminate mites that have contaminated the environment. A potential source of infection for new pets is contaminated bedding or fomites from breeders, pet shops, or in contact with infected animals.[2,25,46] All bedding should be removed and disposed of and cage furniture should be disinfected or discarded.[30] All in-contact animals should also be treated at the same time.

Summary

Wild hedgehogs carry an abundance of ectoparasites and many studies have been performed on tick and flea burdens and their potential as vectors of disease, including zoonoses.[25,46–50] However, none of these recent ectoparasite studies have investigated mite infestations. Earlier studies do exist on levels of mite burden in wild hedgehogs, although there is some confusion over identification of exact mite species.[14] More recent case reports in pet African pygmy hedgehogs have helped to clarify mite species and determine keys for morphologic identification of the species involved.[17,20,29] These reports have shown a wide geographic case distribution. Diagnosis of mite infestation is straightforward, but treatment is recommended with suspicious clinical signs despite negative skin scrapes on microscopy. Treatment options are varied and straightforward, with resolution of clinical signs in most cases if diagnosed early.

CENTRAL NERVOUS SYSTEM LESIONS
Introduction

Nearly 30 years ago, muscle atrophy with progressive ascending paralysis was described in pet African pygmy hedgehogs: wobbly hedgehog syndrome (WHS). Histopathology confirmed a spongy myelinopathy with gross vacuolization and demyelination.[51,52] The original survey investigating WHS queried 676 owners from 2000 to 2005 and found that 10% of their pets had an element of paralysis. Forty-five of these animals were eventually obtained for postmortem examination and 40 were positively diagnosed with WHS. In the remaining 5, 1 had extensive hepatic disease and 4 were found to have central brain neoplasms, without any evidence of the demyelination or vacuolization typical of WHS.[51]

It is reported that neoplasia has been found on postmortem examination in approximately 30% of hedgehogs.[11] A retrospective study found that 29% of formalin-fixed samples from 14 hedgehogs from 1992 to 1996 had neoplastic lesions.[10] Another review found neoplastic masses in 53% of samples from African hedgehogs submitted for histopathology. Of these, 85% were malignant and 8.6% had multiple tumor types. Mammary gland adenocarcinoma, lymphosarcoma, and oral squamous cell carcinoma were found most frequently.[13] In a third study, 105 samples from 100 similarly submitted samples from 2012 to 2017 revealed neoplasia in 60% of cases.[8]

Evaluating these data, the incidence of neoplasia in ill hedgehogs may be nearer to 47%. In these reviews, no primary brain neoplasms were found, likely because of the central nervous system (CNS) not being sampled or submitted for investigation. Therefore, the true incidence of overall neoplasia in *Atelerix* spp could very well be higher than reported. It is likely that central lesions are under-reported in this species and perhaps misdiagnosed as WHS.

Central Brain Neoplasms

As insectivores, African pygmy hedgehogs have a few anatomic differences within the CNS. The olfactory lobe is prominent,[2] which allows their strong sense of smell. The cerebrum is smaller than in other species; it does not extend as far as the cerebellum and the hemispheres do not contain fissures.[53]

In 2006, a report by Graesser and colleagues[51] found that 6.7% (3 of 45) of hedgehogs investigated for WHS actually had primary brain tumors. Histopathologic samples from 762 *Atelerix* spp submitted from 1997 to 2015 to a single institution revealed 12 cases (1.6%) of neoplasia in the brain. Astrocytomas predominated, followed by gangliogliomas and a single case of oligodendroglioma.[54]

Since 2006, a growing number of case reports have been published on CNS neoplasms in pet African hedgehogs (**Table 2**). Astrocytomas (n=5) represent the most reported brain neoplasm[51,55,56] followed by meningiomas (n=2)[51,57] as well as single cases of histiocytic sarcoma[58] and mixed tumor types such as oligoastrocytoma[59] and oligodendroglioma.[60] All reported brain neoplasms in hedgehogs are summarized in **Table 2**.

There has been 1 case report of a 2-year-old male hedgehog with profound ataxia that had an infiltrative mass of the cranium diagnosed on computed tomography (CT). On postmortem, an extraskeletal soft tissue sarcoma that eroded the cranium and invaded the cerebellum and cerebrum was confirmed.[61]

Table 2
Central nervous system neoplasms reported in African pygmy hedgehogs

Type of Neoplasm	Number of Cases	Associated Clinical Signs	Reference
Astrocytoma	13	Lameness, ataxia, falling over, seizures, anorexia, paresis, urinary bladder retention	51,52,54–56
Ganglioglioma	6	Weakness, forelimb rigidity, blindness, ataxia, paresis, tetraplegia	54
Oligodendroglioma and oligoastrocytoma	3	Ataxia, anuria with bladder retention, inappetence, walking in circles, falling to one side	54,59,60
Meningioma	2	Ataxia, anorexia, exophthalmos	51,57
Histiocytic sarcoma	1	Tremors, falling to one side, dysphagia, paresis	58

Data from Refs.[51,52,54–60]

In domestic species, the prevalence of tumors of the CNS is low; reportedly 2% to 4.5% in dogs.[54] Given the higher incidence of neoplasia in African hedgehogs, it is likely that the prevalence of CNS masses is greater as well.

More than half of the CNS tumors reported in hedgehogs were found to be astrocytomas (13 out of 25), predominantly in the cerebrum, whereas they are only found in about 15% of dogs with brain masses.[62] Gangliogliomas represented 24% of brain neoplasms in hedgehogs but are rare in dogs and typically found in the thalamus or brainstem.[62] Four of 6 hedgehogs with gangliogliomas had masses in the brainstem. In dogs and cats, meningiomas are the most common primary brain neoplasm, with an incidence of 45% and 60% respectively.[62] In hedgehogs, meningiomas represented 8% of the central brain tumors discovered.

Oligodendrogliomas also made up 8% of reported CNS neoplasms in hedgehogs. Comparatively, in dogs the prevalence of primary nervous system tumors is 15%, with some breeds showing a higher predilection.[62]

Other Disorders

As with other animals, it can be expected that a variety of disorders can cause neurologic signs as well.[63] A retrospective study of 104 hedgehog cases presented to a veterinary university from 1994 to 2013 identified several disease processes that could present with secondary neurologic signs after progression: otitis externa, hepatic disease, cardiac disease, and musculoskeletal disease such as spondylosis.[1] Histopathology samples from 14 hedgehogs submitted for evaluation from 1992 to 1996 revealed hepatic lipidosis, cardiac disease, encephalitis, and encephalopathy.[10] Another retrospective study evaluating 105 tissues submitted from 100 hedgehogs from 2012 to 2017 identified hepatic lipidosis and cardiomyopathy in pet hedgehogs.[8] Intervertebral disc disease, positively diagnosed through radiography and CT, has been reported to cause ataxia in hedgehogs that progressed to hind limb paresis.[64,65] Infectious diseases such as *Baylisascaris* migration, encephalitides, and paramyxovirus (pneumonia virus of mice) have also shown neurologic disease in pet hedgehogs.[63]

Clinical Signs

Concomitant disease is routinely found on postmortem examination of hedgehogs,[2,10,52] which can make clinical case presentation complex. One study of 12 hedgehogs with suspected WHS compared neuropathologic location with clinical signs. No association was found except for cerebellar lesions, which matched the expected cerebellar and vestibular deficits.[52] Typical signs of neurologic disease include weakness, ataxia, paresis, paralysis, and weight loss (Video 2). Fine tremors, seizures, and blindness can also be seen (Video 3).

Diagnostics and Treatment Options

Almost all of the reported cases of central brain masses were initially diagnosed as WHS on presentation without evidence of this on postmortem.[51,56–60] However, it is emerging that there are some key differences in presentation to guide clinicians.

The average age of clinical onset of WHS is less than 2 years (1–36 months), with a survival time of 15 to 25 months after presentation.[56] However, neurogenic neoplasms typically present in older animals (mean, 3 years) [52,54–56,58–60] and progression is more rapid, with death or euthanasia occurring within 1 to 9 months.[56–59] In addition, urinary bladder retention and anuria have been reported in hedgehogs[55,60] with central neoplasia but not in hedgehogs with WHS alone.[52]

Diagnostic aids rely on imaging, although radiographs are unable to detect CNS neoplasia.[56] Neuroimaging techniques such as MRI remain the gold standard, although CT may be helpful, as in canine and feline medicine,[62] and guided micro-biopsy is an option in these species, although has not been described in the hedgehog.

Treatment options to date have relied on supportive and palliative care. Nonsteroidal and steroidal therapeutics have been trialed with no real improvement in quality-of-life parameters or life span. Radiotherapy for CNS tumors in dogs and cats can be successful, although other limiting side effects may be encountered.[66] At present, this modality is logistically difficult in *Atelerix* spp.

Prognosis

To date, both neoplasia of the CNS and WHS remain fatal diagnoses. By understanding the high potential for concomitant disease as well as differences in presentation, clinical progression, and diagnostics, clinicians can manage owner expectations and ensure that quality-of-life parameters are upheld for these animals. In the future, advances in oncologic therapeutic options and a deeper comprehension of the causes of WHS could improve prognosis.

ACKNOWLEDGMENTS

The authors would like to acknowledge Dr David Couper, Dr Tim Nuttall, and Louise Ross for their help sourcing images for the article, as well as their families and work colleagues for their patience and understanding while collating and writing this article.

DISCLOSURE

The authors have nothing to disclose.

SUPPLEMENTARY DATA

Supplementary data related to this article can be found online at https://doi.org/10. 1016/j.cvex.2020.01.010.

REFERENCES

1. Gardhouse S, Eshar D. Retrospective study of disease occurrence in captive African Pygmy hedgehogs (Atelerix albiventris). Isr J Vet Med 2015;70(1):32–6.
2. Ivey E, Carpenter J. African hedgehogs. In: Quesenberry K, Carpenter J, editors. Ferrets, rabbits and rodents: clinical medicine and surgery. St Louis (MO): Elsevier; 2012. p. 411–27.
3. Simone-Freilicher EA, Hoefer HL. Hedgehog care and husbandry. Vet Clin North Am Exot Anim Pract 2004;7(2):257–67.
4. Hoefer HL. Hedgehogs. Vet Clin North Am Small Anim Pract 1994;24(1):113–20.
5. Heatley JJ. Hedgehogs. In: Mitchell MA, Tully TN, editors. Manual of exotic pet practice. St Louis (MO): W.B. Saunders; 2009. p. 433–55.
6. Johnson D. African Pygmy hedgehogs. In: Meredith A, Johnson-DeLaney C, editors. BSAVA manual of exotic pets. Gloucester (UK): BSAVA; 2010. p. 455.
7. Bexton S. Hedgehogs. In: Mullineaux E, Keeble E, editors. BSAVA manual of wildlife casualties. Cheltenham (England): BSAVA; 2016. p. 117–36.
8. Okada K, Kondo H, Sumi A, et al. A retrospective study of disease incidence in African pygmy hedgehogs (Atelerix albiventris). J Vet Med Sci 2018;80(10): 1504–10.

9. Farres PS, Soler V, Martorell J. Retrospective study of hedgehog diseases in FHCV (2011-2018). in International conference on avian, herpetological and exotic mammal medicine. ICARE, London, 28 April - 2 May, 2019.

10. Raymond JT, White MR. Necropsy and histopathologic findings in 14 African hedgehogs (atelerix albiventris): a retrospective study. J Zoo Wildl Med 1999; 30(2):273–7.

11. Heatley JJ, Mauldin GE, Cho DY. A review of neoplasia in the captive African Hedgehog (Atelerix albiventris). Seminars in Avian and Exotic Pet Medicine 2005;14(3):182–92.

12. Pei-Chi H, Jane-Fang Y, Lih-Chiann W. A Retrospective Study of the Medical Status on 63 African Hedgehogs (Atelerix albiventris) at the Taipei zoo from 2003 to 2011. J Exot Pet Med 2015;24(1):105–11.

13. Raymond JT, Garner MM. Spontaneous Tumours in Captive African Hedgehogs (Atelerix albiventris):a Retrospective Study. J Comp Pathol 2001;124(2–3): 128–33.

14. Brockie RE. The hedgehog mange mite, Caparinia tripilis, in New Zealand. N Z Vet J 1974;22(12):243–7.

15. Gerson L, Boever WJ. Acariasis (Caparinia sp.) in hedgehogs (Erinaceus spp.): diagnosis and treatment. The Journal of Zoo Animal Medicine 1983;14(1):17–9.

16. Keymer IF, Gibson EA, Reynolds DJ. Zoonoses and other findings in hedgehogs (Erinaceus europaeus): a survey of mortality and review of the literature. Vet Rec 1991;128(11):245–9.

17. Iacob O, Iftinca A. The dermatitis by Caparinia tripilis and Microsporum , in african pygmy hedgehog (Atelerix albiventris) in Romania - first report. Rev Bras Parasitol Vet 2018;27(4):584.

18. Reeve N. Malentities and Misfortune. Demography, disease, death. In: Reeve N, editor. Hedgehogs. London: AD Poyser Natural History; 1994. p. 214–48.

19. Moreira A, Troyo A, Calderón-Arguedas O. First report of acariasis by Caparinia tripilis in African hedgehogs, (Atelerix albiventris), in Costa Rica. Rev Bras Parasitol Vet 2013;22(1):155–8.

20. Kim D, Oh DS, Ahn KS, et al. An outbreak of Caparinia tripilis in a colony of African pygmy hedgehogs (Atelerix albiventris) from Korea. Korean J Parasitol 2012; 50(2):151–6.

21. Demkowska-Kutrzepa M, Tomczuk K, Studzińska M, et al. Caparinia tripilis in African hedgehog (Atelerix albiventris). Vet Dermatol 2015;26(1):73–5.

22. Fredes F, Román D. Fauna parasitaria en erizos de tierra africanos (Atelerix albiventris). Parasitología latinoamericana 2004;59(1–2):79–81.

23. Smith JMB, Marples MJ. Trichophyton mentagrophytes var. erinacei. Sabouraudia 1963;3(1):1–10.

24. Isenbugel E, Baumgartner R. Diseases of the Hedgehog. In: Fowler M, editor. Zoo and wild animal medicine: current therapy. Philadelphia: WB Saunders Company; 1993. p. 294–303.

25. Dziemian S, Sikora B, Piłacińska B, et al. Ectoparasite loads in sympatric urban populations of the northern white-breasted and the European hedgehog. Parasitol Res 2015;114(6):2317–23.

26. Thamm S, Kalko E, Wells K. Ectoparasite infestations of Hedgehogs (Erinaceus europaeus) are associated with small-scale landscape structures in an urban–suburban environment. Ecohealth 2009;6(3):404–13.

27. Lennox AM. Emergency and critical care procedures in sugar gliders (Petaurus breviceps), African Hedgehogs (Atelerix albiventris), and prairie dogs (Cynomys spp). Vet Clin North Am Exot Anim Pract 2007;10(2):533–55.

28. Kim K-R, Ahn KS, Oh DS, et al. Efficacy of a combination of 10% imidacloprid and 1% moxidectin against Caparinia tripilis in African pygmy hedgehog (Atelerix albiventris). Parasit Vectors 2012;5(1):158.

29. Eo KY, Kwak D, Kwon OD. Treatment of mange caused by Caparinia tripilis in native Korean wild hedgehogs (Erinaceus amurensis): a case report. Vet Med 2015;60(1):57–61.

30. Romero C, Sheinberg Waisburd G, Pineda J, et al. Fluralaner as a single dose oral treatment for Caparinia tripilis in a pygmy African hedgehog. Vet Dermatol 2017;28(6). 622-e152.

31. Fehr M, Koestlinger S. Ectoparasites in small exotic mammals. Vet Clin North Am Exot Anim Pract 2013;16(3):611–57.

32. Letcher JD. Amitraz as a treatment for acariasis in African Hedgehogs (Atelerix albiventris). The Journal of Zoo Animal Medicine 1988;19(1/2):24–9.

33. Perry S, Sander S, Mitchell M. Integumentary system. In: Mitchell MA, Tully TN, editors. Current therapy in exotic pet practice. St Louis (MO): Elsevier; 2016. p. 17–75.

34. Pantchev N, Hofmann T. Notoedric mange caused by Notoedres cati in a pet African pygmy hedgehog (Atelerix albiventris). Vet Rec 2006;158(2):59–60.

35. Takahashi Y, Haritani K, Sano A, et al. An isolate of Arthroderma benhamiae with Trichophyton mentagrophytes var. erinacei anamorph isolated from a four-toed hedgehog (Atelerix albiventris) in Japan. Nihon Ishinkin Gakkai Zasshi 2002; 43(4):249.

36. Meredith A. Skin diseases and treatment of hedgehogs. In: Paterson S, editor. Skin diseases of exotic pets. Ames (IA): Blackwell Science; 2006. p. 264–74.

37. Carpenter JW, Lindemann D. Diseases of hedgehogs 2015. Available at: https://www.msdvetmanual.com/exotic-and-laboratory-animals/hedgehogs/diseases-of-hedgehogs. Accessed October 24, 2019.

38. Snider TA, Joyner PH, Clinkenbeard KD. Disseminated histoplasmosis in an African pygmy hedgehog. J Am Vet Med Assoc 2008;232(1):74–6.

39. Han J-I, Na K-J. Dermatitis caused by Neosartorya hiratsukae infection in a hedgehog. J Clin Microbiol 2008;46(9):3119.

40. Han J-I, Na K-J. Cutaneous paecilomycosis caused by Paecilomyces variotii in an African Pygmy Hedgehog (Atelerix albiventris). J Exot Pet Med 2010;19(4): 309–12.

41. Gregory MW. Mites of the hedgehog Erinaceus albiventris Wagner in Kenya: observations on the prevalence and pathogenicity of Notoedres oudemansi Fain, Caparinia erinacei Fain and Rodentopus sciuri Fain. Parasitology 1981;82(1): 149–57.

42. Sweatman G. Life history, non-specificity, and revision of the genus Chorioptes, a parasitic mite of herbivores. Can J Zool 1957;35:641–89.

43. Nuttall T. Head of veterinary dermatology. University of Edinburgh, Royal (Dick) School of Veterinary Studies; 2019.

44. Morrisey JK, Carpenter JW. Formulary. In: Quesenberry K, Carpenter JW, editors. Ferrets, rabbits and rodents: Clinical medicine and surgery. St Louis (MO): Elsevier; 2012. p. 566–75.

45. Weishaupt J, Kolb-Mäurer A, Lempert S, et al. A different kind of hedgehog pathway: tinea manus due to Trichophyton erinacei transmitted by an African pygmy hedgehog (Atelerix albiventris). Mycoses 2014;57(2):125–7.

46. Krawczyk AI, van Leeuwen AD, Jacobs-Reitsma W, et al. Presence of zoonotic agents in engorged ticks and hedgehog faeces from Erinaceus europaeus in (sub) urban areas. Parasit Vectors 2015;8(1):210.

47. Földvári G, Rigó K, Jablonszky M, et al. Ticks and the city: Ectoparasites of the Northern white-breasted hedgehog (Erinaceus roumanicus) in an urban park. Ticks Tick Borne Dis 2011;2(4):231–4.

48. Moshaverinia A, Borji H, Kameli M, et al. A survey on parasites of long-eared hedgehog (Hemiechinus auritus) in northeast of Iran. J Parasit Dis 2016;40(4): 1355–8.

49. Hajipour N, Tavassoli M, Gorgani-Firouzjaee T, et al. Hedgehogs (Erinaceus europaeus) as a Source of Ectoparasites in Urban-suburban Areas of Northwest of Iran. J Arthropod Borne Dis 2014;9(1):98–103.

50. Gaglio G, Allen S, Bowden L, et al. Parasites of European hedgehogs (Erinaceus europaeus) in Britain: epidemiological study and coprological test evaluation. Eur J Wildl Res 2010;56(6):839–44.

51. Graesser D, Spraker TR, Dressen P, et al. Wobbly Hedgehog Syndrome in African Pygmy Hedgehogs (Atelerix spp.). J Exot Pet Med 2006;15(1):59–65.

52. Díaz-Delgado J, Whitley DB, Storts RW, et al. The Pathology of Wobbly Hedgehog Syndrome. Vet Pathol 2018;55(5):711–8.

53. D'Agostino J. Insectivores (Insectivora, Macroscelidea, Scandentia). In: Miller RE, Fowler ME, editors. Fowler's zoo and wild animal medicine. St Louis (MO): Elsevier; 2015. p. 275–81.

54. Muñoz-Gutiérrez JF, Garner MM, Kiupel M. Primary central nervous system neoplasms in African hedgehogs. J Vet Diagn Invest 2018;30(5):715–20.

55. Gibson CJ, Parry NM, Jakowski RM, et al. Anaplastic astrocytoma in the spinal cord of an African Pygmy Hedgehog (Atelerix albiventris). Vet Pathol 2008; 45(6):934–8.

56. Nakata M, Miwa Y, Itou T, et al. Astrocytoma in an African Hedgehog (Atelerix albiventris) Suspected Wobbly Hedgehog Syndrome. J Vet Med Sci 2011;73(10): 1333–5.

57. Kondo H, Yamamoto N, Seino N, et al. Cerebral meningioma in an African pygmy hedgehog (Atelerix albiventris). J Exot Pet Med 2019;28(C):56–8.

58. Ogihara K, Suzuki K, Madarame H. Primary Histiocytic Sarcoma of the Brain in an African Hedgehog (Atelerix albiventris). J Comp Pathol 2017;157(4):241–5.

59. Benneter SS, Summers BA, Schulz-Schaeffer WJ, et al. Mixed Glioma (Oligoastrocytoma) in the Brain of an African Hedgehog (Atelerix albiventris). J Comp Pathol 2014;151(4):420–4.

60. Volker I, Schwarze I, Brezina TE, et al. Oligodendroglioma with neuronal differentiation in an 8-month-old African hedgehog (Atelerix albiventris). Tierarztl Prax Ausg K Kleintiere Heimtiere 2016;44(5):348–54.

61. Díaz-Delgado J, Pool R, Hoppes S, et al. Spontaneous multicentric soft tissue sarcoma in a captive African pygmy hedgehog (Atelerix albiventris): case report and literature review. J Vet Med Sci 2017;79(5):889.

62. Higgins RJ, Bollen AW, Dickenson PJ. Tumors of the nervous system. In: Meuten DJ, editor. Tumors in domestic animals. Ames (IA): Wiley Blackwell; 2017. p. 834–91.

63. Turner PV, Brash ML, Smith DA. Hedgehogs. In: Turner PV, Brash ML, Smith DA, editors. Pathology of small mammal pets. Hoboken (NJ): Wiley; 2018. p. 387–416.

64. Raymond JT, Aguilar R, Dunker F, et al. Intervertebral disc disease in african hedgehogs (Atelerix albiventris): four cases. J Exot Pet Med 2009;18(3):220–3.

65. Allison N, Chang TC, Steele KE, et al. Fatal Herpes Simplex Infection in a Pygmy African Hedgehog (Atelerix albiventris). J Comp Pathol 2002;126(1):76–8.

66. Foale R, Demetriou J. Principles of cancer radiotherapy, in small animal oncology. Edinburgh (Scotland): Saunders/Elsevier; 2010. p. 35–6.

67. Leonatti SR. Ornithonyssus bacoti mite infestation in an African pygmy hedge-hog. Exot DVM 2007;9(2):3–4.
68. Helmer PJ, Carpenter JW. Hedgehogs. In: Carpenter JW, editor. Exotic animal formulary. St Louis (MO): Elsevier; 2018. p. 443–58.
69. Staley EC, Staley EE, Behr MJ. Use of permethrin as a miticide in the African hedgehog (Atelerix albiventris). Vet Hum Toxicol 1994;36(2):138.

Salmonellosis in Hedgehogs

Emma Keeble, BVSc (Hons), DECZM (Mammalian), MRCVS[a],*,
Bronwyn Koterwas, BA, BVM&S, MRCVS[b]

KEYWORDS

- African pygmy hedgehog • Salmonellosis • Zoonosis • Carrier status • Resistance

KEY POINTS

- Salmonella is a worldwide zoonosis with recent outbreaks of salmonella infection in humans in the United States being directly associated with owning pet hedgehogs.
- A diagnosis of salmonellosis is based on microscopic, histopathologic, and microbiological findings.
- Multidrug resistance is common in Salmonella bacteria in both human and veterinary medicine.
- Control and eradication may be difficult in a group situation because of the presence of asymptomatic carriers.
- With the worldwide increase in popularity of African pygmy hedgehogs as pets, it is the duty of veterinarians to fully inform hedgehog owners of the potential to contract salmonellosis from their pet and its surroundings.

INTRODUCTION

Salmonella species are gram-negative, motile, rod-shaped facultative anaerobes found ubiquitously in the environment and belonging to the family Enterobacteriaceae. They are resistant to dehydration, but do not survive temperatures higher than 158°F (70°C).[1] Salmonella nomenclature is complex and can be confusing, with scientists using different systems to refer to and communicate about this genus. Classification can be based on several nomenclatural systems that inconsistently divide the genus into species, subspecies, subgenera, groups, subgroups, and serotypes (serovars).[2] The Centers for Disease Control and Prevention currently recognize 2 species within the genus Salmonella: Salmonella bongori and Salmonella enterica. The 2 species are further classified according to serotypes, S bongori having 20 serotypes and S enterica being further divided into 6 subspecies (eg, S enterica subsp enterica).[2] The name

[a] The Dick Vet Rabbit and Exotic Practice, The University of Edinburgh, The Royal (Dick) School of Veterinary Studies, The Roslin Institute, Easter Bush Campus, Midlothian EH25 9RG, UK;
[b] The Dick Vet Rabbit and Exotic Practice, The University of Edinburgh, The Royal (Dick) School of Veterinary Studies, The Roslin Institute, Easter Bush Campus, Midlothian EH25 9RG, UK
* Corresponding author.
E-mail address: emma.keeble@ed.ac.uk

Vet Clin Exot Anim 23 (2020) 459–470
https://doi.org/10.1016/j.cvex.2020.01.011
1094-9194/20/© 2020 Elsevier Inc. All rights reserved.

is usually abbreviated only indicating the serotype, for example, *S enterica* subsp *enterica* ser typhimurium occurs as *S typhimurium*.[3]

There are more than 2400 *S enterica* serotypes all potentially pathogenic; however, animal and human infections are most commonly associated with only a few of these serotypes.[4]

Salmonella is naturally isolated from the intestinal tract of many animal species. Live poultry, reptiles, amphibians, and small nontraditional pets are thought to present a high risk of zoonotic salmonellosis.[5] Infection has been described in many different mammalian, reptilian, and avian species, and all vertebrates are considered susceptible.[4] Salmonella is possibly the most widely occurring zoonosis worldwide, and recent outbreaks of salmonella infection in humans in the United States have been associated with owning pet hedgehogs.[6] *S typhimurium* was isolated; however, a common source has to date not been identified, with pet hedgehogs being purchased from a variety of breeders, pet shops, or online sources.[7] Links have also been made to wild European hedgehog (*Erinaceus europaeus*) reservoirs as a potential source of human salmonella infection in Europe.[8,9]

CAUSE

In pet African pygmy hedgehogs, *S typhimurium*, *S tilene*, and *S enteritica* serovar Stanley have been reported.[10–12] Pet African pygmy hedgehogs could act as a source of infection for other pets, which in turn could infect their human owners. Human zoonotic infection is thought to have occurred from a hedgehog breeding facility where sugar gliders from the same facility had contact with hedgehogs and were sold as pets to a family, and later, the sugar gliders became ill and died. The sugar gliders were found to be positive for *S tilene* after a 4-month-old family member became ill with salmonellosis.[11] In the United States, sale of African pygmy hedgehogs is licensed by the US Department of Agriculture.

In wild African pygmy hedgehogs in Burkina Faso, Africa, 96% of collected fecal samples tested positive for salmonella (*S enterica* ssp *enterica*). These animals were a possible source of infection to livestock via contact with feces and to locals who hunt them as a meat source.[13]

In wild European hedgehogs from the United Kingdom and continental Europe, infection with *Salmonella enteritidis* (phage type [PT]11, PT9a, PT66, and sequence type [ST] 183) has been mostly reported, but *S typhimurium* definitive type 104 and *Salmonella kottbus* are also occasionally isolated.[8,10,14–16] To date, PT66 has only been reported in wild European hedgehogs from Southern and Central Scotland.[9] Overall prevalence of salmonella infection in wild hedgehogs isolated from fecal samples and rectal swabs is reportedly low (3%–3.8%).[9,16] However, this can increase significantly in areas where wild hedgehogs are routinely fed by humans at feeding stations in which up to 71% of sampled animals can be positive carriers.[8] These investigators also question whether feeding stations could be a source of cross-contamination of salmonella between hedgehogs and avian species feeding at the same site. Immunosuppression and stress may also play an important part in the pathogenesis of this disease, with juvenile hedgehogs particularly at risk, leading to high mortalities.

The bacterium can be ubiquitous in the animal's environment because it is shed in feces, leading to contamination of the spines, coat, and the animal's surroundings. Hedgehogs easily spread infection in their environment because they naturally have soft stools and their behavior is such that they will walk through the feces, spreading any infection. The infection is transmitted via the fecal-oral route to in-contact animals and humans. Once ingested, the bacteria colonize the small intestine and adhere to the intestinal mucosa where they multiply and drain to local lymph nodes. From here, localized infection to the liver and spleen may occur, followed by systemic spread to multiple organs, such as the heart, kidney, central nervous system, and joints.[3]

Because this condition may be asymptomatic in carrier animals, any direct contact with pet hedgehogs or indirect contact with their environment (housing, food and water bowls, litter trays, and bedding) must be considered a potential source of infection.[10] In wild European hedgehogs, transmission may occur through ingestion of contaminated foraged carrion and invertebrates, such as maggots and beetles.

Other infections that cause gastroenteritis, pancreatitis, hepatitis, and peritonitis with associated clinical signs of abdominal pain, diarrhea, anorexia, vomiting, and weight loss are differential diagnoses for salmonella infection in hedgehogs.[17] Differential diagnoses include enteric bacterial infections, such as *Klebsiella* sp (zoonotic), *Yersinia pseudotuberculosis* (zoonotic, enlarged mesenteric lymph nodes, hindlimb weakness), coccidiosis, *Capillaria erinacei* (mucoid feces), and intestinal fluke (*Brachylaemus erinacei*) (intermediate hosts are snails, therefore typically seen in wild animals causing bloody diarrhea).[18,19] Alimentary candidiasis (*Candida albicans*) has been described as causing weight loss, depression, and blood in the feces in a pet hedgehog.[20] Cryptosporidium has also been reported in juvenile pet hedgehogs and can be fatal.[21] Diarrhea associated with dietary change should also be considered. Although many of the above infections have been identified on postmortem in wild European hedgehogs, the significance of these infections in pet African pygmy hedgehogs is unclear and may be minimal.[20]

EPIDEMIOLOGY IN HUMAN CASES

Salmonella infection in humans is commonly reported, with most infections originating from contaminated food sources. However, zoonotic salmonella infections from contact with pet animals or wildlife may occur, for example, *S typhimurium* from wild bird contact[22,23] or *S enterica* subspecies *arizonae* from pet reptiles.[24] The potential for zoonotic infection from pets to their owners should always be considered, although the risk is likely to be low.[25]

S tilene was first isolated from a human case in 1960 in Senegal,[26] and the first human infection in the United States with this organism was reported in 1994[25] and linked to the family owning a breeding herd of African pygmy hedgehogs. Subsequent human cases were described in Canada and Japan.[11,12]

A higher incidence in children is likely reflective of a generally poorer level of hygiene in small children and greater risk of exposure through outdoor play from wildlife sources. Ninety percent of cases occurring in humans in the United States have been associated with confirmed direct contact with a pet hedgehog.[10] Immunocompromised humans are at a greater potential risk of salmonella infection from pet hedgehogs and should be discouraged from keeping them as pets.[27]

EPIDEMIOLOGY IN HEDGEHOGS

S typhimurium, *S tilene*, and *S enteritica* serovar Stanley have been isolated from pet African pygmy hedgehogs belonging to affected humans.[10–12] The Salmonella carriage rate in pet African pygmy hedgehogs is unknown.[5] In the United States and Europe, the main species of hedgehog kept as a pet is the African pygmy hedgehog; however, in Europe, *E europaeus* may be kept in captivity as permanent captives/pets if unable to be released into the wild or, more commonly, juvenile animals are housed over winter before release the following spring when the days are warmer. In the United States, pet hedgehogs are reared by breeders, since importation from the wild (Africa) was banned in 1991 because of concerns with foot and mouth virus transmission.[5]

Salmonella is thought to be endemic and widespread in wild European hedgehog (*E europaeus*) populations in the United Kingdom,[18] with 1 survey reporting a 33% incidence of *S enteritidis* PT11 isolated from postmortem samples[14] and another more recent survey reporting a 27% incidence of *S enteritidis* ST183 isolated at postmortem.[9] *S typhimurium* has also been isolated from wild hedgehogs in Norway.[8] Sporadic disease outbreaks may occur in wild hedgehogs and have been reported in juvenile animals housed in wildlife rehabilitation facilities in the United Kingdom.[18] Carrier rates are reportedly higher in young animals, those with clinical diarrhea, and animals in crowded living conditions under stress.[25]

CLINICAL SIGNS

Salmonella infection in pet hedgehogs may be asymptomatic with carrier status common. Subclinically, an infected hedgehog may have a latent infection within the lymph nodes, or it may be a carrier, shedding the pathogen in feces for a short period of time, intermittently, or persistently.[1] However, in some cases, mucoid, green, or bloody diarrhea associated with enterocolitis may develop[17] (**Fig. 1**). *S enteritica* serovar Stanley was the cause of enterocolitis in a 3-week-old pet African pygmy hedgehog.[12] Anorexia, dehydration, lethargy, weight loss, and death have also reported to be associated with this organism.[19,20] Sudden death can occur in peracute cases. In young animals, in particular those being reared by hand, vomiting and regurgitation has been reported,[18] as well as tenesmus and rectal prolapse in advanced cases. Immunosuppressed and juvenile animals may be at greater risk of developing septicemia.[3] In severe cases, septicemia may occur with multisystemic effects, including neurologic signs, tachypnea, and collapse. On postmortem examination, mesenteric lymph node enlargement and abscessation, gastritis, enteritis, peritonitis, pyelonephritis, and intestinal intussusception may be evident.[9]

There are many factors that should be considered when dealing with a salmonella outbreak, such as the virulence of the pathogen, the route of infection, the dose infected, the age and immune status of the host, and stressful situations, such as poor ventilation, overcrowding, concurrent disease, poor nutrition, and recent transport.[3]

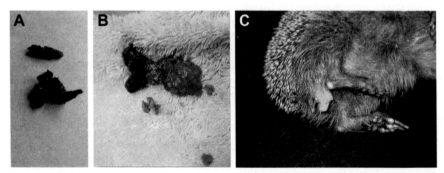

Fig. 1. (*A*) Normal pet hedgehog feces. (*B*) Mucoid hemorrhagic feces associated with salmonella enteritis. (*C*) Mucoid green diarrhea in a European hedgehog (*E europaeus*) with salmonellosis. (*Courtesy of* [*A*] Louise Ross, Edinburgh, Scotland; and [*B, C*] David Couper, BVM&S, Taunton, England.)

A novel clinical presentation has recently been described in adult wild European hedgehogs presenting to a wildlife rehabilitation center over a 7-year period from 2008 to 2015 in Scotland.[9] Affected animals had palpable abdominal masses, which were thought to be enlarged/abscessed mesenteric lymph nodes, and all animals were subsequently euthanized on welfare grounds. In some cases, mesenteric lymph node enlargement was significant (up to 11.5% of body weight). *S enteritidis* (PT66) was isolated in all cases and was always associated with severe lesions and salmonellosis (**Figs. 2** and **3**).

In human cases, diarrhea, pyrexia, headaches, nausea, vomiting, and abdominal cramps may develop 6 to 72 hours after exposure to the bacteria and can persist for 2 to 4 days.[1] Most cases recover without treatment, and systemic illness with associated mortality is rare, but has been reported.[5,10,28] Diarrhea may persist for up to 3 weeks in severe cases.[25] Infection is more serious in the very young or elderly or in immunocompromised individuals, with seizures occurring in severe cases.[12]

DIAGNOSIS

The mainstay of diagnosis in pet hedgehogs has been fecal culture using selective agar media and Salmonella-enriching media.[20] Fresh samples should be used because overgrowth with other enteric bacteria is common and may affect results. In a salmonellosis outbreak, pathologic and histologic examination of carcasses will greatly aid diagnosis and determination of the severity of the infection. Areas of focal pneumonia (catarrhal to purulent bronchopneumonia with fibrosis, atelectasis, and abscesses, resulting from secondary bacterial infection, eg, *Pasteurella multocida* or *Bordetella bronchiseptica*) may also be present in septicemic animals.[19] In these cases, samples should be taken for culture from the affected organs.

In suspect cases whereby culture of the organism from fresh feces is negative or not possible because of sample availability, serologic and immunohistochemical assays may be useful. Enzyme-linked immunosorbent assay for antibody response to salmonella infection tested on blood and tissue is available in other species.[3] and might be useful in acute clinical cases; however, chronic infections are often seronegative.

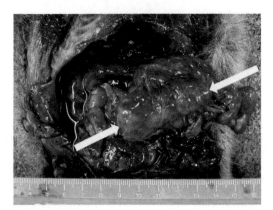

Fig. 2. Enlarged mesenteric lymph node in a hedgehog with *S enteritidis* PT66 infection. White arrows denote the maximum dimensions (6 cm long). (*From* Lawson B, Franklinos LHV, Rodriguez-Ramos Fernandez J, et al. Salmonella Enteritidis ST183: Emerging and endemic biotypes affecting western European hedgehogs (Erinaceus europaeus) and people in Great Britain. Scientific Reports. 2018; 8:2449; with permission.)

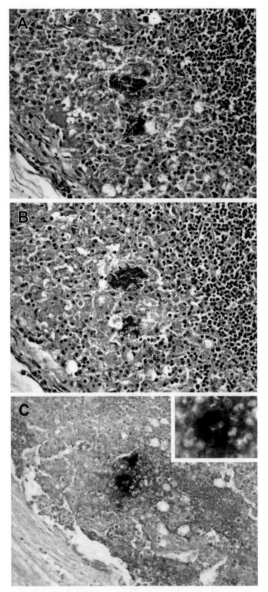

Fig. 3. Histopathology and immunohistochemistry of hedgehog with *S enteritidis* PT66 infection. (*A–C*) Serial sections of mesenteric lymph node from hedgehog XT-1053-15. (*A*) Necrotizing lymphadenitis in subcapsular areas with abundant intralesional bacterial colonies. Hematoxylin and eosin, original magnification ×400. (*B*) The bacteria are gram negative. Gram Twort, original magnification ×400. (*C*) The bacteria show immunoreactivity for *Salmonella* CSA-1. Inset: detail of bacterial immunolabeling. Immunohistochemistry, Ventana, original magnification ×400. (*From* Lawson B, Franklinos LHV, Rodriguez-Ramos Fernandez J, et al. Salmonella Enteritidis ST183: Emerging and endemic biotypes affecting western European hedgehogs (Erinaceus europaeus) and people in Great Britain. Scientific Reports. 2018; 8:2449; with permission.)

Polymerase chain reaction tests are also available for detection of Salmonella DNA from tissue or fecal samples and for further serotype classification.[3]

A diagnosis of salmonellosis (infection causing clinical disease) should ideally be made based on microscopic, histopathologic, and microbiological findings.[9] In the absence of histopathologic examination, salmonella infection is likely in clinical cases with suspicious presenting signs and a positive culture. In cases where Salmonella sp are isolated on fecal culture alone without clinical signs, the significance of the infection is unknown, but that animal is assumed to be a carrier. Any hedgehog exhibiting clinical signs of diarrhea should be barrier nursed, and samples should be taken for salmonella screening. In 1 study, 50% of hedgehogs had diarrhea before human infection and illness occurred.[5] A negative fecal culture does not rule out infection with salmonella because of the carrier status and the possibility of intermittent fecal shedding of this organism.

Salmonella isolates can be further characterized by serotyping, antimicrobial-susceptibility testing, phage typing, and pulsed-field gel electrophoresis laboratory techniques.[5,13]

TREATMENT IN PET HEDGEHOGS

Information on treatment of salmonella infection in pet hedgehogs is sparse and often generic with supportive care and appropriate fluid therapy.[17,29] Probiotics may also be instigated. In mild cases, clinical signs may only last 2 to 4 days and are often self-limiting. Supportive care consisting of fluids, electrolytes, and analgesia may be indicated.[3] Nonsteroidal anti-inflammatory drugs should be avoided in clinical cases because they are associated with adverse gastrointestinal effects, such as mucosal damage. Instead, opiate analgesics could be used, such as buprenorphine (0.01–0.5 mg/kg subcutaneously, intramuscularly every 8–12 hours) and hydromorphone (0.1 mg/kg subcutaneously) or tramadol, an opiate-like agonist (2–4 mg/kg orally every 12 hours).[30]

A risk assessment should be carried out for staff handling salmonella-positive animals, and appropriate personal protective equipment used, such as latex gloves and disposable aprons. Barrier nursing and quarantine protocols should be used to reduce the risk of zoonotic infection to staff and inpatients.

Maintenance fluids in inappetent and debilitated animals should be instigated at 100 mL/kg/d, with supplemental fluid therapy calculated to address dehydration deficits and to replace losses.[20]

Hypothermic hedgehogs should be gently warmed, until normothermic (95.7°F–98.6°F).[20] In general, weak, lethargic, or collapsed African pygmy hedgehogs should be housed at temperatures of 80°F to 85°F if hospitalized.[20]

The prognosis is poor in severely affected animals, with full recovery being rare, and in these cases, euthanasia should be considered on welfare grounds. The risk of disease transmission to in-contact animals and humans should also be considered.

Systemic antimicrobial therapy (eg, amoxicillin) may be indicated in severe acute and potentially life-threatening cases with potential bacteremia, but the risks of creating a carrier status with long-term shedding of the bacteria should always be considered and discussed with the owner first. In such cases, a long-term treatment course of up to 3 weeks should be considered[3]; however, some investigators do not advocate treatment with antibiotics.[1] Antibiotic choice should always be based on culture and sensitivity results, particularly because multidrug resistance is common in Salmonella bacteria in both human and veterinary medicine.[31] Antibiotics that may be useful in confirmed salmonella cases are ampicillin, amoxicillin, quinolones (enrofloxacin, ciprofloxacin, danofloxacin), tetracyclines, erythromycin, clindamycin, streptomycin, gentamicin, and trimethoprim/sulfonamides.[3] Gentamicin should be used with caution in pet hedgehogs because it can be nephrotoxic.[30] For antimicrobial dose rates in pet hedgehogs, see Ref.[30] It should be borne in mind that in severe cases, the uptake of enterally administered drugs may be reduced because of the dilution effect of increased fluid within the gastrointestinal tract and parenterally administered drugs may be preferable.

If clinical signs of disease are present and Salmonella has been isolated from the affected animal, then treatment may be indicated; however, a discussion should take place with the owner regarding the zoonotic risks, potential for development of carrier status, and of creating antibiotic resistance in their pet.[20] It is well documented that animals treated with antimicrobials have prolonged bacterial shedding following treatment.[31]

ANTIMICROBIAL RESISTANCE

Multidrug resistance is common in Salmonella bacteria in both human and veterinary medicine.[1,31] Resistance occurs because of acquisition of antibiotic-resistant plasmids and genetic mutations. Antimicrobial resistance has been reported in hedgehog isolates (**Table 1**).

PREVENTION

Veterinary advice to pet hedgehog owners to reduce the risk of salmonella infection is essential and should be provided to all hedgehog owners as a written document at first point of contact and ideally at the point of sale from breeders. It should be assumed that any pet hedgehog could be a potential carrier for salmonella.[32] Elderly, young, or immunocompromised people should ideally avoid contact with pet hedgehogs because they may be at higher risk of infection.[5,27] Prevention of disease centers on good hygienic practices[33] (**Box 1**).

Table 1			
Reported antimicrobial resistance to Salmonella isolates			
Salmonella Isolate	**Species Reported**	**Antimicrobial Resistance Reported**	**Reference**
S kottbus	Wild European hedgehog (E europaeus)	Ampicillin, streptomycin, sulfonamide, trimethoprim/ sulfamethoxazole, nalidixic acid, and tetracycline.	Molina-Lopez et al,[16] 2015
S enteritidis	Wild European hedgehog (E europaeus)	Rare	Lawson et al,[9] 2018
S enteritidis	Human isolates	Ampicillin, chloramphenicol, gentamicin, sulfonamide, tetracycline, and spectinomycin	Lawson et al,[9] 2018

Data from Lawson B, Franklinos LHV, Rodriguez-Ramos Fernandez J, et al. Salmonella Enteritidis ST183: Emerging and endemic biotypes affecting western European hedgehogs (Erinaceus europaeus) and people in Great Britain. Scientific Reports. 2018; 8:2449; and Molina-Lopez RA, Vidal A, Obon E, et al. Multidrug-resistant Salmonella enterica Serovar Typhimurium Monophasic Variant 4,12:i:- Isolated from Asymptomatic Wildlife in a Catalonian Wildlife Rehabilitation Center, Spain. J Wildl Dis. 2015; 51(3):759-763.

> **Box 1**
> **General veterinary advice to pet hedgehog owners to avoid salmonella infection**
>
> - Hands should be washed thoroughly with warm water and soap after handling pet hedgehogs, after handling their food and water dishes, or after any contact with their environment and especially before human food preparation or eating.[11]
>
> - Children should be supervised by an adult when washing hands to ensure it is done properly.
>
> - Kissing or cuddling pet hedgehogs as well as carrying them inside clothing should always be avoided.[5]
>
> - Keep pet hedgehogs away from food preparation or storage areas, such as the kitchen.
>
> - The hedgehog's environment should be cleaned regularly with an appropriate disinfectant (such as dilute sodium hypochlorite),[34] and all waste should be bagged and properly disposed.
>
> - Cleaning should ideally take place outdoors to avoid contamination within the house.
>
> - Water and food bowls as well as toys and housing items should be regularly disinfected.
>
> - Kitchen sinks or baths should not be used to clean any hedgehog items.
>
> *Data from* Refs.[5,11,34]

Hedgehogs should be carefully monitored for signs of illness and changes to fecal color and consistency. If there are any suspicious clinical signs, immediate veterinary advice should be sought. Breeders should be extra careful and use good hygienic practice with appropriate personal protective equipment, such as wearing separate overalls when feeding and cleaning hedgehogs and diligent hand-washing practices. Children should not be allowed into breeding facilities.[11] It should be noted that infection has been diagnosed in very young infants, and in these cases, there was no direct contact with hedgehogs, indicating that the infection spread indirectly.[11] Practices such as housing pet hedgehogs in the bedroom and bathing them in the family bathtub or sink have been linked with human zoonotic infections and should be avoided.[5] The authors do not recommend African pygmy hedgehogs as children's pets, because of the risk of salmonellosis. If children are present within a household, direct adult supervision is essential.

CONTROL

Control and eradication may be difficult in a group situation (eg, breeding colony) because of the presence of asymptomatic carriers. A comprehensive preventative control program should be drawn up by the veterinarian in consultation with the owner, particularly in group situations, and should be primarily based on good hygiene practice, personal protective clothing, and appropriate disinfection. In a breeding situation, the owner should be encouraged to work closely with an exotic pet veterinary specialist to evaluate the salmonella status of their animals.[5] The salmonella status should be determined via pooled fecal samples, and new animals entering the collection should be screened before introduction to the group. Regular screening at appropriate time intervals (eg, quarterly) should be instigated. Bear in mind that a negative culture result does not exclude infection with salmonella; it just indicates that at the time of sampling the animal was not shedding the bacteria in its feces. A positive result without clinical signs indicates carrier status and is a potential risk for infection of in-contact animals and humans. Stress may also play a part in development of clinical disease and shedding of the bacteria in carrier animals. Balancing social groups, reducing stocking density, careful introduction of new animals to a social group, optimizing husbandry, ensuring a nutritionally balanced diet, and providing environmental enrichment are all key to ensuring a healthy population or individual animal.[3] Concurrent disease may also predispose an animal to salmonellosis, and any ill animal should ideally be isolated, and barrier nursed.

SUMMARY

A One Health approach is essential when investigating human salmonella outbreaks with collaboration between public and animal health organizations.[5] In the face of an outbreak in humans, questions regarding contact with pet hedgehogs should always be asked. It is important that the risks of salmonella infection from pet hedgehog ownership are fully highlighted and explained to all in-contact parties, from breeder to seller to pet owner, along the chain. Increased awareness of the zoonotic risk from pet hedgehogs among public and animal health officials as well as veterinarians and health care providers is essential, with education provided to all on appropriate prevention and control measures to prevent future outbreaks.[9]

DISCLOSURE

The authors have nothing to disclose.

REFERENCES

1. Pignon C, Mayer J. Zoonoses of ferrets, hedgehogs, and sugar gliders. Vet Clin North Am Exot Anim Pract 2011;14(3):533–49.
2. Brenner FW, Villar RG, Angulo FJ, et al. Salmonella nomenclature. J Clin Microbiol 2000;38(7):2465.
3. Ketz-Riley CJ. Salmonellosis and shigellosis. In: Fowler M, Miller E, editors. Zoo and wild animal medicine. Philadelphia: Saunders, Elsevier Science; 2003. p. 686–9.
4. Mitchell M, Tully T. Zoonotic diseases. In: Quesenberry K, Carpenter J, editors. Ferrets, rabbits and rodents: clinical medicine and surgery. St Louis (MO): Elsevier; 2012. p. 557–65.
5. Anderson TC, Marsden-Haug N, Morris JF, et al. Multistate outbreak of human salmonella typhimurium infections linked to pet hedgehogs–United States, 2011-2013. Zoonoses Public Health 2017;64(4):290–8.
6. Miller SG. Pet hedgehogs are the latest source of salmonella outbreak. 2019 July 17. 2019. Available at: https://www.livescience.com/64601-pet-hedgehog-salmonella.html. Accessed July 17, 2019.
7. Prevention, C.f.D.C.a.. Multistate outbreak of salmonella infections linked to hedgehogs. 2019. Available at: https://www.cdc.gov/media/releases/2019/s0531-salmonella-hedgehogs.html. Accessed July 17, 2019.
8. Handeland K, Refsum T, Johansen BS, et al. Prevalence of Salmonella typhimurium infection in Norwegian hedgehog populations associated with two human disease outbreaks. Epidemiol Infect 2002;128(3):523–7.
9. Lawson B, Franklinos LHV, Rodriguez-Ramos Fernandez J, et al. Salmonella enteritidis ST183: emerging and endemic biotypes affecting western European hedgehogs (Erinaceus europaeus) and people in Great Britain. Sci Rep 2018; 8(1):2449.

10. Prevention, C.f.D.C.a.. Outbreak of salmonella infections linked to hedgehogs, investigation notice. 2019. Available at: https://www.cdc.gov/salmonella/typhimurium-01-19/index.html. Accessed July 17, 2019.

11. Craig C, Styliadis S, Woodward D, et al. African pygmy hedgehog–associated Salmonella tilene in Canada. Can Commun Dis Rep 1997;23(17):129.

12. Ichimi R, Yoshino A, Higashigawa M. Salmonella Stanley bacteremia transmitted from a pet hedgehog. Pediatr Int 2018;60(6):606–7.

13. Kagambega A, Lienemann T, Aulu L, et al. Prevalence and characterization of Salmonella enterica from the feces of cattle, poultry, swine and hedgehogs in Burkina Faso and their comparison to human Salmonella isolates. BMC Microbiol 2013;13(1):253.

14. Keymer IF, Gibson EA, Reynolds DJ. Zoonoses and other findings in hedgehogs (Erinaceus europaeus): a survey of mortality and review of the literature. Vet Rec 1991;128(11):245–9.

15. Nauerby B, Pedersen K, Dietz HH, et al. Comparison of Danish isolates of Salmonella enterica Serovar enteritidis PT9a and PT11 from Hedgehogs (Erinaceus europaeus) and humans by plasmid profiling and pulsed-field gel electrophoresis. J Clin Microbiol 2000;38(10):3631.

16. Molina-Lopez RA, Vidal A, Obón E, et al. Multidrug-resistant Salmonella enterica Serovar Typhimurium monophasic variant 4,12:i:- isolated from asymptomatic wildlife in a Catalonian Wildlife Rehabilitation Center, Spain. J Wildl Dis 2015;51(3):759–63.

17. Johnson D. African Pygmy Hedgehogs. In: Meredith A, Johnson-DeLaney C, editors. BSAVA manual of exotic pets. Goucester (UK): BSAVA; 2010. p. 455.

18. Bexton S. Hedgehogs. In: Mullineaux E, Keeble E, editors. BSAVA manual of wildlife casualties. Cheltenham (England): BSAVA; 2016. p. 117–36.

19. Isenbugel E, Baumgartner R. Diseases of the Hedgehog. In: Fowler M, editor. Zoo and wild animal medicine: current therapy. Philadelphia: WB Saunders Company; 1993. p. 294–303.

20. Ivey E, Carpenter J. African hedgehogs. In: Quesenberry K, Carpenter J, editors. Ferrets, rabbits and rodents: clinical medicine and surgery. St Louis (MO): Elsevier; 2012. p. 411–27.

21. Graczyk TK, Cranfield MR, Dunning C, et al. Fatal cryptosporidiosis in a juvenile captive African hedgehog (Ateletrix albiventris). J Parasitol 1998;84(1):178.

22. Lawson B, de Pinna E, Horton RA, et al. Epidemiological evidence that garden birds are a source of human salmonellosis in England and Wales. PLoS One 2014;9(2):e88968.

23. Alley M, Connolly JH, Fenwick SG, et al. An epidemic of salmonellosis caused by Salmonella typhimurium DT160 in wild birds and humans in New Zealand. N Z Vet J 2002;50(5):170–6.

24. Aiken A, Lane C, Adak G. Risk of Salmonella infection with exposure to reptiles in England, 2004-2007. Euro Surveill 2010;15(22):11–8.

25. Centers for Disease Control and Prevention (CDC). African pygmy hedgehog-associated salmonellosis–Washington, 1994. MMWR Morb Mortal Wkly Rep 1995;44(24):462–3.

26. Le Minor L, Pinhede N, Kerrest J, et al. A new serotype of Salmonella, S tilene. Bull Soc Pathol Exot 1960;53:777–8.

27. Riley PY, Chomel BB. Hedgehog zoonoses. Emerg Infect Dis 2005;11(1):1–5.

28. Marsden-Haug N, Meyer S, Bidol S, et al. Notes from the field: multistate outbreak of human salmonella typhimurium infections linked to contact with pet hedgehogs—United States, 2011-2013. JAMA 2013;309(14):1456.

29. Barbiers R. Insectivora (hedgehogs, tenrecs, shrews, moles) and Dermoptera (flying lemurs). In: Fowler ME, Miller RE, editors. Fowler's Zoo and wild animal medicine. Philadelphia: Saunders, Elsevier Science; 2003. p. 308.

30. Fritz A. What's with the recent hedgehog Salmonella outbreak? DVM 360, May 2019, p. 40. Gale Academic Onefile. Available at: https://link.gale.com/apps/doc/A591847236/AONE?u=ed_itw&sid=AONE&xid=85f70815. Accessed August 19, 2019.

31. Wray C, Wray A. Salmonella in domestic animals. Oxford (England): CABI Pub; 2000.

32. Fritz A. What's with the recent hedgehog Salmonella outbreak?(NEWS: exotic medicine). DVM 360 2019;50(5):40.

33. Daly RF, House J, Stanek D, et al. Public veterinary medicine: public health compendium of measures to prevent disease associated with animals in public settings. J Am Vet Med Assoc 2017;251(11):1269–92.

34. Barker J, Naeeni M, Bloomfield SF. The effects of cleaning and disinfection in reducing Salmonella contamination in a laboratory model kitchen. J Appl Microbiol 2003;95(6):1351–60.

Moving?

Make sure your subscription moves with you!

To notify us of your new address, find your **Clinics Account Number** (located on your mailing label above your name), and contact customer service at:

Email: journalscustomerservice-usa@elsevier.com

800-654-2452 (subscribers in the U.S. & Canada)
314-447-8871 (subscribers outside of the U.S. & Canada)

Fax number: 314-447-8029

Elsevier Health Sciences Division
Subscription Customer Service
3251 Riverport Lane
Maryland Heights, MO 63043

*To ensure uninterrupted delivery of your subscription, please notify us at least 4 weeks in advance of move.

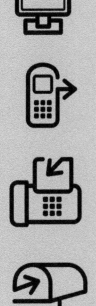

Printed and bound by CPI Group (UK) Ltd, Croydon, CR0 4YY

03/10/2024

01040481-0004